Molecular Oncology Diagnostics

Editor

FEI DONG

CLINICS IN LABORATORY MEDICINE

www.labmed.theclinics.com

Editor-In-Chief
MILENKO JOVAN TANASIJEVIC

September 2022 • Volume 42 • Number 3

ELSEVIER

1600 John F. Kennedy Boulevard • Suite 1800 • Philadelphia, Pennsylvania, 19103-2899

http://www.theclinics.com

CLINICS IN LABORATORY MEDICINE Volume 42, Number 3
September 2022 ISSN 0272-2712, ISBN-13: 978-0-323-84936-4

Editor: Taylor Hayes
Developmental Editor: Ann Gielou M. Posedio

Reprints. For copies of 100 or more, of articles in this publication, please contact the Commercial Reprints Department, Elsevier Inc., 360 Park Avenue South, New York, New York 10010-1710. Tel. 212-633-3874, Fax: 212-633-3820, E-mail: reprints@elsevier.com.

Clinics in Laboratory Medicine (ISSN 0272-2712) is published quarterly by Elsevier Inc., 360 Park Avenue South, New York, NY 10010-1710. Months of issue are March, June, September, and December. Business and Editorial offices: 1600 John F. Kennedy Blvd., Suite 1800, Philadelphia, PA 19103-2899. Periodicals postage paid at NewYork, NY and additional mailing offices. Subscription prices are $283.00 per year (US individuals), $753.00 per year (US institutions), $100.00 per year (US students), $363.00 per year (Canadian individuals), $776.00 per year (Canadian institutions), $100.00 per year (Canadian students), $404.00 per year (international individuals), $776.00 per year (international institutions), $185.00 (international students). Foreign air speed delivery is included in all Clinics subscription prices. All prices are subject to change without notice. POSTMASTER: Send address changes to *Clinics in Laboratory Medicine*, Elsevier Health Sciences Division, Subscription Customer Service, 3251 Riverport Lane, Maryland Heights, MO 63043. **Customer Service: 1-800-654-2452 (US). From outside of the US and Canada, call 1-314-447-8871. Fax: 1-314-447-8029. E-mail: journalscustomerservice-usa@elsevier.com (for print support) or journalsonlinesupport-usa@elsevier.com (for online support).**

Clinics in Laboratory Medicine is covered in *EMBASE/Exerpta Medica, MEDLINE/PubMed (Index Medicus), Cinahl, Current Contents/Clinical Medicine, BIOSIS and ISI/BIOMED.*

Contributors

EDITOR-IN-CHIEF

MILENKO JOVAN TANASIJEVIC, MD, MBA
Vice Chair for Clinical Pathology and Quality, Department of Pathology, Director of Clinical Laboratories, Brigham and Women's Hospital, Dana-Farber Cancer Institute, Associate Professor of Pathology, Harvard Medical School, Boston, Massachusetts, USA

EDITOR

FEI DONG, MD
Associate Pathologist, Brigham and Women's Hospital, Assistant Professor, Harvard Medical School, Boston, Massachusetts, USA

AUTHORS

DARA AISNER, MD, PhD
Professor, Department of Pathology, University of Colorado, Aurora, Colorado, USA

KAJIA CAO, PhD
Division of Genomic Diagnostics, Department of Pathology and Laboratory Medicine, Children's Hospital of Philadelphia, Philadelphia, Pennsylvania, USA

OZGE CEYHAN-BIRSOY, PhD
Department of Pathology and Laboratory Medicine, Memorial Sloan Kettering Cancer Center, New York, New York, USA

ALANNA J. CHURCH, MD
Associate Director, Laboratory for Molecular Pediatric Pathology (LaMPP), Department of Pathology, Boston Children's Hospital, Assistant Professor of Pathology, Harvard Medical School, Boston, Massachusetts, USA

ADRIAN M. DUBUC, PhD, FACMG
Assistant Professor in Pathology, Harvard Medical School, Assistant Director of Cytogenetics, Brigham and Women's Hospital, BWH Center for Advanced Molecular Diagnostics (CAMD), Boston, Massachusetts, USA

ADAM S. FISCH, MD, PhD
Clinical Fellow in Head and Neck Pathology, Massachusetts General Hospital, Instructor of Pathology, Harvard Medical School, Boston, Massachusetts, USA

QIONG GAN, MD, PhD
Department of Anatomic Pathology, The University of Texas MD Anderson Cancer Center, Houston, Texas, USA

TATYANA GINDIN, MD, PhD
Clinical Associate Professor, Department of Pathology, NYU Grossman School of
Medicine, New York, New York, USA

TASOS GOGAKOS, MD, PhD
Center for Integrated Diagnostics, Department of Pathology, Massachusetts General
Hospital, Harvard Medical School, Boston, Massachusetts, USA

MEHENAZ HANBAZAZH, MD
Assistant Professor, Department of Pathology, Faculty of Medicine, University of Jeddah,
Jeddah, Saudi Arabia; Division of Genomic Diagnostics and Bioinformatics, Department
of Pathology, The University of Alabama at Birmingham, Birmingham, Alabama, USA

SHUKO HARADA, MD
Professor, Division of Genomic Diagnostics and Bioinformatics, Department of
Pathology, The University of Alabama at Birmingham, Birmingham, Alabama, USA

CHRISTOPHER B. HERGOTT, MD, PhD
Hematopathologist, Brigham and Women's Hospital, Clinical and Research Fellow in
Pathology, Harvard Medical School, Boston, Massachusetts, USA

SUSAN J. HSIAO, MD, PhD
Assistant Professor, Department of Pathology and Cell Biology, Columbia University
Medical Center, New York, New York, USA

ANNETTE S. KIM, MD, PhD
Associate Professor, Department of Pathology, Brigham and Women's Hospital, Harvard
Medical School, Boston, Massachusetts, USA

ERIC Q. KONNICK, MD, MS
Associate Professor, Associate Director, Genetics and Solid Tumors Laboratory,
Department of Laboratory Medicine and Pathology, University of Washington, Brotman-
Baty Institute for Precision Medicine, University of Washington, Seattle, Washington, USA

MARILYN M. LI, MD
Division of Genomic Diagnostics, Department of Pathology and Laboratory Medicine,
Department of Pediatrics, Children's Hospital of Philadelphia, Perelman School of
Medicine, University of Pennsylvania, Philadelphia, Pennsylvania, USA

CHRISTINA H. LOCKWOOD, PhD
Professor, Director, Genetics and Solid Tumors Laboratory, Department of Laboratory
Medicine and Pathology, University of Washington, Brotman-Baty Institute for Precision
Medicine, University of Washington, Seattle, Washington, USA

ALEXANDER C. MACKINNON, MD, PhD
Professor, Division of Genomic Diagnostics and Bioinformatics, Department of
Pathology, The University of Alabama at Birmingham, Birmingham, Alabama, USA

DIANA MORLOTE, MD
Assistant Professor, Division of Genomic Diagnostics and Bioinformatics, Department of
Pathology, The University of Alabama at Birmingham, Birmingham, Alabama, USA

VALENTINA NARDI, MD
Department of Pathology, Massachusetts General Hospital, Harvard Medical School,
Boston, Massachusetts, USA

ZEHRA ORDULU, MD
Department of Pathology, Immunology and Laboratory Medicine, University of Florida, Gainesville, Florida, USA; Department of Pathology, Massachusetts General Hospital, Harvard Medical School, Boston, Massachusetts, USA

VERA PAULSON, MD, PhD
Assistant Professor, Associate Director, Genetics and Solid Tumors Laboratory, Department of Laboratory Medicine and Pathology, University of Washington, Brotman-Baty Institute for Precision Medicine, University of Washington, Seattle, Washington, USA

LAUREN L. RITTERHOUSE, MD, PhD
Assistant Professor, Harvard Medical School, Associate Director, Center for Integrated Diagnostics, Department of Pathology, Massachusetts General Hospital, Boston, Massachusetts, USA

SOMAK ROY, MD, FCAP
Associate Professor, Department of Pathology, Cincinnati Children's Hospital Medical Center, Cincinnati, Ohio, USA

SINCHITA ROY-CHOWDHURI, MD, PhD
Department of Anatomic Pathology, The University of Texas MD Anderson Cancer Center, Houston, Texas, USA

JEFFREY SCHUBERT, PhD
Division of Genomic Diagnostics, Department of Pathology and Laboratory Medicine, Children's Hospital of Philadelphia, Philadelphia, Pennsylvania, USA

LYNETTE SHOLL, MD
Associate Professor, Department of Pathology, Brigham and Women's Hospital, Boston, Massachusetts, USA

TARA SPENCE, MSc, PhD
Cytogeneticist and Molecular Geneticist, Director of Cytogenomics Laboratory, Vancouver General Hospital, Vancouver Coastal Health, Vancouver, British Columbia, Canada

NICHOLAS WILLARD, DO
Assistant Professor, Department of Pathology, University of Colorado, Aurora, Colorado, USA

JINHUA WU, PhD
Division of Genomic Diagnostics, Department of Pathology and Laboratory Medicine, Children's Hospital of Philadelphia, Philadelphia, Pennsylvania, USA

Contents

> The genetic testing of solid tumors has evolved rapidly. With an ever-increasing number of clinically significant and/or actionable gene alterations in addition to increasing biologic, gene, or mutation-specific therapies, single-target testing is no longer suitable for many modern oncology patients. This review explores panel-based testing, including its history and evolution from prior testing modalities. We also discuss its current usefulness, as best exemplified by lung cancer, and other special considerations including a summary of the pros and cons of panel implementation and use. Lastly, we discuss the successes and challenges of panel-based testing and explore future directions.

> Molecular diagnostics inhabit an increasingly central role in characterizing hematopoietic malignancies. This brief review summarizes the genomic targets important for many major categories of hematopoietic neoplasia by focusing on disease pathogenesis. In myeloid disease, recurrent mutations in key functional classes drive clonal hematopoiesis, on which additional variants can specify clinical presentation and accelerate progression. Lymphoblastic leukemias are frequently initiated by oncogenic fusions that block lymphoid maturation while, in concert with additional mutations, driving proliferation. The links between genetic aberrations and lymphoma patient outcomes have been clarified substantially through the clustering of genomic profiles. Finally, the addition of next-generation sequencing strategies to cytogenetics is refining risk stratification for plasma cell myeloma. In all categories, molecular diagnostics shed light on the unique mechanistic underpinnings of each individual malignancy, thereby empowering more rational, personalized care for these patients.

> Pediatric neoplasms have unique demands, including triaging of small biopsies for multiple testing modalities, and a pediatric cancer genome that is notably different from the adult cancer genome. Pediatric cancers are more likely to be driven by gene fusions and typically have a lower tumor mutational burden. Clinically relevant unique molecular targets exist within pediatric cancers, with important implications for diagnosis, prognosis,

and treatment selection. Hence, assays and interpretation workflows must be designed thoughtfully to support molecular tumor profiling for children with cancer, including accommodation of small samples, detection of gene fusions, and consideration of potential germline associations.

Qiong Gan and Sinchita Roy-Chowdhuri

Proper treatment of the patient with cancer depends on an accurate diagnosis of the tumor and is further directed by prognostic and more recently therapeutic molecular signatures in the era of precision medicine. Molecular oncology testing provides diagnostic, prognostic, and therapeutic information derived from the tumor genome. The aim of this review is to provide valuable information to laboratories for choosing optimal clinical specimens for molecular oncology testing by evaluating the strengths and weaknesses of different sample types from the procurement, processing, and pre-analytic selection matching to different test platforms.

Mehenaz Hanbazazh, Diana Morlote, Alexander C. Mackinnon, and Shuko Harada

Molecular testing is now considered the standard of care to screen for disease, confirm the diagnosis, guide management, and use target therapy. Currently, several testing strategies are being used. One of the most common strategies is single-gene testing, which is often conducted for known mutations, such as BRAF in melanoma and EGFR in lung cancer. Subsequently, next-generation sequencing (NGS), which tests many genes simultaneously, was developed using targeted gene panels, whole-exome, or whole-genome sequencing. Ordering the best diagnostic tool and choosing between single-gene testing and NGS depends on several factors. In this review, we discuss different single-gene testing methodologies and the impact of using them in comparison to NGS/multigene panel.

Tatyana Gindin and Susan J. Hsiao

This article covers analytical principles of cancer next generation sequencing (NGS). Cancer samples require special considerations due to the cancer-specific applications of testing, as well as cancer sample specific issues, including low input, low tumor purity, or fixation-related artifacts. Laboratories typically use a combination of approaches around specimen processing, assay design, and bioinformatics analysis to allow for successful detection of actionable biomarkers. Examples of these approaches for cancer NGS testing are discussed and reviewed here.

Clinical bioinformatics plays a key role in the implementation of clinical next-generation sequencing (NGS) testing infrastructure. Bioinformatics workflows in a clinical laboratory are complex and therefore need to be validated as part of an end-to-end NGS assay validation before clinical use. The validation cohort should be representative of the types of samples, types of variants, lower limits of detection of the assay, as well as sequence context of the panel. When validating an NGS bioinformatics pipeline, the pipeline validation lifecycle should be adhered to. Software containers and modern software automation tools can allow the building of a scalable and reliable clinical bioinformatics infrastructure and can be implemented in clinical bioinformatics operations in a phased way depending on the size and skillset of the bioinformatics team.

Because the clinical impact of cancer genomics is being increasingly recognized, tumor sequencing will likely continue to expand in breadth and scope. Therefore, it is vital for laboratory professionals to adopt the Association for Molecular Pathology, American Society of Clinical Oncology, and College of American Pathologists guidelines and create a standardized system of classification and nomenclature for somatic variants. Combining robust bioinformatics pipelines with thorough data analysis is necessary to efficiently and reproducibly identify and assess the impact of clinically relevant variants.

Oncogenic gene rearrangements have been exponentially significant for clinical management of cancer, from diagnosis to therapy and disease monitoring. Testing algorithms should be created with caution, and sample type, accessibility to testing method, turnaround time, and economic aspects should be taken into consideration. Herein, different molecular technologies for detecting these gene rearrangements are discussed and the benefits and limitations of each method are highlighted.

Accurate detection of copy number alterations (CNAs) has become increasingly important in clinical oncology for the purpose of diagnosis, prognostication, and disease management. Cytogenetic approaches for the detection of CNAs, including karyotype, fluorescence in situ hybridization (FISH), and chromosomal microarray, remain mainstays in clinical laboratories. Yet, with rapidly decreasing costs and improved accuracy of CNA detection using emerging technologies such as next-generation sequencing and optical genome mapping, we are approaching a new era of cytogenomics and molecular oncology. The aim of this review is

CLINICS IN LABORATORY MEDICINE

SERIES OF RELATED INTEREST

Surgical Pathology Clinics
Available at: https://www.surgpath.theclinics.com/

THE CLINICS ARE NOW AVAILABLE ONLINE!
Access your subscription at:
www.theclinics.com

CLINICS IN LABORATORY MEDICINE

Molecular Oncology Diagnostics

FORTHCOMING ISSUES

December 2022
Current Topics in Molecular Diagnostics and Precision Medicine
Gregory J. Tsongalis, Editor

March 2023
Artificial Intelligence in the Clinical Laboratory: Current Practice and Emerging Opportunities
Jason Baron, Editor

June 2023
Point of Care Testing
Linoj Samuel, Editor

RECENT ISSUES

June 2022
Covid-19 Molecular Testing and Clinical Correlates
Sanjat Kanjilal and Yi-Wei Tang, Editors

March 2022
Detection of SARS-CoV-2 Antibodies in Diagnosis and Treatment of COVID-19
Gulnaz P Simmons and Peter H. Schur, Editors

December 2021
Updates in Blood Banking and Transfusion Medicine
Suzanne R. Thibodeaux, Editor

SERIES OF RELATED INTEREST

Surgical Pathology Clinics
Available at: https://www.surgpath.theclinics.com

THE CLINICS ARE NOW AVAILABLE ONLINE!
Access your subscription at:
www.theclinics.com

Preface

The Medical Practice of Molecular Oncology Diagnostics

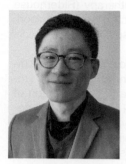

Fei Dong, MD
Editor

Molecular diagnostics is a rapidly changing field. In a short period of time, molecular diagnostics for applications in cancer has evolved from a loose collection of investigational ancillary tests to redefine pathologic disease classification and usher in the era of precision medicine. Today, molecular testing, including the targeted sequencing of cancer genomes, is standard of care for confirming pathologic diagnosis, predicting clinical risk, and guiding the use of conventional and molecularly targeted therapies for most life-threatening human cancers.

The growing complexity of molecular applications, technology, and interpretation necessitates regular updates to help health care providers stay informed about standard clinical practices in molecular medicine. This special collection of review articles addresses the clinical challenges in molecular oncology diagnostics from expert molecular pathologists and geneticists who actively practice in the field. The issue is organized into four parts:

Part 1 provides updates in the clinical utility of molecular diagnostics, including the use of molecular testing to guide therapy selection in solid tumors (Willard, Sholl, and Aisner) and in the systematic classification of hematopoietic neoplasms (Hergott and Kim) with special considerations for molecular testing in pediatric cancers (Fisch and Church).

Part 2 focuses on the analytical aspects of clinical molecular testing. This section addresses issues that molecular diagnosticians face on a daily basis, including the selection of pathologic specimens (Gan and Roy-Chowdhuri), the principles of single-gene testing (Hanbazazh, Morlote, Mackinnon, and Harada) compared with multigene next-generation sequencing panels (Gindin and Hsiao), informatics pipelines that support

Clin Lab Med 42 (2022) xiii–xiv
https://doi.org/10.1016/j.cll.2022.06.001
0272-2712/22/© 2022 Published by Elsevier Inc.

the analysis of complex sequencing data (Roy), and best practices in clinical interpretation and reporting (Schubert, Wu, Li, and Cao).

Part 3 describes how laboratories use a variety of current and emerging molecular methods to detect structural alterations in cancer, such as gene rearrangements (Ordulu and Nardi) and copy number alterations (Spence and Dubuc), and the strengths and limitations of different molecular technologies used for this indication.

Part 4 highlights current and emerging hot topics in molecular oncology diagnostics, including biomarkers that predict response to cancer immunotherapy (Ritterhouse and Gogakos), molecular testing performance for cell free nucleic acids (Paulson, Konnick, and Lockwood), and strategies to identify cancer-predisposing germline variants (Ceyhan-Birsoy).

Multiple themes emerge in this collection of expert reviews. Molecular oncology diagnostics is a diverse field with multiple testing modalities, and the strengths and limitations of different molecular methods are highly complementary. The selection of molecular testing is complex and multifactorial, and the optimal testing strategy depends on clinical history, pathologic diagnosis, tissue availability, and pretest probability of clinically actionable molecular targets. An increasing volume of molecular data brings challenges in clinical interpretation but also opportunities to enhance patient care.

The purpose of this collection is to provide unique perspectives into molecular diagnostics and to aid pathologists, geneticists, and other clinicians in the field of medical oncology. I hope that the articles will also introduce imaginative young people, students, scientists, and resident physicians, to the world of molecular diagnostics, made possible by incredible scientific advances and the desire to help patients in need. Consider joining us in a riveting and rewarding career in molecular pathology, medical genetics, laboratory medicine, or bioinformatics. Ultimately, our collective expertise in molecular diagnostics is needed to fulfill the promise of precision medicine.

Fei Dong, MD
Brigham and Women's Hospital
75 Francis Street, Cotran 3, Boston, MA 02115, USA

E-mail address:
fdong1@bwh.harvard.edu

Panel Sequencing for Targeted Therapy Selection in Solid Tumors

Nicholas Willard, DO[a],*, Lynette Sholl, MD[b], Dara Aisner, MD, PhD[a]

KEYWORDS

- Next-generation sequencing (NGS) • Panel • Solid tumor • Targeted • Sequencing
- Therapy

KEY POINTS

- Panel-based testing via next-generation sequencing offers many advantages in identifying clinically relevant alterations over single-target techniques.
- Lung cancer serves as a prime example of the growing usefulness of panel-based testing, but this is increasingly being expanded to other tumor types.
- May nuanced considerations exist when implementing panel-based testing, including personnel training, bioinformatics, and reimbursement.

INTRODUCTION

Over the past 1 to 2 decades, molecular diagnostics has shifted from a focus on single gene or even single mutation target testing toward panel-based testing in many human diseases. In cancer management in particular, panel-based strategies provide a more effective strategy for the identification of the growing number of tumor and germline variants that have diagnostic, prognostic, and predictive usefulness. Within the realm of solid tumors, panel-based testing has gained traction in clinical practice, both owing to an ever-increasing number of therapeutically relevant targets, as well as greater assay accessibility and increasingly streamlined workflows. Next-generation sequencing (NGS) has largely driven this revolution because it permits massively parallel sequencing of a customizable number of genes and gene targets with relatively good analytical sensitivity. For the purposes of this review, panel-based testing is defined as the aggregation of genomic regions of interest into a single assay. This practice is in contrast with the interrogation of single exons and/or genes via standalone tests run in parallel or sequentially. We explore panel-based testing, including its history, current usefulness, and special

[a] Department of Pathology, University of Colorado, 12705 East Montview Boulevard BioScience 2, Room 4105, Aurora, CO 80045, USA; [b] Department of Pathology, Brigham and Women's Hospital, 75 Francis Street, Boston, MA 02115, USA
* Corresponding author.
E-mail address: Nicholas.willard@childrenscolorado.org

Clin Lab Med 42 (2022) 309–323
https://doi.org/10.1016/j.cll.2022.04.004
0272-2712/22/© 2022 Elsevier Inc. All rights reserved.
labmed.theclinics.com

considerations. We also show examples of the successes and challenges of panel-based sequencing and discuss potential future directions.

HISTORY

Within the realm of molecular diagnostics and in many laboratories, Sanger sequencing remains the gold standard for the evaluation of (most commonly) single exons within single genes. Developed by Fredrich Sanger in 1977, this technology uses the incorporation of chain-terminating dideoxynucleotides by the DNA polymerase during in vitro DNA replication.[1] This process permits an analysis of the various-sized products via gel or capillary electrophoresis with subsequent sequence assembly and variant identification. Although Sanger sequencing has stood the test of time in cancer genetics, it is somewhat laborious and suffers from relatively poor analytical sensitivity, often requiring 15% to 20% or more mutant alleles for reliable detection.[1–3] Quantitative polymerase chain reaction (PCR) techniques such as SYBR green and TaqMan overcome the issue of limited analytical sensitivity, routinely generating reliable results for specimens containing 1% to 5% mutant alleles; however, their application is constrained to specific alterations of interest, thus limiting their usefulness in the interrogation of broader genomic regions.[4] Analytical sensitivity can be further enhanced using platforms such as droplet digital PCR, which can reliably detect mutant alleles in the 0.1% to 0.5% range, with the potential for further improvement depending on input type.[5] Other testing strategies permit for good analytical sensitivity and greater magnitude of multiplexibility, including mass spectrophotometry-based assays or primer extension methods that distinguish between wild-type and mutant alleles based on product mass (Seqenom) or size analysis (Snapshot).[6,7] These techniques typically demonstrate analytical sensitivity in the 5% to 10% mutant allele range. However, these too are limited by a need for a priori knowledge of the variants of interest and fall short when interrogating tumor suppressor genes or when looking for variants other than single nucleotide substitutions. In contrast with these targeted approaches, NGS offers the capability to achieve nearly limitless target multiplexing, albeit requiring more resources (**Fig. 1**).

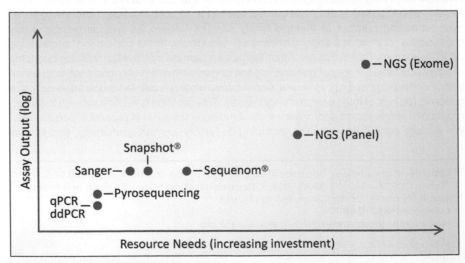

Fig. 1. Resource needs versus assay output.

Given the ever-growing investment in biomarker-driven precision oncology, the number of clinically relevant genomic alterations in solid tumors has increased steadily. Many common solid tumors are now recognized to contain oncogenic drivers or tumor suppressor gene alterations that have implications for diagnostic classification, prognostication, and, importantly, prediction of targeted therapy sensitivity or resistance. At this critical inflection point in the history of cancer medicine, it is difficult to rationalize the ongoing use of targeted single gene assays alone in clinical diagnostics, except for when specimen limitations preclude a more comprehensive analysis. This is due to a multitude of reasons including, but not limited to, potential costs, low throughput, technologist time, and the greater likelihood of tissue depletion when doing piecemeal testing. Although targeted testing remains useful for specific circumstances (such as specimen limitations), increasingly, the benefits of panel-based testing outweigh the concerns and resource needs (**Table 1**).

LUNG CANCER AS A PARADIGM

No other solid tumor better epitomizes the usefulness of panel-based testing than non-small cell lung cancer (NSCLC). Lung cancer is the leading cause of cancer deaths both in the United States and worldwide.[8] Studies exploring the genomic landscape of NSCLC over the last 2 decades have identified multiple driver alterations in multiple genes (15, 16, 17), including missense mutations, insertions–deletions, copy number alterations, and structural variants, such as those leading to gene fusions. Many of these specific variants predict response to one or more targeted therapies. Given the diversity of alterations predicting response to a wide array of therapies (**Table 2**), there is growing evidence that panel-based testing is not only appropriate from the standpoint of comprehensive clinical sensitivity, but is often the most financially and logistically viable approach.[9]

The first gene of clinical relevance to be identified as a driver in NSCLC was epidermal growth factor gene family member *EGFR*, encoding the epidermal growth factor receptor, a crucial receptor tyrosine kinase that signals in lung development and homeostasis. Early clinical trials of the EGFR tyrosine kinase inhibitors erlotinib and gefitinib in unselected patients with NSCLC led to disappointing results, with no apparent survival benefit over cytotoxic chemotherapy.[10] However, case reports described impressive responses to these drugs in certain patients—most commonly women of Asian descent with limited to no history of smoking—but otherwise the reason for these discrepant results was unclear.[11,12] Focused sequencing of the *EGFR* tyrosine kinase domain in cohorts of patients with lung cancer who responded to EGFR tyrosine kinase inhibitors revealed the presence of highly recurrent mutations that led to constitutive downstream signaling (the oncogenic driver) that correlated with a sensitivity to these targeted inhibitors (the Achilles heel).[12,13] Subsequently, transcriptional profiling efforts identified gene fusion events as another class of oncogenic driver alteration in NSCLC, starting with discovery of fusions in the receptor tyrosine kinase gene *ALK* in 2007.[14] Fortuitously, *ALK* fusions were readily detectable using fluorescence in situ hybridization and were also shown to predict response to crizotinib, an existing tyrosine kinase inhibitor developed against hepatocyte growth factor receptor (encoded by *MET*). Crizotinib was quickly repurposed for use in *ALK*-rearranged lung cancers and approved for this indication only 3 years after these alterations were discovered.[15]

These developments prompted the first ever guideline for molecular biomarker testing for lung cancer. Published in 2013, the College of American Pathologists, the International Association for the Study of Lung Cancer, and the Association for

Table 1
Advantages and disadvantages of panel next generation sequencing in clinical laboratories

	Pros	Cons
Technical parameters/ performance characteristics	• Analytical sensitivity of NGS greater than Sanger and comparable to PCR • Detects multiple classes of variants permitting improved clinical sensitivity relative to single gene assays • Ease of data visualization permits detection of artifacts, phasing of variants, and variant quantitation	• Achieving sensitivity comparable to standalone digital techniques (eg, droplet digital PCR) requires high sequencing depth and error correction • Significant dependence on bioinformatics processes and personnel
Clinical usefulness	• Broad scope of coverage • Clinical biomarkers can be built into a panel in anticipation of future actionability and turned on when needed for reporting • Facilitates data aggregation to inform design of clinical trials of precision therapies • Supports biomarker discovery relative to therapeutic outcomes • Ease of detection of multiple classes of alterations improves interpretation of biologic/clinical relevance ○ For example, inference of biallelic inactivation of tumor suppressor genes • Narrows the gap between introduction of biomarker in the research setting and reporting in a diagnostic laboratory	• May be perceived by payors as outside of the realm of clinical usefulness, thus jeopardizing reimbursement • Data analysis may be laborious and time consuming • Distinction between biologically relevant variants and passenger mutations can be time-consuming and associated with interpretive uncertainty and inconsistency
Germline variant detection	• Variant quantification can be used to aid in inference of somatic vs germline status (in tumor only testing) • Can facilitate screening for hereditary diseases • Detection of incidental germline findings, when communicated properly	• Tumor-only testing requires potentially unreliable inference of germline events based on variant allele fraction and population databases • Paired tumor–germline analysis drives up sequencing costs

(*continued on next page*)

Table 1 (*continued*)		
	Pros	**Cons**
	to the patient, can facilitate risk reduction practices for patient and family members	• For tests that return germline results, dedicated germline pipeline and curation expert are needed • Patient consent and access to genetic counseling are required when laboratories return germline results
Tissue use	• A single large panel assay may require less tissue than multiple targeted assays in aggregate • Comprehensive panel testing reduces the need to conserve tissue for further and potential future testing • Amplicon-based NGS may accept extremely limited input, achieving a balance between tissue use and clinical sensitivity when material is scant	• Up-front panel sequencing may require more tissue than any individual single gene assay
Staff use	• Consolidation of multiple genomic targets in a single assay reduces number of individual testing platforms required in the laboratory, permitting more focused technical expertise • Reducing number of clinical platforms creates time and labor savings around staff training and competency • Laboratory management can focus on validation and maintenance of a more confined set of instruments	• Overall demands on staff time and attention may be greater, requiring more training and closer supervision • Greater automation may drive down technical staff engagement with the process and lead to inattention
Cost effectiveness	• Technical cost per base is consistently dropping; the cumulative cost per analyte is vastly in favor of NGS panel-based testing	• Overall cost per sample is higher when larger NGS panels are performed • Reimbursement of expansive panels remains a topic of contention • Precision techniques and high throughput drive

(*continued on next page*)

Table 1
(continued)

	Pros	Cons
		need for additional capital investment in robotic platforms
Turnaround time	• A single comprehensive panel test may require less time to complete than multiple sequential targeted tests	• At present, panel sequencing typically has a longer turnaround time than individual targeted assays • Relatively inflexible technical considerations for hybrid capture NGS drives longer overall assay time relative to alternative methods • The amount of information generated can be difficult to navigate, leading to delays in reporting time, particularly in inexperienced hands
Bioinformatics requirements	• Customizable data analysis enables optimization of individual assays based on the laboratory needs • Bioinformatic processes can largely be automated • Commercial pipeline solutions are readily available for labs lacking specialized bioinformatics expertise	• Qualified bioinformatics personnel that can build, modify, and troubleshoot pipelines can be both costly and scarce • Resources to ensure longitudinal access to informatics platform are necessary, and pipelines may not be easily portable
Data management/ computation	• A robust data warehouse allows for data mining, including the incidence of variants in different disease types • Linking of aggregated results to outcomes data facilitates interpretation of rare variants • Facilitates target discovery approaches (eg, what markers modulate responsiveness to targeted therapy) • Many commercial products are available to help facilitate this as well as provide interinstitutional data	• Requires significant software and hardware computational bandwidth • Data storage is associated with high costs • Local institutions may lack the resources to support secure, accessible data storage • Cloud-based infrastructure/storage may not be acceptable to medical institutions owing to concerns over health information security

Table 2
Selected somatic targets and tumor-types and therapies for solid tumors

Biomarker	Tumor Type (approved)	Tumor Type (emerging)[a]	Therapies
EGFR 'sensitizing mutations'	NSCLC		Erlotinib, gefitinib, osimertinib
EGFR ex20ins	NSCLC		Amivantamab-vmjw
ALK rearrangement	NSCLC	Pan-solid tumor	Alectinib, crizotinib
ROS1 rearrangement	NSCLC	Pan-solid tumor	Entrectinib, crizotinib
RET rearrangement	NSCLC, thyroid	Pan-solid tumor	Selpercatinib, pralesetinib
MET exon 14 splice mutation	NSCLC		Capmatinib, tepotinib, crizotinib
MET amplification		NSCLC	Capmatinib, tepotinib, crizotinib
BRAF p.V600 E	NSCLC, melanoma, CRC, thyroid	Pan-solid tumor	Dabrafanib + trametinib
NTRK1/2/3 rearrangement	Pan-solid tumor		Entrectinib, larotrectinib
ERBB2 exon 20 mutation		NSCLC	Trastuzumab–deruxtecan[a]
KRAS p.G12 C mutation	NSCLC	Pan-solid tumor	Adagrasib,[a] sotorasib
PIK3CA hotspot mutations	Breast		Alpelisib
ERBB2 (HER2) amplification	Breast, GEJ	CRC	Trastuzumab Pertuzumab Trastuzumab–deruxtecan[a]
FGFR2 fusion	Intrahepatic cholangiocarcinoma, urothelial		Erdafitinib Pemigatinib Infagratinib
FGFR3 mutations (exons 7, 10 hotspots)	Urothelial		Erdafitinib
IDH1 p.R132X mutation	Intrahepatic cholangiocarcinoma	Glioma chondrosarcoma	Ivositinib
KIT exon 11, 13, 14, 17 mutations	GIST		Imatinib Sunitinib
PDGFRA p.D842 V mutation	GIST		Avapritinib
Mismatch repair deficiency/ microsatellite instability	Pan-solid tumor		Pembrolizumab
Tumor mutation burden	Pan-solid tumor		Pembrolizumab

Abbreviations: CRC, colorectal carcinoma; GEJ, gastroesophageal junction carcinoma; GIST, gastrointestinal stromal tumor; NSCLC, non small cell lung carcinoma.
[a] Emerging tumor types may not indicate efforts to seek FDA approval for that indication.

Molecular Pathology recommended routine profiling for *EGFR* and *ALK* gene alterations in NSCLC, stating, "The major, evidence-based recommendations are to test for *EGFR* mutations and *ALK* fusions in all patients with advanced stage adenocarcinoma, regardless of sex, race, or smoking history, and to prioritize *EGFR* and *ALK* testing over other molecular predictive tests."[16] At this point in history, panel-based NGS testing was not widely available and was largely considered to be for research purposes only. Indeed, the testing guidelines in 2013 emphasized the appropriate test type and performance characteristics (sensitive molecular methods for *EGFR* mutational profiling; fluorescence in situ hybridization for *ALK*) but gave little airtime to more comprehensive testing strategies.

These early discoveries motivated a number of tumor profiling efforts that have since defined the genetic landscape of lung cancer; we now know that approximately two-thirds of nonsquamous non-small cell lung carcinomas (predominantly adenocarcinomas) are characterized by individual mitogenic pathway driver events that occur in a predominantly mutually exclusive fashion, but whose biology may be modified by the presence of facilitative alterations in tumor suppressor genes or parallel progrowth pathways. Since the 2013 guidelines, targetable driver gene alterations have been identified in NSCLC in *ROS1*, *BRAF*, *MET*, *RET*, *KRAS*, *ERBB2* (HER2), and *NTRK1/2/3*, among others.[17] Based on superior survival benefits when compared to cytotoxic chemotherapy, at least one, and in most cases multiple, selective inhibitors have been approved by the US Food and Drug Administration (FDA) as first- or second-line therapies for patients whose lung tumors harbor specific alterations in these genes.[18–20] In light of this complexity, it is clear that standalone single-gene assays are unlikely to suffice for NSCLC testing. Targeted assays that have been optimized for hotspot point mutations and small indels will be insensitive to the more diverse spectrum of oncogenic alterations observed in certain targets (eg, *MET*, *EGFR* exon 20).[21,22] Targeted fusion testing strategies (fluorescence in situ hybridization, reverse transcriptase PCR) can be difficult to multiplex to a level that offers optimal clinical sensitivity and demand a completely unique parallel workflow from NGS-based molecular testing. In contrast, NGS-based techniques can reliably detect the majority of the clinically relevant alterations, particularly if DNA and RNA strategies are combined.[23]

In 2018, the College of American Pathologists/International Association for the Study of Lung Cancer/Association for Molecular Pathology guidelines were revised to include mandatory testing for *EGFR*, *ALK*, and *ROS1* with optional inclusion of *ERBB2*, *MET*, *BRAF*, *KRAS*, and *RET* testing for those laboratories that perform NGS panels.[24] This expert consensus promoted the use of NGS-based methods while also acknowledging that the technology at the time still had made limited entry into clinical diagnostics and could be cost prohibitive for many laboratories. Since 2018, comprehensive NGS-based panel testing has been widely commercialized and test reimbursement has become more favorable (as discussed elsewhere in this article), thus lifting some of the logistical and economic restraints on more widespread adoption. Although the College of American Pathologists/International Association for the Study of Lung Cancer/Association for Molecular Pathology molecular testing guidelines have not yet been updated at the time of this writing, other organizations (American Society of Clinical Oncology, National Comprehensive Cancer Network) have emphasized the need for comprehensive testing in the clinical management of patients with lung cancer and the recommended use of NGS approaches when possible.[25–27]

It is worth noting that these guidelines also suggest the use of assays with 5% or greater analytical sensitivity for the detection of heterogeneous resistance mutations such as *EGFR* p.T790 M in the setting of progression on early generation tyrosine kinase inhibitors. When dealing with resistance (sub)clones, it is clear that traditional Sanger sequencing is not sensitive enough to reliably detect variants such as *EGFR* p.T790M. Furthermore, newer generation EGFR inhibitors are associated with fewer secondary *EGFR* variants and more bypass pathway mechanisms of resistance, including mutations, copy number, and structural variants in genes within parallel signaling pathways.[28] Similar complexity has been observed in resistance patterns arising following targeted therapies for the range of other oncogenic drivers seen in lung cancer.[29] Thus, for the purposes of the optimal characterization of targeted therapy resistance both for sensitivity and breadth, panel-based NGS strategies are strongly preferred.

EXTRAPOLATION TO OTHER CANCER TYPES

Beyond lung cancer, we are now seeing usefulness for panel sequencing for a rapidly growing number of other tumor types. At present, relatively few genomic targets may be required to select a patient for relevant therapies for some tumor types (eg, *PIK3CA* hotspot mutations in breast cancer; *FGFR2* and *FGFR3* alterations in bladder cancer; *FGFR2* and *IDH1* alterations in cholangiocarcinoma) (see **Table 2**),[30] and although some FDA-approved companion diagnostics have included panel-based NGS tests, many drugs are paired with unique targeted assays that are highly focused on a small number of specific alterations.[31] Practically, however, many laboratories serve a diverse population of patients with cancer and cannot support the panoply of companion diagnostic assays created by different manufacturers using a diversity of techniques, platforms, and extraction methodologies. Therefore, a more comprehensive NGS-based strategy is preferable; this testing can be designed to report uniformly on all the gene targets covered by the baiting strategy, or results can be bioinformatically filtered to be disease specific. The former allows for a greater breadth of mutation detection and the potential for unexpected targetable findings, whereas the latter allows for the simplification of reporting. Using NSCLC as the paradigm, it is reasonable to expect that, over time, a similar diversity of low-frequency yet clinically vital alterations will be recognized in multiple tumor types.

In addition to the increasingly ubiquitous adoption of short read sequencing for mutation detection, technical and bioinformatic processes have unveiled a broader application of NGS panel testing. This process includes an assessment of broader mutational patterns to inform diagnosis and therapy, in many cases by using computationally derived variables that are uniquely possible in larger panels. Tumor mutational burden has been recognized as a potential surrogate for tumor neoantigenic load and predicting response to immune checkpoint blockade and indeed has been approved by the FDA for use as a biomarker of response to the anti–programmed cell death-1 therapy pembrolizumab across all solid tumors.[32] Mismatch repair deficiency detection by NGS performs comparably with the detection of mismatch repair protein loss by immunohistochemistry or microsatellite instability by PCR.[33–35] Indeed, the ability to examine a wide spectrum of microsatellite loci has the potential to optimize the detection of mismatch repair deficiency in a tumor-type–specific fashion.[35] Mutational signatures, derived from the substitution type and adjacent base context for any individual mutation, have the potential for powerful additional disease characterization.[36,37] In particular, signatures that point to tumor etiology, such as ultraviolet light and tobacco, can be identified in NGS panels and have the potential to refine the primary diagnosis.[38] Specifically, NGS panels that capture several hundred genes (or approximately 0.7 Mb of content) are typically sufficient for the purposes of tumor mutational burden,[39] mismatch repair, and other mutational signature detection assuming appropriate bioinformatic strategies are used; there is no need to develop a separate assay.

COST AND REIMBURSEMENT

Multiple factors contribute to the assessment of overall cost when considering NGS-based testing, and decisions about whether and how to adopt such approaches can be challenging. As with any fiscal analysis in laboratory medicine, an evaluation of fixed costs, indirect costs, capital expenditures, projection of testing volumes, and clinical reimbursement requires careful analysis. Beyond the typical concerns, some considerations regarding cost are relatively unique to NGS. One such consideration is the rapid evolution of sequencing technologies, leading to an ever-increasing demand for more genomic information per patient. Capital equipment purchases to meet current volume and panel size standards can be outpaced rapidly by clinical interest in larger panels, even if such interest outpaces clinically proven actionability. Despite evolving interest in more extensive genomic profiling, to date there is little evidence of the clinical usefulness of technologies, such as whole exome sequencing or whole genome sequencing for most adult patients with cancer. Instrumentation can become obsolete in 5 years or less, which is far less time than typical laboratory platform lifecycle considerations for major capital expenditures.[40]

Assay complexity is another factor that can create unique considerations, because it engenders a need for a workforce of highly trained personnel and/or advanced robotic equipment to automate the more complex elements of library preparation. The labor-intensive nature of the work, combined with expensive reagents and consumables, leads to a high average operating cost per test. Estimating an actual cost per test is challenging at best; numerous variables (such as batch size and the specific instrument platform used if multiple are available within the laboratory) can impact internal costs dramatically. An often underestimated cost to maintain NGS testing not commonly encountered in typical laboratory medicine environments is in bioinformatics and data management. The identification and retention of bioinformatics personnel is a significant challenge, and alternatives to this model, such as pay-per-case bioinformatics from commercial software as a service provider, warrant consideration. Several studies have identified the challenges of costing or microcosting NGS testing, and inevitably, unanticipated costs are likely.

Given the resource-intensive nature of this testing paradigm, many health systems are challenged with a build-versus-buy decision. Choosing to build an infrastructure to support NGS testing likely needs a concurrent commitment to subsidize operational costs over time, because the reimbursement landscape of this testing is challenging. Insourcing testing does provide specific advantages, however, including the ability to adapt testing to specimen types not accepted by large reference laboratories, data governance benefits, and, importantly, the connection between treating provider and laboratory.

The billing, coding, and reimbursement landscape for molecular diagnostics remains vexing, despite an overhaul in the Current Procedural Terminology coding for these services.[41] In 2012, Current Procedural Terminology codes previously geared around specific laboratory technical procedures were replaced by analyte-specific codes to generate increased transparency around which genetic testing is performed. Codes for panel-based testing, termed genomic sequencing procedures, were implemented; in oncology testing, these codes are based on the number of genes interrogated and whether the tested sample is a solid tumor or hematolymphoid neoplasm. This new paradigm for billing has created a new round of challenges; payers cite the number of genes tested as an insufficient measure of whether the right genes are tested. Because the smallest panel codes are for 5 to 50 genes, payers have similarly opposed coverage of panel testing; many tumor types have on-label indications related to fewer than 5 biomarkers. Similarly, concerns about the coverage of larger scale genomic testing are centered on the lack of clear clinical usefulness. Medicare and private payer coverage for panel-based billing codes has lagged significantly compared with the timeline of clinical adoption.[42]

Despite these challenges, payers are increasingly recognizing that roadblocks to effective genomic testing ultimately have adverse implications for therapy selection and patient outcomes.[43]

FUTURE AVENUES

Given the expanding role of molecular characterization in the management of patients with cancers, sequencing panels are increasingly essential, not just for the detection of targetable oncogenic driver alterations, but also to uncover more complex aspects of tumor biology. With increasingly widespread access to the laboratory and computation infrastructure to support comprehensive tumor molecular profiling, more patients can be expected to have access to a breadth of tumor and germline mutational information that may modify treatment and management decisions. At present, most of the mutational information generated by panel assays containing hundreds of gene targets does not influence cancer diagnosis or therapeutic selection, but preliminary evidence does suggest that several tumor suppressor genes have prognostic implications and may possibly influence response to targeted therapies in some contexts.[44–50] The future of molecular diagnostics almost certainly will involve the integration of results across not only DNA-based sequencing panels, but also transcriptomic and methylomic assays. This process will likely require the implementation of more sophisticated computational algorithms and artificial intelligence layered on the currently largely manual variant interpretation process carried out in most laboratories.[51,52] Algorithms that incorporate signature analyses can further validate the role of specific mutations, such as POLE ultramutation signature in the context of *POLE* mutations, and signature 3 or homologous recombination signatures in the context of *BRCA* or other homologous recombination pathway gene alterations.[53–56] These signatures may have important implications for the prediction of response to targeted therapies including immune checkpoint blockade and poly-ADP ribose polymerase inhibitors, respectively. For this information to be leveraged optimally for patient care, the tumor and germline profiles will need to be distilled into succinct, digestible reports and interpreted by clinicians with a solid understanding of genomics as it applies to cancer management in different disease contexts. The future of oncology precision medicine will surely rely on enhanced cross-disciplinary communication and updated training modalities to ensure up-to-date knowledge and adoption of broader testing across the board. Molecular diagnosticians and treating clinicians will increasingly rely on robust bioinformatics infrastructure and incorporation of big data to inform their practice; this practice goes hand in hand with the technical revolution in sequencing afforded by panel testing.

CLINICS CARE POINTS

Panel-based testing for cancer genomic biomarkers offers benefits beyond single gene assays related to completeness of biomarker detection, conservation of tumor tissue, and potential economic benefit.

DISCLOSURE

Dr L. Sholl reports consulting income from Genentech and Lilly, and research funds from Genentech. Dr D. Aisner reports consulting income from Takeda, Sanofi-Genzyme, Loxo Oncology, and Blueprint Medicines.

REFERENCES

1. Sanger F, Coulson AR. A rapid method for determining sequences in DNA by primed synthesis with DNA polymerase. J Mol Biol 1975;94(3):441–8.
2. Rehm HL, Bale SJ, Bayrak-Toydemir P, et al. ACMG clinical laboratory standards for next-generation sequencing. Genet Med 2013;15(9):733–47.
3. Tsiatis AC, Norris-Kirby A, Rich RG, et al. Comparison of Sanger sequencing, pyrosequencing, and melting curve analysis for the detection of KRAS mutations: diagnostic and clinical implications. J Mol Diagn 2010;12(4):425–32.
4. Sheikine Y, Rangachari D, McDonald DC, et al. EGFR testing in advanced non–small-cell lung cancer, a mini-review. Clinical Lung Cancer 2016;17(6):483–92.
5. Cabel L, Proudhon C, Romano E, et al. Clinical potential of circulating tumour DNA in patients receiving anticancer immunotherapy. Nat Rev Clin Oncol 2018; 15(10):639–50.
6. MacConaill LE, Garcia E, Shivdasani P, et al. Prospective enterprise-level molecular genotyping of a cohort of cancer patients. J Mol Diagn 2014;16(6):660–72.
7. Su Z, Dias-Santagata D, Duke M, et al. A platform for rapid detection of multiple oncogenic mutations with relevance to targeted therapy in non-small-cell lung cancer. J Mol Diagn 2011;13(1):74–84.
8. Sung H, Ferlay J, Siegel RL, et al. Global cancer statistics 2020: GLOBOCAN estimates of incidence and mortality worldwide for 36 cancers in 185 countries. CA Cancer J Clin 2021;71(3):209–49.
9. Steuten L, Goulart B, Meropol NJ, Pritchard D, Ramsey SD. Cost effectiveness of multigene panel sequencing for patients with advanced non-small-cell lung cancer. JCO Clin Cancer Inform 2019;3:1–10.
10. Fukuoka M, Yano S, Giaccone G, et al. Multi-institutional randomized phase II trial of gefitinib for previously treated patients with advanced non-small-cell lung cancer (The IDEAL 1 Trial) [corrected]. J Clin Oncol 2003;21(12):2237–46.
11. Bareschino MA, Schettino C, Troiani T, Martinelli E, Morgillo F, Ciardiello F. Erlotinib in cancer treatment. Ann Oncol 2007;18(Suppl 6):vi35–41.
12. Lynch TJ, Bell DW, Sordella R, et al. Activating mutations in the epidermal growth factor receptor underlying responsiveness of non–small-cell lung cancer to gefitinib. N Engl J Med 2004;350(21):2129–39.
13. Paez JG, Janne PA, Lee JC, et al. EGFR mutations in lung cancer: correlation with clinical response to gefitinib therapy. Science 2004;304(5676):1497–500.
14. Soda M, Choi YL, Enomoto M, et al. Identification of the transforming EML4-ALK fusion gene in non-small-cell lung cancer. Nature 2007;448(7153):561–6.
15. Solomon BJ, Mok T, Kim DW, et al. First-line crizotinib versus chemotherapy in ALK-positive lung cancer. N Engl J Med 2014;371(23):2167–77.
16. Lindeman NI, Cagle PT, Beasley MB, et al. Molecular testing guideline for selection of lung cancer patients for EGFR and ALK tyrosine kinase inhibitors: guideline from the College of American Pathologists, International Association for the Study of Lung Cancer, and Association for Molecular Pathology. J Mol Diagn 2013;15(4):415–53.
17. Konig D, Savic Prince S, Rothschild SI. Targeted therapy in advanced and metastatic non-small cell lung cancer. An update on treatment of the most important

actionable oncogenic driver alterations. Cancers (Basel) 2021;13(4). https://doi.org/10.3390/cancers13040804.

18. Shaw AT, Riely GJ, Bang YJ, et al. Crizotinib in ROS1-rearranged advanced non-small-cell lung cancer (NSCLC): updated results, including overall survival, from PROFILE 1001. Ann Oncol 2019;30(7):1121–6.

19. Vansteenkiste JF, Van De Kerkhove C, Wauters E, Van Mol P. Capmatinib for the treatment of non-small cell lung cancer. Expert Rev Anticancer Ther 2019;19(8): 659–71.

20. Drilon A, Laetsch TW, Kummar S, et al. Efficacy of larotrectinib in TRK fusion-positive cancers in adults and children. N Engl J Med 2018;378(8):731–9.

21. Arcila ME, Nafa K, Chaft JE, et al. EGFR exon 20 insertion mutations in lung adenocarcinomas: prevalence, molecular heterogeneity, and clinicopathologic characteristics. Mol Cancer Ther 2013;12(2):220–9.

22. Socinski MA, Pennell NA, Davies KD. MET exon 14 skipping mutations in non-small-cell lung cancer: an overview of biology, clinical outcomes, and testing considerations. JCO Precis Oncol 2021. https://doi.org/10.1200/PO.20.00516.

23. Benayed R, Offin M, Mullaney K, et al. High yield of RNA sequencing for targetable kinase fusions in lung adenocarcinomas with no mitogenic driver alteration detected by DNA sequencing and low tumor mutation burden. Clin Cancer Res 2019;25(15):4712–22.

24. Lindeman NI, Cagle PT, Aisner DL, et al. Updated molecular testing guideline for the selection of lung cancer patients for treatment with targeted tyrosine kinase inhibitors: guideline from the College of American Pathologists, the International Association for the Study of Lung Cancer, and the Association for Molecular Pathology. J Mol Diagn 2018;20(2):129–59.

25. Ettinger DS, Wood DE, Aisner DL, et al. NCCN guidelines insights: non-small cell lung cancer, version 2.2021. J Natl Compr Canc Netw 2021;19(3):254–66.

26. Network NCC. Non-small cell lung cancer. Accessed January 1, 2022.

27. Mosele F, Remon J, Mateo J, et al. Recommendations for the use of next-generation sequencing (NGS) for patients with metastatic cancers: a report from the ESMO Precision Medicine Working Group. Ann Oncol 2020;31(11): 1491–505.

28. Leonetti A, Sharma S, Minari R, Perego P, Giovannetti E, Tiseo M. Resistance mechanisms to osimertinib in EGFR-mutated non-small cell lung cancer. Br J Cancer 2019;121(9):725–37.

29. Rotow J, Bivona TG. Understanding and targeting resistance mechanisms in NSCLC. Nat Rev Cancer 2017;17(11):637–58.

30. Mo HR, Catherine. Biomarker-driven targeted therapies in solid tumor malignancies. J Hematol Oncol Pharm 2021;11(2):84–91.

31. Keeling P, Clark J, Finucane S. Challenges in the clinical implementation of precision medicine companion diagnostics. Expert Rev Mol Diagn 2020;20(6): 593–9.

32. Chan TA, Yarchoan M, Jaffee E, et al. Development of tumor mutation burden as an immunotherapy biomarker: utility for the oncology clinic. Ann Oncol 2019; 30(1):44–56.

33. Nowak JA, Yurgelun MB, Bruce JL, et al. Detection of mismatch repair deficiency and microsatellite instability in colorectal adenocarcinoma by targeted next-generation sequencing. J Mol Diagn 2017;19(1):84–91.

34. Middha S, Zhang L, Nafa K, et al. Reliable pan-cancer microsatellite instability assessment by using targeted next-generation sequencing data. JCO Precis Oncol 2017. https://doi.org/10.1200/PO.17.00084.

35. Long DR, Waalkes A, Panicker VP, Hause RJ, Salipante SJ. Identifying optimal loci for the molecular diagnosis of microsatellite instability. Clin Chem 2020; 66(10):1310–8.

36. Alexandrov LB, Nik-Zainal S, Wedge DC, Campbell PJ, Stratton MR. Deciphering signatures of mutational processes operative in human cancer. Cell Rep 2013; 3(1):246–59.

37. Alexandrov LB, Nik-Zainal S, Wedge DC, et al. Signatures of mutational processes in human cancer. Nature 2013;500(7463):415–21.

38. Lawrence L, Kunder CA, Fung E, Stehr H, Zehnder J. Performance characteristics of mutational signature analysis in targeted panel sequencing. Arch Pathol Lab Med 2021;145(11):1424–31.

39. Vega DM, Yee LM, McShane LM, et al. Aligning tumor mutational burden (TMB) quantification across diagnostic platforms: phase II of the Friends of Cancer Research TMB Harmonization Project. Ann Oncol 2021;32(12):1626–36.

40. van Nimwegen KJM, van Soest RA, Veltman JA, et al. Is the $1000 genome as near as we think? A cost analysis of next-generation sequencing. Clin Chem 2016;62(11):1458–64.

41. Sireci AN, Patel JL, Joseph L, et al. Molecular Pathology economics 101: an overview of molecular diagnostics coding, coverage, and reimbursement: a report of the association for molecular Pathology. J Mol Diagn 2020;22(8):975–93.

42. Hsiao SJ, Sireci AN, Pendrick D, et al. Clinical utilization, utility, and reimbursement for expanded genomic panel testing in adult oncology. JCO Precision Oncol 2020;(4):1038–48.

43. Pennell NA, Mutebi A, Zhou Z-Y, et al. Economic impact of next-generation sequencing versus single-gene testing to detect genomic alterations in metastatic non–small-cell lung cancer using a decision analytic model. JCO Precision Oncol 2019;3:1–9.

44. Aisner DL, Sholl LM, Berry LD, et al. The impact of smoking and TP53 mutations in lung adenocarcinoma patients with targetable mutations—the Lung Cancer Mutation Consortium (LCMC2). Clin Cancer Res 2018;24(5):1038–47.

45. Liu SY, Bao H, Wang Q, et al. Genomic signatures define three subtypes of EGFR-mutant stage II-III non-small-cell lung cancer with distinct adjuvant therapy outcomes. Nat Commun 2021;12(1):6450.

46. Chua KP, Teng YHF, Tan AC, et al. Integrative profiling of T790M-negative EGFR-mutated NSCLC reveals pervasive lineage transition and therapeutic opportunities. Clin Cancer Res 2021;27(21):5939–50.

47. Skoulidis F, Goldberg ME, Greenawalt DM, et al. STK11/LKB1 mutations and PD-1 inhibitor resistance in KRAS-mutant lung adenocarcinoma. Cancer Discov 2018;8(7):822–35.

48. Ricciuti B, Arbour KC, Lin JJ, et al. Diminished efficacy of programmed death-(ligand)1 inhibition in STK11- and KEAP1-mutant lung adenocarcinoma is affected by KRAS mutation status. J Thorac Oncol 2021. https://doi.org/10.1016/j.jtho.2021.10.013.

49. Schoenfeld AJ, Bandlamudi C, Lavery JA, et al. The genomic landscape of SMARCA4 alterations and associations with outcomes in patients with lung cancer. Clin Cancer Res 2020;26(21):5701–8.

50. Alessi JV, Ricciuti B, Spurr LF, et al. SMARCA4 and other SWItch/sucrose nonfermentable family genomic alterations in NSCLC: clinicopathologic characteristics and outcomes to immune checkpoint inhibition. J Thorac Oncol 2021;16(7):1176–87.

51. Zeng J, Shufean MA. Molecular-based precision oncology clinical decision making augmented by artificial intelligence. Emerg Top Life Sci 2021;5(6):757–64.

52. Asada K, Kaneko S, Takasawa K, et al. Integrated analysis of whole genome and epigenome data using machine learning technology: toward the establishment of precision oncology. Front Oncol 2021;11:666937. https://doi.org/10.3389/fonc.2021.666937.

53. Watkins PJ, Gorrod JW. Studies on the in vitro biological N-oxidation of trimethoprim. Eur J Drug Metab Pharmacokinet 1987;12(4):245–51.

54. Takamatsu S, Brown JB, Yamaguchi K, et al. Utility of homologous recombination deficiency biomarkers across cancer types. JCO Precis Oncol 2021. https://doi.org/10.1200/PO.21.00141.

55. Stover EH, Fuh K, Konstantinopoulos PA, Matulonis UA, Liu JF. Clinical assays for assessment of homologous recombination DNA repair deficiency. Gynecol Oncol 2020;159(3):887–98.

56. Kroeze LI, de Voer RM, Kamping EJ, et al. Evaluation of a hybrid capture–based pan-cancer panel for analysis of treatment stratifying oncogenic aberrations and processes. J Mol Diagn 2020;22(6):757–69.

Molecular Diagnostic Testing for Hematopoietic Neoplasms
Linking Pathogenic Drivers to Personalized Diagnosis

Christopher B. Hergott, MD, PhD[a,b], Annette S. Kim, MD, PhD[a,b],*

KEYWORDS

- Molecular diagnostics • Next-generation sequencing • Leukemia • Lymphoma
- Myeloma • Myeloid • Lymphoid

KEY POINTS

- Molecular diagnostics play a central role in the evaluation of hematopoietic malignancies.
- The molecular profiles of myeloid, lymphoid, and plasmacytic neoplasms can provide key diagnostic, prognostic, and therapeutic information while elucidating underlying biology.
- Next-generation sequencing technologies have empowered more personalized tumor characterization and individualized therapy.

INTRODUCTION

Once relegated to investigational or ancillary roles, nucleic acid-based molecular tests have become essential for the diagnosis and management of most hematologic malignancies. Molecular assays can offer improved analytical sensitivity, wide and customizable target breadth, and operational scalability/automation. However, their greatest strength lies in the ability to directly illuminate genetic alterations that drive disease pathogenesis. These insights allow diagnosticians to use a powerful, personalized approach to disease characterization, predict future disease behavior, and provide targets for therapy in some cases.[1–3] Recognizing these advances, the World Health Organization (WHO) and other organizations continue to expand the number of molecular alterations used as primary diagnostic criteria in their classifications of hematopoietic tumors.[4] Meanwhile, a pipeline of new molecular technologies

[a] Department of Pathology, Brigham and Women's Hospital, 75 Francis Street, Boston, MA 02115, USA; [b] Harvard Medical School, Boston, MA 02115, USA
* Corresponding author.
E-mail address: askim@bwh.harvard.edu

Clin Lab Med 42 (2022) 325–347
https://doi.org/10.1016/j.cll.2022.04.005
0272-2712/22/© 2022 Elsevier Inc. All rights reserved.

labmed.theclinics.com

continually narrows the gap between mechanistic insights and their application to patient care. In other words, the days of molecular diagnostics in an auxiliary role are behind us.

This review aims to provide a concise overview of the genetic alterations most important to detect in several major categories of adult hematopoietic neoplasia. For myeloid neoplasms, lymphoblastic leukemia/lymphoma, a selection of B and T cell lymphomas, and plasma cell neoplasms, we will focus on aberrations with diagnostic or prognostic importance and outline key techniques used for their detection. Although not a comprehensive review, this discussion should offer a guideline for building a minimal panel of genetic targets in the routine evaluation of these disease categories and provide a logical testing framework based on their pathogenic mechanisms.

MYELOID NEOPLASIA
Clonal Hematopoiesis

Human aging is accompanied by an accumulation of somatic mutations in nearly all tissues.[5–7] Although most of these variants are benign and transient, a distinct subset occurring in stem/progenitor cells can provide a durable fitness advantage, permitting progressive clonal expansion. In the hematopoietic system, this is referred to as clonal hematopoiesis (CH) and is most often detected by next-generation DNA sequencing (NGS).[8] The presence of detectable CH is strongly associated with advancing age (<1% of individuals aged younger than 40 years; >10% of individuals aged older than 70 years),[9] prior chemotherapy, chronic inflammation, and other conditions that augment expansion of mutant clones.[9–11] Although most patients with CH will not develop a hematologic malignancy, its presence is associated with a significantly increased risk of developing chronic myeloid neoplasms and/or acute myeloid leukemia (AML) in subsequent years.[8,12–14] Intriguingly, the adverse effects of CH lie not only in the development of subsequent myeloid neoplasms but also from an increased risk of atherosclerotic cardiovascular disease and other inflammatory conditions, driven in part by cytokines emanating from CH-derived leukocytes.[15–17] Thus, the timely detection of CH in otherwise healthy individuals can provide valuable information on risk for both neoplastic and nonneoplastic disorders.

A relatively restricted subset of mutations predominates among patients with CH (**Fig. 1**). In age-related CH, genes involved in epigenetic regulation (*DNMT3A*, *TET2*,

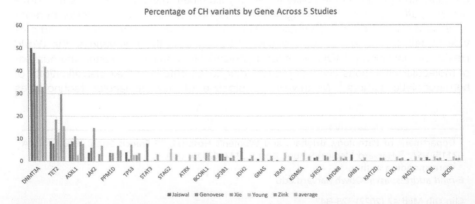

Fig. 1. Frequency (%) of CH variants by gene across 5 studies with fitted average line.[9,14,18–20]

and *ASXL1*) are among the most commonly mutated. Spliceosome gene mutations (*SRSF2, SF3B1*) are especially increased in individuals aged older than 70 years. *PPM1D* and *TP53* variants are enriched in therapy-related CH.[10,14,18–21] Although less prevalent than CH-associated sequence variants, myeloid-biased somatic copy number variants can also be detected in healthy individuals (termed mosaic chromosomal alterations) and may cooperate with mutations in pathogenesis through loss of heterozygosity.[22–24]

Although these mutations reflect changes characteristic of stem cells selected for survival, they are also among the most common mutations detected in myelodysplastic syndrome (MDS) (discussed in more detail in the Myelodysplastic Syndrome Section below).[22] This suggests CH-associated mutations likely serve as a mutational "foundation" on which additional genetic lesions accumulate in patients who progress to frank myeloid malignancy and should be included in any myeloid-directed mutation panel.

Myelodysplastic Syndrome and Secondary Acute Myeloid Leukemia

Evidence from multiple large patient cohorts has converged on a clinicopathologic model in which patients with CH (clonal mutation(s) without overt hematologic abnormalities) can progress to a clonal cytopenia of undetermined significance (CCUS; clonal mutation(s) plus cytopenia(s), without morphologic dysplasia) and ultimately frank MDS (clonal mutation(s), cytopenia(s), and morphologic dysplasia).[23] Although the molecular features of these diseases often overlap, MDS exhibits a higher burden of mutations in general, consistent with progression from the other conditions. Unsurprisingly, multiple mutations and higher mutant allele fractions are associated with increased risk of progression.[12] Stratifying the risk conferred by individual mutations is more complex but CH-associated variants enriched in MDS patients (compared with stable CH patients) are generally thought to confer higher risk of progression. Among these are mutations in *IDH1*, *IDH2*, and the splicing factors *U2AF1*, *SF3B1*, and *SRSF2*, as well as *TP53* and *PPM1D* in association with therapy-related myeloid neoplasms.[10,12,13,24]

The mutational profile of MDS builds on CH-associated variants and adds additional, disease-associated mutation classes that are rarer in CH. These include mutations in additional epigenetic modifiers (eg, *EZH2*, *IDH1*), splicing factors (as above, and *ZRSR2*), transcription factors (eg, *RUNX1*, *ETV6*, *GATA2*), cohesin complex components (eg, *STAG2*, *SMC1A*, *SMC3*, *RAD21*), and signaling mediators (*CBL*, *N/KRAS*, *FLT3*, *PTPN11*).[22,25–27] Similar to the progression from CH/CCUS to MDS, distinct constellations of MDS-associated mutations increase the risk of transformation to AML (termed "secondary AML;" sAML). Mutations in *TP53* (especially biallelic alterations), transcription factors, and signaling mediators seem reliably associated with progression, whereas *SF3B1* mutations confer a more favorable prognosis in MDS (and frequent presence of ringed sideroblasts).[22,26,28–30] Conversely, 8 MDS-associated mutations are highly specific for the appropriate designation of sAML, even if the antecedent neoplasm was undiagnosed: *SRSF2, SF3B1, U2AF1, ZRSR2, ASXL1, EZH2, BCOR*, or *STAG2*.[31]

Recurrent copy number variants and other cytogenetic abnormalities also comprise cardinal genetic changes in MDS/sAML. These can be detected by traditional karyotype and/or fluorescence in situ hybridization (FISH) studies. A subset of cytogenetic abnormalities appearing recurrently in MDS (**Table 1**) can provide presumptive molecular evidence of MDS even in the absence of frank morphologic dysplasia (although +8, del(20q), and −Y are insufficient for diagnosis). For example, the WHO has separated MDS with isolated del(5q) as a distinct subcategory—the only

Table 1
Myelodysplastic syndrome and acute myeloid leukemia genetic prognostic table from World Health Organization (WHO)/European LeukemiaNet (ELN)[32,33]

Chromosomal Abnormality	Prognosis^	Frequency MDS	Frequency t-MDS	Chromosomal/Molecular Abnormality	Prognosis^	Frequency AML
Unbalanced				**Balanced**		
Loss chr Y**	Very good	5%		t(15;17)(q22q11-12); PML::RARA	Favorable^	13%
del(11q)	Very good	3%		t(8;21)(q22;q22.1); RUNX1::RUNX1T1	Favorable	7%
[normal karyotype]	Good	50%		inv(16)(p13.1;q22) or t(16;16)(p13.1;q22); CBFB::MYH11	Favorable	5
del(5q)	Good	10%	20%	**Mutations**		
del(20q)*	Good	5-8%		Mutated NPM1 without FLT3-ITD or with FLT3-ITD^low	Favorable	
del(12p)	Good	3%		Biallelic CEBPA	Favorable	
[double, including del(5q)]	Good			**Balanced**		
del(7q)	Intermediate	10%#	50%#	t(9;11)(p21.3;q23.3); MLLT3::KMT2A	Intermediate	2%
gain chr 8*	Intermediate	10%		[cytogenetic abnormalities not classified as favorable or adverse]	Intermediate	
gain chr 19	Intermediate			**Mutations**		
iso(17q)	Intermediate	2-5%	25-30%	Mutated NPM1 and FLT3-ITD^high	Intermediate	
[single or double abnormalities, not specified in other subgroups]	Intermediate			Wild-type NPM1 without FLT3-ITD or with FLT3-ITD^low	Intermediate	
[2 or more independent but non-complex clones]	Intermediate			**Unbalanced**		
del13q		3%		Loss chr 5 or del(5q)	Adverse	
del(9q)		1-2%		Loss chr 7	Adverse	
loss chr 7	Poor	10%#	50%#	loss chr 17 or abn(17p)	Adverse	
idic(X)(q13)		1-2%		**Balanced**		
Balanced				t(6;9)(p23;q34.1); DEK::NUP214	Adverse	1%
inv(3)(q21.3q26.2)/t(3;3)(q21.3q26.2)	Poor	1%		t(v;11q23.3); KMT2A rearranged	Adverse	4%##
t(6;9)(p23;q34.1)		1%		t(9;22)(q34.1;q11.2); BCR::ABL1	Adverse	1%
t(2;11)(p21;q23.3)		1%		inv(3)(q21.3q26.2)/t(3;3)(q21.3q26.2); GATA2, MECOM	Adverse	1%
t(1;3)(p36.3;q21.2)		1%		[complex karyotype]	Adverse	
t(3;21)(q26.2;q22.1)			2%	[monosomal karyotype]	Adverse	
t(11;16)(q23.2;p13.3)			3%	**Mutations**		
[double including loss chr 7 or del(7q)]	Poor			Wild-type NPM1 and FLT3-ITD^high	Adverse	
[complex, 3 abnormalities]	Poor			Mutated RUNX1**	Adverse	
[complex, >3 abnormalities]	Very poor			Mutated ASXL1**	Adverse	
				Mutated TP53	Adverse	

^Prognostic designations, in alternating shading colors (no shading for genetic abnormalities not covered in the respective prognostic scoring systems), per the Comprehensive Cytogenetic Scoring System (CCSS) for MDS[ref] and the European LeukemiaNet risk stratification for AML.[ref] Note, the ELN stratification does not include PML::RARA and WHO prognosis is applied.

*Insufficient as a sole cytogenetic abnormality to make a presumptive diagnosis of MDS.

#Frequency in MDS and t-MDS combined for del(7q) and loss chr 7.

##This frequency includes t(9;11) cases.

**These mutations are considered adverse prognosis in the absence of a favorable-risk AML subtype. Note, unlike the NPM1 and CEBPA, these genes represent provisional categories in the 2017 WHO classification of AML.

Abbreviations: AML - acute myeloid leukemia, chr - chromosome, MDS - myelodysplastic syndrome, t-MDS - therapy-related MDS cytogenetically defined subset of MDS listed to date—reflecting its favorable prognosis and sensitivity to lenalidomide therapy.[4,34]

Myeloproliferative Neoplasms and Mastocytosis

Although we have focused thus far on the CH-MDS-sAML progression axis due to its genomic complexity, myeloid-directed molecular diagnostics must also account for myeloproliferative neoplasms (MPNs). Most famous among these is chronic myeloid leukemia (CML), characterized by a t(9;22) (q34;q11.2) BCR::ABL1 translocation detectable by karyotype, FISH, and/or quantitative polymerase chain reaction. Karyotype can be helpful in detecting secondary genomic abnormalities that help define accelerated-phase disease.[4] Sanger or next-generation sequencing can identify key resistance mutations in the ABL1 kinase domain (eg, p.T315I) among patients developing resistance to targeted tyrosine kinase inhibitors (eg, imatinib) and prompt transition to an alternative inhibitor (eg, dasatinib, nilotinib).[35]

Other MPNs may arise from a background of CH, with distinct subclonal mutations enriched in different neoplasms. The diagnosis of chronic neutrophilic leukemia (CNL) can be aided by inclusion of CSF3R mutations in a myeloid-directed sequencing panel. Although activating CSF3R mutations can appear in other myeloid neoplasms, its detection in patients with unexplained, marked neutrophilia can strongly support the diagnosis (83%–100% of CNL cases harbor a CSF3R mutation, including hotspot p.T618I).[36] Pathogenic mutations in JAK2, MPL, and CALR are shared in differing proportions by polycythemia vera, essential thrombocythemia, and primary myelofibrosis despite their often-divergent clinical manifestations.[37] Although these mutations (particularly JAK2) may also be found in CH/MDS, their detection in MPNs can qualify patients for treatment with a targeted inhibitor (eg, ruxolitinib).[38,39] In many MPN cases, the overall pattern of mutations can be more prognostically significant than the WHO-defined morphologic category alone.[40] Therefore, we recommend using a broader myeloid panel to establish the genomic context in which JAK2, CALR, or MPL mutations are found. Finally, mast cell neoplasms are characterized by activating mutations in the KIT oncogene (eg, p.D816V). In contrast to cutaneous mastocytosis, KIT mutations in systemic mastocytosis/mast cell leukemia commonly manifest as a late subclonal events in a background of CH.[41,42] KIT mutation status should be examined in any patient with symptoms suspicious for a mast cell disorder, both to support the diagnosis and potentially qualify the patient for KIT-targeted therapy (eg, avapritinib).[43] A summary of key molecular targets for MPNs is depicted in **Fig. 2**.

Myelodysplastic/Myeloproliferative Neoplasms

As the name suggests, myelodysplastic/MPNs share clinicopathologic features with both MDS and MPNs. These disorders exhibit substantial genomic overlap with MDS, although enrichments for specific mutational patterns may support their diagnosis.[44] Chronic myelomonocytic leukemia harbors CH/MDS-associated mutations; in fact, mutations in ASXL1, TET2, or SRSF2 are founding driver mutations in 90% of cases, whereas RAS signaling pathway mutations may drive a more proliferative, clinically aggressive phenotype.[44-48] Juvenile myelomonocytic leukemia exhibits a characteristic mutation pattern involving the RAS/RAF/MEK/ERK pathway (eg, PTPN11, NRAS, KRAS, NF1, CBL, RIT1) and some of these mutations may be germline-encoded (in association with Noonan syndrome or neurofibromatosis).[49] MDS/MPN with ring sideroblasts and thrombocytosis exhibits recurrent mutations in SF3B1 and JAK2 (less commonly CALR), reflecting the "dysplastic with ring sideroblasts" influence of the former with the proliferative influence of the latter.[50] BCR::ABL1-negative atypical CML (aCML) and unclassifiable MDS/MPN exhibit

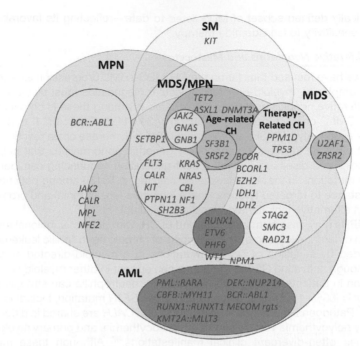

Fig. 2. Venn diagram of mutations associated with chronic myeloid neoplasia.

weaker distinctions from the broader mutational spectra of chronic myeloid neoplasms, although there may be a mild enrichment for *SETBP1* mutations in aCML.[51] In a more general sense, many overlap neoplasms may represent a spectrum of related diseases for which genomic characterization cannot provide sharp discrimination (see **Fig. 2**).[52,53]

De Novo Acute Myeloid Leukemia/Acute Myeloid Leukemia with Recurrent Genetic Abnormalities

Primary or "de novo" AML refers to myeloid leukemia arising in the absence of an antecedent myeloid neoplasm, without a mutational pattern strongly linked with sAML, and without prior exposure to leukemogenic therapies.[31,54] Despite partial overlap with mutations found in sAML, de novo AML cases enrich a unique set of recurrent mutations and chromosomal aberrations that can be detected by targeted sequencing, cytogenetic studies, and/or fusion transcript amplification (summarized in **Table 1**). In this group, recurrent somatic mutations in *NPM1*, *CEBPA* (biallelic), and *RUNX1* comprise discrete diagnostic and prognostic subtypes in the WHO classification and should be included in any myeloid-directed sequencing panel.[4] Germline-encoded mutations in *CEBPA*, *RUNX1*, and other genes can also drive MDS or AML.[55] However, these may be challenging to distinguish from somatic-origin mutations if blast frequency is high and concurrent, "nontumor" tissue is absent. Referral of these patients and their families to genetic counseling should be considered when clinical suspicion is high.

Genomic characterization has begun to directly influence risk stratification for AML patients, exemplified most notably by the 2017 European Leukemia Net (ELN) Guidelines detailed in **Table 1**. This classification stratifies AML into favorable, intermediate, and adverse genetic risk categories that strongly associate with patient outcomes.[34]

PRECURSOR LYMPHOID NEOPLASMS
B-Lymphoblastic Leukemia/Lymphoma

The genomic landscape of B-lymphoblastic leukemia/lymphoma (B-ALL) is complex and key driving alterations vary with patient age (**Fig. 3**).[56,57] Gross chromosomal changes, pathogenic gene fusions, copy number changes, and pathogenic sequence variants can all contribute to pathogenesis. Therefore, well-validated cytogenetic/FISH techniques, targeted mutation panels, and RNA-seq-based fusion detection can all serve important roles in a rigorous molecular diagnostics platform for B-ALL.[58] Conceptually, B-ALL arises from founder alterations that confer enhanced proliferation in B lymphoid progenitors and prevent B cell maturation, aided by cooperating mutations that disable key tumor suppressors and enhance proliferative signaling pathways.[59]

Key diagnostic subtypes of B-ALL are generally segregated by their founding genetic lesions (see **Fig. 3**), often including oncogenic gene fusions involving transcription factors or large-scale aneuploidy. These foundational genetic categories correspond with differing patient epidemiology and outcomes.[56] For example, B-ALL with hyperdiploid genome (>50 chromosomes), *ETV6::RUNX1* fusion, or rearrangements involving *DUX4* associate with a favorable prognosis; near-haploid cytogenetics (24–30 chromosomes), *NUTM1* fusions, and some *ZNF384* rearrangements

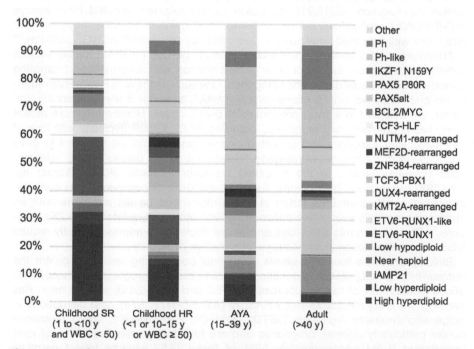

Fig. 3. B-ALL subtypes by age. AYA, adolescent and young adult; HR, high risk; Ph, Philadelphia chromosome; SR, standard risk; WBC, white blood cell count. (Inaba H, Mullighan CG. Pediatric acute lymphoblastic leukemia. Haematologica 2020;105(11):2524-2539; https://doi.org/10.3324/haematol.2020.247031.)

are considered intermediate-prognosis; and cases with low-hypodiploid genomes (31–39 chromosomes), *TCF3::HLF* fusion, *TCF3::PBX1* fusion, or *MEF2D* rearrangements correspond with adverse outcomes.[59]

B-ALL with *BCR::ABL1* fusion ("Philadelphia chromosome-positive" B-ALL) is a special case, traditionally associated with a poor prognosis but amenable to therapy with tyrosine kinase inhibitors (TKIs, eg, dasatinib). When used in concert with glucocorticoids, TKI therapy can obviate the need for cytotoxic induction chemotherapy in some patients, underscoring the importance of early detection of this pathogenic fusion.[60] *BCR::ABL1*-like B-ALL, a provisional entity in the 2016 WHO Classification,[4] harbors a transcriptional profile that resembles *BCR::ABL1* B-ALL but lacks this pathogenic fusion. Instead, these cases harbor a multiplicity of alternate fusions, particularly involving *CRLF2*, *ABL1* (non-*BCR* partners), and other kinases. Despite association with an adverse prognosis, recent studies suggest a reliance on JAK/STAT signaling and potential sensitivity to TKIs targeting *ABL1* or *JAK2* in some of these cases.[61]

Rearrangements involving *KMT2A* also confer a poor prognosis in B-ALL. Strikingly, *KMT2A* fusions can drive increased rates of lineage-discordant antigen expression and mutational profiles, lineage plasticity, and frank lineage switch to AML (particularly under therapeutic pressure).[62] This plasticity may complicate diagnosis in the absence of swift molecular diagnostics.

Finally, B-ALL with intrachromosomal amplification of chromosome 21 comprises a distinct subtype with predilection for pediatric patients and high risk of relapse following standard therapy but improved prognosis with intensive chemotherapy.[56,63] Although this amplification can appear in conventional cytogenetics if associated with gross abnormalities of chromosome 21 (eg, germline ring chromosome 21 or Robertsonian translocation rob(15;21)), detection usually requires targeted FISH assays (*ETV6::RUNX1* probes can suffice, showing copy gains of *RUNX1*), copy number array, or a well-validated copy number detection algorithm within an NGS platform.[64]

Advances in NGS have also illuminated disease biology for B-ALL cases without detectable pathogenic fusions or other gross chromosomal abnormalities, prompting consideration for future diagnostic categories. One such example is *PAX5*. Rearrangements and intragenic amplifications involving *PAX5*, a master B-lineage transcription factor, are detected in a small proportion of B-ALL cases. However, a more recent study has suggested point mutations, including *PAX5* p.P80R (typically with loss of heterozygosity), associate with activated kinase signaling and are sufficient to drive oncogenesis.[56,65] Similarly, whole-gene deletion, intragenic deletions, and heterozygous missense lesions in the lymphoid transcription factor *IKZF1* (Ikaros; eg, p.N159Y) can perturb DNA-binding function and drive oncogenesis.[66] In contrast, intragenic deletions of *ERG* (often in *DUX4*-rearranged cases) associate with an improved prognosis even when cooccurring with otherwise-deleterious *IKZF1* deletions.[67] These intragenic alterations and single nucleotide variants generally require NGS and/or chromosomal microarrays for sensitive detection.

Building on these founding events, additional cooperating lesions augment the outgrowth of B-ALL, disabling genetic barriers to disease progression. These alterations include loss of tumor suppressors *TP53* and *CDKN2A/B*, alterations in Ras pathway signaling mediators (eg, *KRAS*, *NRAS*, *PTPN11*, *NF1*), and disruptions in epigenetic/chromatin regulators (*SETD2*, *WHSC1*, *CREBBP*).[56,68] *TP53* mutations confer particularly adverse prognoses and are found in greater than 91% of low-hypodiploid B-ALL. Approximately 50% of these *TP53* variants reflect germline origin/Li Fraumeni syndrome.[69] Detection of these progression-associated mutations can further characterize disease behavior and stratify risk.

T-Lymphoblastic Leukemia/Lymphoma

T-lymphoblastic leukemia/lymphoma (T-ALL) arises from the coordinated accumulation of genetic lesions that drive overexpression of lymphoid transcription factors, impair T cell differentiation, activate kinase signaling, enhance proliferation, and disrupt tumor suppression mechanisms (**Fig. 4**).[70] Key to initiating this pathogenesis is aberrant overexpression of oncogenic transcription factors, usually driven by pathogenic rearrangements (often with T cell receptor gene enhancers). T-ALL categorization is based on these distinct genetic profiles, which in turn reflect the stages of T cell ontogeny from which the leukemias are thought to arise (ie, early T cell precursor, early cortical, and late cortical).[61,70] Activating mutations in *NOTCH1* comprise an orthogonal pillar of T-ALL pathogenesis across all subtypes, aided by frequently co-occurring mutations in *FBXW7* that further augment NOTCH1 signaling.[70–73]

Early T cell precursor ALL (ETP-ALL) is of particular importance from a diagnostic standpoint. Emphasized as a separate subcategory in the WHO 2016 classification,[4] ETP-ALL arises from CD4/CD8 double-negative, early T progenitors not yet committed irreversibly to T cell fate. These cases share overlapping immunophenotypic and molecular features with hematopoietic stem cells and myeloid precursors. In contrast with other forms of T-ALL, ETP-ALL harbors fewer alterations in *NOTCH1* and *CDKN2A*, frequent aberrant expression of the transcription factor *LYL1,* and mutation patterns more closely resembling myeloid neoplasia (eg, *RUNX1, FLT3, DNMT3A, NRAS, IDH1/2*).[70,74–76] Later stages of ETP-ALL may involve translocations of *MYB* or *NUP214* and mutations in the *JAK3/IL7R/STAT5B* axis, *ETV6*, and *EZH2* (see **Fig. 4**).[76–78] Given the poor prognosis and immunophenotypic complexity associated with ETP-ALL, these genetic features are especially important to include in any molecular diagnostic evaluation of T-ALL.[77,78]

In contrast, early cortical T-ALL is characterized by overexpression of *HOX11A*, with recurrent translocations involving *TLX3* and *TLX1* (early-phase) and *NKX2-1/5* (later-phase). Key associated alterations are seen in *RB1, PHF6, BCL11B,* and *CDKN1B,* among others. The late cortical stage-derived leukemias are characterized by *TAL1*

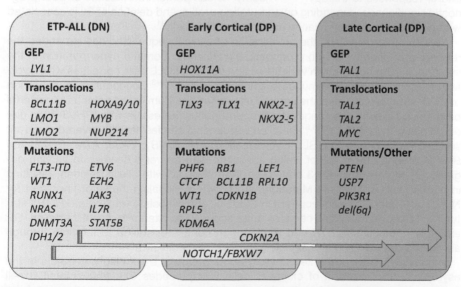

Fig. 4. Illustration of key events in T-ALL with associated mutated genes. DN, double negative (CD4–/CD8–), DP, double positive (CD4+/CD8+), GEP, gene expression profiling.

overexpression, often manifesting as rearrangements involving *TAL1*, *TAL2*, and *MYC*. In this last category, mutations in *PTEN*, *USP7*, and *PIK3R1* are highly recurrent progression-associated events, as is del(6q). Across all categories, loss of tumor suppressor *CDKN2A* disrupts control of cell cycle progression and contributes to disease progression.[70,74–76,78–83]

LYMPHOMA AND PLASMA CELL NEOPLASIA

The wide diversity of discrete mature B and T cell lymphomas, each with their own complex genomic landscapes, precludes comprehensive coverage in this brief overview. A singularly focused, thorough review on lymphoma genomics has been published elsewhere.[84] Here, we discuss particularly illustrative examples of the central role molecular techniques can play in diagnosis and/or prognostication for lymphoma and define the molecular alterations most important for rigorous disease characterization.

Chronic Lymphocytic Leukemia/Small Lymphocytic Lymphoma

Chronic lymphocytic leukemia (CLL) is a chronic lymphoproliferative disorder characterized by circulating, clonal mature B cells that may also involve lymph nodes, spleen, or other extramedullary tissues (small lymphocytic lymphoma [SLL] representing noncirculating, lymphomatous disease).[4] Significant heterogeneity in disease aggressiveness, including varying predisposition among patients toward transformation to more aggressive lymphomas, prompted efforts to link genetic features of CLL/SLL with patient outcomes (summarized in **Table 2**).[85] Among the first prognostically significant alterations discovered were cytogenetic changes detectable by karyotype, FISH, or chromosomal microarrays. Isolated deletions involving chromosome 13q14 (including microRNAs *miR-16–1* and *miR-15a*) are reliably associated with a more favorable prognosis, whereas deletions in 11q (*ATM* and *BIRC3*) or 17p (*TP53*) or the presence of a complex karyotype correspond with poorer patient outcomes and/or responses to therapy.[89,90] Trisomy 12 can confer intermediate or poor prognostic significance, depending on comutation profile, and deletion of 6q is associated with plasmacytoid differentiation and intermediate risk.[91]

As with other disorders, the proliferation of clinical sequencing has expanded the repertoire of alterations with prognostic significance. Somatic hypermutation in the immunoglobulin heavy chain variable region (*IGHV*) of CLL cells correlates with favorable response to chemoimmunotherapy and survival.[92,93] Concomitant identification of *IGHV* subtypes by the same sequencing assay has illuminated potentially powerful prognostic associations (ranging from spontaneous regression with *IGHV3-30* to dire outcomes with *IGHV3-21*).[86,87] Detailed sequencing studies have uncovered recurrent somatic mutations in CLL/SLL involving *NOTCH1*, *SF3B1*, *TP53*, *ATM*, *POT1*, and *BIRC3* (among others), all of which associate with poorer outcomes to varying degrees.[4,85] Mutations in *TP53* and *ATM* often cooccur with allelic deletion, resulting in biallelic loss of function. Mutations in *MYD88*, a signaling mediator important for NF-κB activation, are also recurrent in CLL/SLL and associate with mutated *IGHV* status.[94–96] Specific mutations can also drive acquired resistance to novel therapies. For example, mutations in *BTK* and *PLCG2* can confer resistance to ibrutinib through abrogated drug binding and signaling bypass, respectively.[97]

Intriguingly, many of the key drivers found in CLL/SLL are also detectable in the asymptomatic expansion of clonal B cells that precedes CLL (monoclonal B cell lymphocytosis) and even in a fraction of individuals with no detectable hematologic abnormalities.[98–100] This suggests CLL-associated genetic alterations may arise in

Table 2
Table of prognostically relevant alterations in chronic lymphocytic leukemia

	Prognosis	Frequency	Unmutated	Mutated
Cytogenetic				
del(13q14); *mir-16–1/miR-15a*[a]	Good	50%	48%	65%
SHM				
Mutated (<98% homology)	Good	50%–70%		
IGHV				
IGHV3-72, IGHV3-30	Good	13%[b]		
IGHV4-34	Good	11%[b]		
Cytogenetic				
trisomy 12	Intermediate	20%	19%	15%
del(6q21)[a]	Intermediate	3%–8%		
IGHV				
IGHV3-23	Intermediate	13%		
Cytogenetic				
del(11q23); *ATM/BIRC3*[a]	Poor	20%	27%	4%
del(17p13); *TP53*[a]	Poor	10%	35%	7%
SHM				
Unmutated (≥98% homology)	Poor	30%–50%		
IGHV				
IGHV3-21	Poor	0–5%[b]		
IGHV1-69)	Poor	13%[b]		
Mutations				
SF3B1[a]	Poor	~25%	25%–30%	15%–20%
TP53	Poor	~10%	10%–15%	~5%
NOTCH1[a]	Poor	10%	10%–15%	<5%
ATM[a]	Poor	5%–10%	20%–25%	5%–10%
MYD88[a]	Poor	~5%	0%	5%–10%
BIRC3	Poor	~5	5%–10%	<5%
POT1	Poor	5%–10%	~10%	~5%

[a] Frequency is significantly different between unmutated and mutated cases.
[b] Frequency listed for Southern European populations[86,87]; other frequencies are estimated from the WHO[4] and Landau et al.[88]

the precursor state, similar to the paradigm linking CH with subsequent myeloid malignancy.

Diffuse Large B Cell Lymphoma, Not Otherwise Specified

Diffuse large B cell lymphoma (DLBCL), not otherwise specified, the most common adult lymphoma, can arise through transformation of antecedent lower-grade lymphomas (similar to CLL/SLL or follicular lymphoma) or present de novo. DLBCL exhibits a complex landscape of genetic alterations, including somatic mutations, copy number alterations, and structural variants (summarized in **Fig. 5**).

Traditionally, risk stratification for DLBCL has involved inference of cell-of-origin ("germinal center-like" vs less favorable "activated B cell-like" phenotypes), derived from gene expression data, and associated immunophenotypes.[84,101] More recently, genomic analysis of large patient cohorts by 2 groups added granularity to these

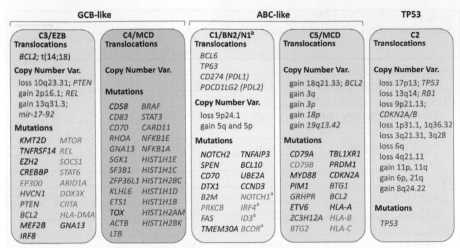

Fig. 5. DLBCL genomic subtypes. Genes found only in Schmitz and colleagues[102] in blue; genes found only in Chapuy and colleagues[103] in brown; genes found in both in black. [a]Schmitz and colleagues describes an N1 subtype characterized by NOTCH1 mutation, which is mutually exclusive of the NOTCH2-driven BN2 subtype. Because there is no analogous Chapuy and colleagues subtype, they are combined in C1. BN2, BCL6/NOTCH2, C, cluster, EZB–EZH2/BCL2, MCD, MYD88/CD79 B; N1, NOTCH1.

prognostic categories.[102,103] One such scheme separates DLBCL cases into 5 clusters of genetic signatures, each enriched with distinct patterns of alterations (summarized in **Fig. 5**).[103] These include 2 groups with relatively favorable outcomes (Cluster 1 (marginal zone-like) and Cluster 4), one with intermediate prognoses (Cluster 2, *TP53*-associated with complex karyotype), and 2 associated with poorer outcomes (Cluster 3 (follicular lymphoma-like) and Cluster 5). Clusters 3 and 4 associate with germinal center cell of origin while Clusters 1 and 5 resemble the activated B cell category. A parallel study identified 4 distinct genetic subtypes, with groups enriched for *BCL6* fusions/*NOTCH2* mutations or *BCL2* fusions/*EZH2* mutations exhibiting more favorable prognoses than those with *MYD88*/*CD79B* comutation or *NOTCH1* mutation (see **Fig. 5**).[102] Despite their differing schema, there is reassuringly extensive overlap between the DLBCL subtypes and both studies affirm known relationships between specific genetic alterations and prognosis, including the unfavorable influences of *MYC* rearrangement, *TP53* mutations/deletions, and deletions involving *CDKN2A/B*, *PTEN*, or *RB1*, among many others.[84]

Angioimmunoblastic T Cell Lymphoma

Among mature T cell lymphomas, angioimmunoblastic T cell lymphoma (AITL) is of particular interest for molecular diagnostics because it encompasses genetic alterations involved in both CH and T cell-specific neoplasia. Derived from CD4-positive T follicular helper cells, this aggressive nodal lymphoma is enriched among aged adults and is frequently associated with features of systemic inflammation (eg, hypergammaglobulinemia, hemolytic anemia, skin rash, fever).[104] Strikingly, genomic profiling of AITL has revealed mutations in epigenetic regulators also frequently observed in CH/myeloid neoplasia, including *TET2* and *DNMT3A*.[105–107] Recurrently accompanying these changes are mutations in the small GTPase *RHOA* (predominantly p.G17V), epigenetic regulator *IDH2*, and T cell signaling costimulator *CD28*.[108–110] Gene fusions resulting in enhanced T cell receptor signaling are also observed (*CTLA4::CD28*, more rarely *ITK::SYK*).[111,112] Among numerous copy number variants, trisomy 5 and gains involving 13q22.3 have been associated with adverse patient outcomes.[113]

The presence of CH-associated mutations in AITL suggests AITL may arise from a clonal hematopoietic stem cell (**Fig. 6**). Indeed, mutations in *TET2* and *DNMT3A* detected in T cell lymphomas of follicular helper origin have also been detected in the same patients' circulating myeloid cells, consistent with a shared origin in multipotent stem/progenitor cells.[114] Multiple AITL patients have developed myeloid neoplasia carrying the same CH-associated mutations, now accompanied by additional myeloid malignancy-associated alterations. These results suggest that the foundational mutations in "lineage-restricted" neoplasms can occur before lineage specification with disease manifestations shaped by subsequently acquired alterations. Supporting this paradigm more broadly, CH-related mutations (particularly in *TET2*) have been identified in other T and natural killer (NK) cell lymphomas and germline *TET2* variants have been linked to a predisposition to developing lymphoma.[115–121]

Plasma Cell Myeloma

Plasma cell myeloma multiple myeloma (MM) is a clonal proliferation of neoplastic plasma cells.[4] Similar to that of sAML and CLL, the pathogenesis of myeloma reflects a clinicopathologic progression from asymptomatic premalignancy monoclonal gammopathy of undetermined significance (MGUS) to smoldering myeloma (SMM) to florid disease (MM) or even leukemic disease (plasma cell leukemia).[4,122] Each step in this malignant progression is accompanied by the acquisition of additional genetic aberrations, many with prognostic implications, now illuminated more fully with the addition of NGS mutation profiling to traditional cytogenetics.[123]

Genetic alterations present in the earliest stages of disease (eg, MGUS) are thought to represent founder/initiating events and can be segregated into subtypes with numerical chromosomal abnormalities and those driven by translocations.[123] Hyperdiploid clones (N ≥ 48) typically contain trisomies of many odd-numbered chromosomes (eg, 3, 5, 7, 9, 11, 15, 19, 21) and relatively fewer balanced

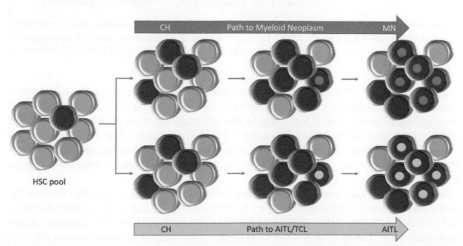

Fig. 6. Clonal relationship between clonal hematopoiesis and angioimmunoblastic T cell lymphoma.

Table 3
Molecular-cytogenetic abnormalities in myeloma

Genomic Event	Gene	Frequency	Prognosis
Clonal drivers			
Translocations	t(4;14)/*IGH::FGFR3/MMSET*	15%	Adverse
	t(6;14)/*IGH::CCND3*	2%	Neutral
	t(11;14)/*IGH::CCND1*	15%	Neutral*
	t(14;16)/*IGH::MAF*	5%	Neutral/Adverse
	t(14;20)/*IGH::MAFB*	1%	Adverse
Numerical changes	Hyperdiploidy (gains in 3, 5, 7, 9, 11, 15, 19, 21)	50%	Favorable
	Del13q (*RB1, DIS3, mir-15a, mir-16–1*)	40%	Neutral
Subclonal/progression events			
Chromosomal gains	1q (*MCL1, CKS1B, ANP32E,* or *BCL9* candidates)	40%	Adverse
	8q (*MYC*)	15%	Neutral
	11q (*CCND1*)	15%	Neutral
Chromosomal losses (including hypodiploidy)	1p (*CDKN2C* or *FAM46 C* candidates)	30%	Adverse
	12p (*CD27*)	15%	Adverse
	4q (*TRAF3*)	10%	Not Determined
	16q (*CYLD* or *WWOX* candidates)	30%	Neutral
	17p (*TP53*)	10%	Adverse
Translocations	*MYC* (often complex)	15%	Adverse
Somatic mutations	MAPK pathway: *KRAS, NRAS, BRAF*	45%	Neutral
	NF-κB pathway: *CYLD, TRAF3, LBT, NIK*	15%	Neutral
	RNA metabolism: *DIS3, FAM46C*	15%	Neutral
	DNA repair pathway: *TP53, ATM, ATR*	10%	Adverse
	Plasma cell differentiation: *IRF4, PRDM1*	10%	Favorable

Adapted from Manier S, Salem KZ, Park J, Landau DA, Getz G, Ghobrial IM. Genomic complexity of multiple myeloma and its clinical implications. *Nat Rev Clin Oncol.* 2017;14(2):100-113. https://doi.org/10.1038/nrclinonc.2016.122.

rearrangements.[124] Prognoses for hyperdiploid cases are generally more favorable than that for hypodiploid cases (although not as favorable as normal karyotype) and even a single trisomy 3 or 5 may negate the relatively adverse prognosis associated with t(4;14)/*IGH::FGFR3/MMSET* fusions.[123,125–127] However, this favorable outlook is negatively impacted when *MYC* rearrangements are acquired as secondary alterations, often in the context of complex, chromothripsis/chromoplexy-related changes.[128,129]

Recurrent balanced rearrangements are detectable by FISH and often involve the *IGH* enhancer locus. These include t(4;14)/*IGH::FGFR3/MMSET*, t(6;14)/*IGH::CCND3*, t(11;14)/*IGH::CCDN1*, t(14;16)/*IGH::MAF*, and t(14;20)/*IGH::MAFB*, among others (summarized in **Table 3**) and tend to cooccur with additional mutations in the *IGH* fusion partners.[130] *CCND1::IGH* fusions are associated with small, CD20-positive lymphoplasmacytoid cells and confer adverse outcomes when cooccurring with *CCND1* mutations (neutral otherwise).[128] *IGH::MAF* fusions are also associated with a poor prognosis, at least partly through driving APOBEC3A/B-mediated hypermutation.[128] *IGH::MAFB* fusion exhibits an unusual prognostic profile, with recent evidence suggesting a protective effect in early MGUS/SMM but an adverse effect in florid myeloma.[123,131] *IGH::FGFR3/MMSET* fusions overexpress *MMSET* invariably (driving methylation of histone H3K36) and *FGFR3* in a large subset of cases (driving survival/proliferative signaling). Although these latter fusions are linked with poor outcomes, they may also confer improved responses to proteasome inhibitor therapy.[132] Plasma cell clones often acquire copy number changes during progression, most notably gains in chromosome 1q and deletions in 17p, 13q, or 1p. 1q gains exert an adverse prognostic effect most frequently in high-risk translocation cases, including those with *IGH::FGFR3/MMSET* fusions.[133] In contrast, losses in 17p (including *TP53*) and 1p (including *CDKN2C*) confer poor outcomes in all subtypes and are frequent progression events.[134,135] Deletion of 13q (including *RB1*) is considered neutral with respect to prognosis. Reflecting the prognostic importance of many of these alterations, the widely used Revised International Staging System includes adverse cytogenetic alterations (any of *IGH::MAF*, *IGH::MAFB*, *IGH::FGFR3/MMSET*, del(17p), or 1q gain) to help define "high risk" patients and prompt more aggressive therapy.[130]

This prognostic paradigm is now evolving to include the mutational profiling made possible by NGS. For example, mutations in B cell differentiation factor *IRF4* seem to associate with favorable outcomes and are associated with t(11;14) translocations. Mutations in *TP53* (often cooccurring with del(17p)), *ATM*, and *ATR* confer an adverse prognostic impact.[123,136] Although mutations in the RAS/MAPK (eg, *KRAS*, *NRAS*, *BRAF*) and NF-κB signaling (eg, *TRAF3*, *LTB*) pathways are commonly detected among myeloma patients and associate with specific cytogenetic abnormalities, they seem to exert little independent prognostic influence.[136] Despite this complexity, new algorithms are being developed to stratify risk more precisely through the addition of genomic data to other established risk factors.[136] In addition, mutations in components of the CRL4^CRBN E3 ubiquitin ligase complex and its degradation targets (eg, *CRBN*, *CUL4B*, *IRF4*, *IKZF1*) have been linked to disease refractory to immunomodulatory drugs.[137–139] Thus, molecular diagnostics for myeloma, similar to that for myeloid and lymphoid disease, will play an increasingly central role in guiding patient management in addition to its traditional diagnostic role.

CLINICS CARE POINTS

- Myeloid neoplasms are often founded by early mutations driving clonal hematopoiesis, on which additional alterations specify clinical manifestation and accelerate progression.

- Foundational alterations in lymphoblastic leukemias, enriched for oncogenic fusions, augment cell survival and proliferation while inhibiting lymphoid maturation.

- Constellations of mutations possess stronger predictive power than individual variants for many lymphomas.

- Next-generation sequencing is refining risk stratification for plasma cell neoplasms beyond traditional, cytogenetic categories.

- Molecular and genetic lesions are identified in precursor (asymptomatic) states and serve as the foundation for future clinical disease (clonal hematopoiesis to myelodysplastic syndrome or angioimmunoblastic T cell lymphoma, monoclonal B cell lymphocytosis to chronic lymphocytic leukemia, monoclonal gammopathy of undetermined significance to multiple myeloma).

DISCLOSURE

A.S. Kim consulted for LabCorp, Inc, and receives research funding from the Multiple Myeloma Research Foundation.

REFERENCES

1. Stone RM, Mandrekar SJ, Sanford BL, et al. Midostaurin plus chemotherapy for acute myeloid leukemia with a FLT3 mutation. N Engl J Med 2017;377(5): 454–64.
2. Malcovati L, Stevenson K, Papaemmanuil E, et al. SF3B1-mutant MDS as a distinct disease subtype: a proposal from the International Working Group for the Prognosis of MDS. Blood 2020;136(2):157–70.
3. Mendoza H, Tormey CA, Rinder HM, et al. The utility and limitations of B- and T-cell gene rearrangement studies in evaluating lymphoproliferative disorders. Pathology 2020;53(2):157–65.
4. Swerdlow SH, Campo E, Harris NL, et al. WHO Classification of Tumours of Haematopoietic and Lymphoid Tissues; 2017.
5. Hoang ML, Kinde I, Tomasetti C, et al. Genome-wide quantification of rare somatic mutations in normal human tissues using massively parallel sequencing. Proc Natl Acad Sci 2016;113(35):9846–51.
6. Martincorena I. Somatic mutation and clonal expansions in human tissues. Genome Med 2019;11(1):35.
7. Steensma DP, Ebert BL. Clonal hematopoiesis as a model for premalignant changes during aging. Exp Hematol 2020;83:48–56.
8. Jaiswal S, Ebert BL. Clonal hematopoiesis in human aging and disease. Science 2019;366(6465):eaan4673.
9. Jaiswal S, Fontanillas P, Flannick J, et al. Age-related clonal hematopoiesis associated with adverse outcomes. N Engl J Med 2014;371(26):2488–98.
10. Bolton KL, Ptashkin RN, Gao T, et al. Cancer therapy shapes the fitness landscape of clonal hematopoiesis. Nat Genet 2020;52(11):1219–26.
11. Dharan NJ, Yeh P, Bloch M, et al. HIV is associated with an increased risk of age-related clonal hematopoiesis among older adults. Nat Med 2021;27(6): 1006–11.
12. Abelson S, Collord G, Ng SWK, et al. Prediction of acute myeloid leukaemia risk in healthy individuals. Nature 2018;559(7714):400–4.
13. Desai P, Mencia-Trinchant N, Savenkov O, et al. Somatic mutations precede acute myeloid leukemia years before diagnosis. Nat Med 2018;24(7):1015–23.
14. Genovese G, Kähler AK, Handsaker RE, et al. Clonal hematopoiesis and blood-cancer risk inferred from blood DNA sequence. N Engl J Med 2014;371(26): 2477–87.
15. Jaiswal S, Natarajan P, Silver AJ, et al. Clonal hematopoiesis and risk of atherosclerotic cardiovascular disease. N Engl J Med 2017;377(2):111–21.
16. Kim PG, Niroula A, Shkolnik V, et al. Dnmt3a-mutated clonal hematopoiesis promotes osteoporosis. J Exp Med 2021;218(12):e20211872.
17. Hecker JS, Hartmann L, Rivière J, et al. CHIP and hips: clonal hematopoiesis is common in patients undergoing hip arthroplasty and is associated with autoimmune disease. Blood 2021;138(18):1727–32.
18. Xie M, Lu C, Wang J, et al. Age-related cancer mutations associated with clonal hematopoietic expansion. Nat Med 2014;20(12):1472–8.

19. Zink F, Stacey SN, Norddahl GL, et al. Clonal hematopoiesis, with and without candidate driver mutations, is common in the elderly. Blood 2017;130(6): 742–52.
20. Young AL, Challen GA, Birmann BM, et al. Clonal haematopoiesis harbouring AML-associated mutations is ubiquitous in healthy adults. Nat Commun 2016; 7(1):12484.
21. Feusier JE, Arunachalam S, Tashi T, et al. Large-scale identification of clonal hematopoiesis and mutations recurrent in blood cancers. Blood Cancer Discov 2021;2(3):226–37.
22. Kennedy JA, Ebert BL. Clinical implications of genetic mutations in myelodysplastic syndrome. J Clin Oncol 2017;35(9):968–97.
23. DeZern AE, Malcovati L, Ebert BL. CHIP, CCUS, and other acronyms: definition, implications, and impact on practice. Am Soc Clin Oncol Educ Book 2019;39: 400–10.
24. Gibson CJ, Lindsley RC, Tchekmedyian V, et al. Clonal hematopoiesis associated with adverse outcomes after autologous stem-cell transplantation for lymphoma. J Clin Oncol 2017;35(14):1598–605.
25. Saygin C, Godley LA. Genetics of myelodysplastic syndromes. Cancers 2021; 13(14):3380.
26. Papaemmanuil E. Consortium on behalf of the CMD working group of the ICG, Gerstung M, et al. Clinical and biological implications of driver mutations in myelodysplastic syndromes. Blood 2013;122(22):3616–27.
27. Khalife-Hachem S, Saleh K, Pasquier F, et al. Molecular landscape of therapy-related myeloid neoplasms in patients previously treated for gynecologic and breast cancers. Hemasphere 2021;5(9):e632.
28. Takahashi K, Jabbour E, Wang X, et al. Dynamic acquisition of FLT3 or RAS alterations drive a subset of patients with lower risk MDS to secondary AML. Leukemia 2013;27(10):2081–3.
29. Mossner M, Jann JC, Wittig J, et al. Mutational hierarchies in myelodysplastic syndromes dynamically adapt and evolve upon therapy response and failure. Blood 2016;128(9):1246–59.
30. Bernard E, Nannya Y, Hasserjian RP, et al. Implications of TP53 allelic state for genome stability, clinical presentation and outcomes in myelodysplastic syndromes. Nat Med 2020;26(10):1549–56.
31. Lindsley RC, Mar BG, Mazzola E, et al. Acute myeloid leukemia ontogeny is defined by distinct somatic mutations. Blood 2015;125(9):1367–76.
32. Schanz J, Tüchler H, Solé F, et al. New comprehensive cytogenetic scoring system for primary myelodysplastic syndromes (MDS) and oligoblastic acute myeloid leukemia after MDS derived from an international database merge. J Clin Oncol 2012;30(8):820–9.
33. Döhner H, Estey E, Grimwade D, et al. Diagnosis and management of AML in adults: 2017 ELN recommendations from an international expert panel. Blood 2017;129(4):424–47.
34. List A, Dewald G, Bennett J, et al. Lenalidomide in the myelodysplastic syndrome with chromosome 5q deletion. N Engl J Med 2006;355(14):1456–65.
35. Soverini S, Hochhaus A, Nicolini FE, et al. BCR-ABL kinase domain mutation analysis in chronic myeloid leukemia patients treated with tyrosine kinase inhibitors: recommendations from an expert panel on behalf of European LeukemiaNet. Blood 2011;118(5):1208–15.
36. Maxson JE, Gotlib J, Pollyea DA, et al. Oncogenic CSF3R mutations in chronic neutrophilic leukemia and atypical CML. N Engl J Med 2013;368(19):1781–90.

37. McClure RF, Ewalt MD, Crow J, et al. Clinical significance of DNA variants in chronic myeloid neoplasms a report of the association for molecular pathology. J Mol Diagn 2018;20(6):717–37.
38. Kiladjian JJ, Zachee P, Hino M, et al. Long-term efficacy and safety of ruxolitinib versus best available therapy in polycythaemia vera (RESPONSE): 5-year follow up of a phase 3 study. Lancet Haematol 2020;7(3):e226–37.
39. Ortmann CA, Kent DG, Nangalia J, et al. Effect of mutation order on myeloproliferative neoplasms. N Engl J Med 2015;372(7):601–12.
40. Grinfeld J, Nangalia J, Baxter EJ, et al. Classification and personalized prognosis in myeloproliferative neoplasms. N Engl J Med 2018;379(15):1416–30.
41. Jawhar M, Schwaab J, Schnittger S, et al. Additional mutations in SRSF2, ASXL1 and/or RUNX1 identify a high-risk group of patients with KIT D816V+ advanced systemic mastocytosis. Leukemia 2016;30(1):136–43.
42. Jawhar M, Schwaab J, Schnittger S, et al. Molecular profiling of myeloid progenitor cells in multi-mutated advanced systemic mastocytosis identifies KIT D816V as a distinct and late event. Leukemia 2015;29(5):1115–22.
43. Gotlib J, Radia DH, George TI, et al. Pure pathologic response is associated with improved overall survival in patients with advanced systemic mastocytosis receiving avapritinib in the phase I explorer study. Blood 2020;136(Supplement 1):37–8.
44. Patnaik MM, Lasho TL. Genomics of myelodysplastic syndrome/myeloproliferative neoplasm overlap syndromes. Hematology 2020;2020(1):450–9.
45. Patnaik MM, Itzykson R, Lasho TL, et al. ASXL1 and SETBP1 mutations and their prognostic contribution in chronic myelomonocytic leukemia: a two-center study of 466 patients. Leukemia 2014;28(11):2206–12.
46. Elena C, Gallì A, Such E, et al. Integrating clinical features and genetic lesions in the risk assessment of patients with chronic myelomonocytic leukemia. Blood 2016;128(10):1408–17.
47. Meggendorfer M, Haferlach T, Alpermann T, et al. Specific molecular mutation patterns delineate chronic neutrophilic leukemia, atypical chronic myeloid leukemia, and chronic myelomonocytic leukemia. Haematologica 2014;99(12):e244-6.
48. Savona MR, Malcovati L, Komrokji R, et al. An international consortium proposal of uniform response criteria for myelodysplastic/myeloproliferative neoplasms (MDS/MPN) in adults. Blood 2015;125(12):1857–65.
49. Stieglitz E, Taylor-Weiner AN, Chang TY, et al. The genomic landscape of juvenile myelomonocytic leukemia. Nat Genet 2015;47(11):1326–33.
50. Patnaik MM, Tefferi A. Refractory anemia with ring sideroblasts (RARS) and RARS with thrombocytosis: "2019 Update on Diagnosis, Risk-stratification, and Management. Am J Hematol 2019;94(4):475–88.
51. Piazza R, Valletta S, Winkelmann N, et al. Recurrent SETBP1 mutations in atypical chronic myeloid leukemia. Nat Genet 2013;45(1):18–24.
52. Zhang H, Wilmot B, Bottomly D, et al. Genomic landscape of neutrophilic leukemias of ambiguous diagnosis. Blood 2019;134(11):867–79.
53. Kim AS, Hergott CB. Are you a lumper or a splitter? Embrace the genomic spectrum of neutrophilic myeloid neoplasms. Hematologist 2019;17(1). https://doi.org/10.1182/hem.v17.1.10150.
54. Network CGAR, Ley TJ, Miller C, et al. Genomic and epigenomic landscapes of adult de novo acute myeloid leukemia. N Engl J Med 2013;368(22):2059–74. https://doi.org/10.1056/nejmoa1301689.

55. Godley LA. Germline mutations in MDS/AML predisposition disorders. Curr Opin Hematol 2020;28(2):86–93.
56. Roberts KG, Mullighan CG. The biology of B-progenitor acute lymphoblastic leukemia. Cold Spring Harb Perspect Med 2020;10(7):a034835.
57. Inaba H, Mullighan CG. Pediatric acute lymphoblastic leukemia. Haematologica 2020;105(11):0.
58. Brown LM, Lonsdale A, Zhu A, et al. The application of RNA sequencing for the diagnosis and genomic classification of pediatric acute lymphoblastic leukemia. Blood Adv 2020;4(5):930–42.
59. Iacobucci I, Kimura S, Mullighan CG. Biologic and therapeutic implications of genomic alterations in acute lymphoblastic leukemia. J Clin Med 2021;10(17): 3792.
60. Foà R, Vitale A, Vignetti M, et al. Dasatinib as first-line treatment for adult patients with Philadelphia chromosome–positive acute lymphoblastic leukemia. Blood 2011;118(25):6521–8.
61. Roberts KG, Yang YL, Payne-Turner D, et al. Oncogenic role and therapeutic targeting of ABL-class and JAK-STAT activating kinase alterations in Ph-like ALL. Blood Adv 2017;1(20):1657–71.
62. Haddox CL, Mangaonkar AA, Chen D, et al. Blinatumomab-induced lineage switch of B-ALL with t(4:11)(q21;q23) KMT2A/AFF1 into an aggressive AML: pre- and post-switch phenotypic, cytogenetic and molecular analysis. Blood Cancer J 2017;7(9):e607.
63. Heerema NA, Carroll AJ, Devidas M, et al. Intrachromosomal amplification of Chromosome 21 is associated with inferior outcomes in children with acute lymphoblastic leukemia treated in contemporary standard-risk children's oncology group studies: a report from the children's oncology group. J Clin Oncol 2013;31(27):3397–402.
64. Garcia DRN, Arancibia AM, Ribeiro RC, et al. Intrachromosomal amplification of chromosome 21 (iAMP21) detected by ETV6/RUNX1 FISH screening in childhood acute lymphoblastic leukemia: a case report. Revista Brasileira De Hematologia E Hemoterapia 2013;35(5):369–71.
65. Gu Z, Churchman ML, Roberts KG, et al. PAX5-driven subtypes of B-progenitor acute lymphoblastic leukemia. Nat Genet 2019;51(2):296–307.
66. Li JF, Dai YT, Lilljebjörn H, et al. Transcriptional landscape of B cell precursor acute lymphoblastic leukemia based on an international study of 1,223 cases. Proc Natl Acad Sci 2018;115(50):201814397.
67. Clappier E, Auclerc MF, Rapion J, et al. An intragenic ERG deletion is a marker of an oncogenic subtype of B-cell precursor acute lymphoblastic leukemia with a favorable outcome despite frequent IKZF1 deletions. Leukemia 2014; 28(1):70–7.
68. Comeaux EQ, Mullighan CG. TP53 mutations in hypodiploid acute lymphoblastic leukemia. Cold Spring Harb Perspect Med 2017;7(3):a026286.
69. Qian M, Cao X, Devidas M, et al. TP53 germline variations influence the predisposition and prognosis of B-Cell acute lymphoblastic leukemia in children. J Clin Oncol 2018;36(6):591–9.
70. Belver L, Ferrando A. The genetics and mechanisms of T cell acute lymphoblastic leukaemia. Nat Rev Cancer 2016;16(8):494–507.
71. O'Neil J, Grim J, Strack P, et al. FBW7 mutations in leukemic cells mediate NOTCH pathway activation and resistance to γ-secretase inhibitors. J Exp Med 2007;204(8):1813–24.

72. Pear WS, Aster JC, Scott ML, et al. Exclusive development of T cell neoplasms in mice transplanted with bone marrow expressing activated Notch alleles. J Exp Med 1996;183(5):2283–91.

73. Weng AP, Ferrando AA, Lee W, et al. Activating mutations of NOTCH1 in human T cell acute lymphoblastic leukemia. Science 2004;306(5694):269–71.

74. Ferrando AA, Neuberg DS, Staunton J, et al. Gene expression signatures define novel oncogenic pathways in T cell acute lymphoblastic leukemia. Cancer Cell 2002;1(1):75–87.

75. Girardi T, Vicente C, Cools J, et al. The genetics and molecular biology of T-ALL. Blood 2017;129(9):1113–23.

76. Zhang J, Ding L, Holmfeldt L, et al. The genetic basis of early T-cell precursor acute lymphoblastic leukaemia. Nature 2012;481(7380):157–63.

77. Wang P, Peng X, Deng X, et al. Diagnostic challenges in T-lymphoblastic lymphoma, early T-cell precursor acute lymphoblastic leukemia or mixed phenotype acute leukemia. Medicine 2018;97(41):e12743.

78. Coustan-Smith E, Mullighan CG, Onciu M, et al. Early T-cell precursor leukaemia: a subtype of very high-risk acute lymphoblastic leukaemia. Lancet Oncol 2009;10(2):147–56.

79. Hebert J, Cayuela JM, Berkeley J, et al. Candidate tumor-suppressor genes MTS1 (p16INK4A) and MTS2 (p15INK4B) display frequent homozygous deletions in primary cells from T- but not from B-cell lineage acute lymphoblastic leukemias. Blood 1994;84(12):4038–44.

80. Mullighan CG, Goorha S, Radtke I, et al. Genome-wide analysis of genetic alterations in acute lymphoblastic leukaemia. Nature 2007;446(7137):758–64.

81. Remke M, Pfister S, Kox C, et al. High-resolution genomic profiling of childhood T-ALL reveals frequent copy-number alterations affecting the TGF-β and PI3K-AKT pathways and deletions at 6q15-16.1 as a genomic marker for unfavorable early treatment response. Blood 2009;114(5):1053–62.

82. Vlierberghe PV, Ambesi-Impiombato A, Keersmaecker KD, et al. Prognostic relevance of integrated genetic profiling in adult T-cell acute lymphoblastic leukemia. Blood 2013;122(1):74–82.

83. Fattizzo B, Rosa J, Giannotta JA, et al. The physiopathology of T- cell acute lymphoblastic leukemia: focus on molecular aspects. Front Oncol 2020;10:273.

84. Shanmugam V, Kim AS. Genomic medicine, a practical guide 2019. p. 253–315. https://doi.org/10.1007/978-3-030-22922-1_16.

85. Bosch F, Dalla-Favera R. Chronic lymphocytic leukaemia: from genetics to treatment. Nat Rev Clin Oncol 2019;16(11):684–701.

86. Donisi PM, Lorenzo ND, Riccardi M, et al. Pattern and distribution of immunoglobulin VH gene usage in a cohort of B-CLI patients from a northeastern region of Italy. Diagn Mol Pathol 2006;15(4):206–15.

87. Dal-Bo M, Giudice ID, Bomben R, et al. B-cell receptor, clinical course and prognosis in chronic lymphocytic leukaemia: the growing saga of the IGHV3 subgroup gene usage. Br J Haematol 2011;153(1):3–14.

88. Landau DA, Tausch E, Taylor-Weiner AN, et al. Mutations driving CLL and their evolution in progression and relapse. Nature 2015;526(7574):525–30.

89. Döhner H, Stilgenbauer S, Benner A, et al. Genomic aberrations and survival in chronic lymphocytic leukemia. N Engl J Med 2000;343(26):1910–6.

90. Zenz T, Kröber A, Scherer K, et al. Monoallelic TP53 inactivation is associated with poor prognosis in chronic lymphocytic leukemia: results from a detailed genetic characterization with long-term follow-up. Blood 2008;112(8):3322–9.

91. Balatti V, Bottoni A, Palamarchuk A, et al. NOTCH1 mutations in CLL associated with trisomy 12. Blood 2012;119(2):329–31.
92. Crombie J, Davids MS. IGHV mutational status testing in chronic lymphocytic leukemia. Am J Hematol 2017;92(12):1393–7.
93. Gaidano G, Rossi D. The mutational landscape of chronic lymphocytic leukemia and its impact on prognosis and treatment. Hematology 2017;2017(1):329–37.
94. Qin SC, Xia Y, Miao Y, et al. MYD88 mutations predict unfavorable prognosis in Chronic Lymphocytic Leukemia patients with mutated IGHV gene. Blood Cancer J 2017;7(12):651.
95. Martínez-Trillos A, Pinyol M, Navarro A, et al. Mutations in TLR/MYD88 pathway identify a subset of young chronic lymphocytic leukemia patients with favorable outcome. Blood 2014;123(24):3790–6.
96. Martínez-Trillos A, Navarro A, Aymerich M, et al. Clinical impact of MYD88 mutations in chronic lymphocytic leukemia. Blood 2016;127(12):1611–3.
97. Ahn IE, Underbayev C, Albitar A, et al. Clonal evolution leading to ibrutinib resistance in chronic lymphocytic leukemia. Blood 2017;129(11):1469–79.
98. Ojha J, Secreto C, Rabe K, et al. Monoclonal B-cell lymphocytosis is characterized by mutations in CLL putative driver genes and clonal heterogeneity many years before disease progression. Leukemia 2014;28(12):2395–8.
99. Agathangelidis A, Ljungström V, Scarfò L, et al. Highly similar genomic landscapes in monoclonal B-cell lymphocytosis and ultra-stable chronic lymphocytic leukemia with low frequency of driver mutations. Haematologica 2018;103(5):865–73.
100. Niroula A, Sekar A, Murakami MA, et al. Distinction of lymphoid and myeloid clonal hematopoiesis. Nat Med 2021;27(11):1921–7.
101. Alizadeh AA, Eisen MB, Davis RE, et al. Distinct types of diffuse large B-cell lymphoma identified by gene expression profiling. Nature 2000;403(6769):503–11.
102. Schmitz R, Wright GW, Huang DW, et al. Genetics and pathogenesis of diffuse large B-Cell lymphoma. N Engl J Med 2018;378(15):1396–407.
103. Chapuy B, Stewart C, Dunford AJ, et al. Molecular subtypes of diffuse large B cell lymphoma are associated with distinct pathogenic mechanisms and outcomes. Nat Med 2018;24(5):679–90.
104. Lunning MA, Vose JM. Angioimmunoblastic T-cell lymphoma: the many-faced lymphoma. Blood 2017;129(9):1095–102.
105. Couronné L, Bastard C, Bernard OA. TET2 and DNMT3A mutations in human T-Cell lymphoma. N Engl J Med 2012;366(1):95–6.
106. Odejide O, Weigert O, Lane AA, et al. A targeted mutational landscape of angioimmunoblastic T-cell lymphoma. Blood 2014;123(9):1293–6.
107. Tiacci E, Venanzi A, Ascani S, et al. High-risk clonal hematopoiesis as the origin of AITL and NPM1-mutated AML. N Engl J Med 2018;379(10):981–4.
108. Chiba S, Sakata-Yanagimoto M. Advances in understanding of angioimmunoblastic T-cell lymphoma. Leukemia 2020;34(10):2592–606.
109. Zang S, Li J, Yang H, et al. Mutations in 5-methylcytosine oxidase TET2 and RhoA cooperatively disrupt T cell homeostasis. J Clin Invest 2017;127(8):2998–3012.
110. Ng SY, Brown L, Stevenson K, et al. RhoA G17V is sufficient to induce autoimmunity and promotes T-cell lymphomagenesis in mice. Blood 2018;132(9):935–47.
111. Yoo HY, Kim P, Kim WS, et al. Frequent CTLA4-CD28 gene fusion in diverse types of T-cell lymphoma. Haematologica 2016;101(6):757–63.

112. Attygalle AD, Feldman AL, Dogan A. ITK/SYK translocation in angioimmuno-blastic T-cell lymphoma. Am J Surg Pathol 2013;37(9):1456–7.

113. Fujiwara S i, Yamashita Y, Nakamura N, et al. High-resolution analysis of chromosome copy number alterations in angioimmunoblastic T-cell lymphoma and peripheral T-cell lymphoma, unspecified, with single nucleotide polymorphism-typing microarrays. Leukemia 2008;22(10):1891–8.

114. Lewis NE, Petrova-Drus K, Huet S, et al. Clonal hematopoiesis in angioimmuno-blastic T-cell lymphoma with divergent evolution to myeloid neoplasms. Blood Adv 2020;4(10):2261–71.

115. Pastoret C, Desmots-Loyer F, Drillet G, et al. Linking the KIR phenotype with STAT3 and TET2 mutations to identify chronic lymphoproliferative disorders of NK cells. Blood 2021;137(23):3237–50.

116. Olson TL, Cheon H, Xing JC, et al. Frequent somatic TET2 mutations in chronic NK-LGL leukemia with distinct patterns of cytopenias. Blood 2021;138(8): 662–73.

117. Almeida AC da S, Abate F, Khiabanian H, et al. The mutational landscape of cutaneous T cell lymphoma and Sézary syndrome. Nat Genet 2015;47(12): 1465–70.

118. Arber DA, Orazi A, Hasserjian R, et al. The 2016 revision to the World Health Organization classification of myeloid neoplasms and acute leukemia. Blood 2016; 127(20):2391–405.

119. Shimoda K, Shide K, Kameda T, et al. TET2 mutation in adult T-cell leukemia/lymphoma. J Clin Exp Hematop 2015;55(3):145–9.

120. Palomero T, Couronné L, Khiabanian H, et al. Recurrent mutations in epigenetic regulators, RHOA and FYN kinase in peripheral T cell lymphomas. Nat Genet 2014;46(2):166–70.

121. Spegarova JS, Lawless D, Mohamad SMB, et al. Germline TET2 loss of function causes childhood immunodeficiency and lymphoma. Blood 2020;136(9): 1055–66.

122. Rajkumar SV. Multiple myeloma: 2020 update on diagnosis, risk-stratification and management. Am J Hematol 2020;95(5):548–67.

123. Manier S, Salem KZ, Park J, et al. Genomic complexity of multiple myeloma and its clinical implications. Nat Rev Clin Oncol 2017;14(2):100–13.

124. Fonseca R, Debes-Marun CS, Picken EB, et al. The recurrent IgH translocations are highly associated with nonhyperdiploid variant multiple myeloma. Blood 2003;102(7):2562–7.

125. Chretien ML, Corre J, Lauwers-Cances V, et al. Understanding the role of hyper-diploidy in myeloma prognosis: which trisomies really matter? Blood 2015; 126(25):2713–9.

126. Smadja NV, Bastard C, Brigaudeau C, et al. Hypodiploidy is a major prognostic factor in multiple myeloma. Blood 2001;98(7):2229–38.

127. Wier SV, Braggio E, Baker A, et al. Hypodiploid multiple myeloma is characterized by more aggressive molecular markers than non-hyperdiploid multiple myeloma. Haematologica 2013;98(10):1586–92.

128. Walker BA, Wardell CP, Murison A, et al. APOBEC family mutational signatures are associated with poor prognosis translocations in multiple myeloma. Nat Commun 2015;6(1):6997.

129. Maura F, Bolli N, Angelopoulos N, et al. Genomic landscape and chronological reconstruction of driver events in multiple myeloma. Nat Commun 2019;10(1): 3835.

130. Sonneveld P, Avet-Loiseau H, Lonial S, et al. Treatment of multiple myeloma with high-risk cytogenetics: a consensus of the International Myeloma Working Group. Blood 2016;127(24):2955–62.

131. Ross FM, Chiecchio L, Dagrada G, et al. The t(14;20) is a poor prognostic factor in myeloma but is associated with long-term stable disease in monoclonal gammopathies of undetermined significance. Haematologica 2010;95(7):1221–5.

132. Avet-Loiseau H, Leleu X, Roussel M, et al. Bortezomib plus dexamethasone induction improves outcome of patients with t(4;14) myeloma but not outcome of patients with del(17p). J Clin Oncol 2010;28(30):4630–4.

133. Avet-Loiseau H, Li C, Magrangeas F, et al. Prognostic significance of copy-number alterations in multiple myeloma. J Clin Oncol 2009;27(27):4585–90.

134. Drach J, Ackermann J, Fritz E, et al. Presence of a p53 gene deletion in patients with multiple myeloma predicts for short survival after conventional-dose chemotherapy. Blood 1998;92(3):802–9.

135. Hebraud B, Leleu X, Lauwers-Cances V, et al. Deletion of the 1p32 region is a major independent prognostic factor in young patients with myeloma: the IFM experience on 1195 patients. Leukemia 2014;28(3):675–9.

136. Walker BA, Boyle EM, Wardell CP, et al. Mutational spectrum, copy number changes, and outcome: results of a sequencing study of patients with newly diagnosed myeloma. J Clin Oncol 2015;33(33):3911–20.

137. Bolli N, Biancon G, Moarii M, et al. Analysis of the genomic landscape of multiple myeloma highlights novel prognostic markers and disease subgroups. Leukemia 2018;32(12):2604–16.

138. Bustoros M, Sklavenitis-Pistofidis R, Park J, et al. Genomic profiling of smoldering multiple myeloma identifies patients at a high risk of disease progression. J Clin Oncol 2020;38(21):2380–9.

139. Kortüm KM, Mai EK, Hanafiah NH, et al. Targeted sequencing of refractory myeloma reveals a high incidence of mutations in CRBN and Ras pathway genes. Blood 2016;128(9):1226–33.

Special Considerations in the Molecular Diagnostics of Pediatric Neoplasms

Adam S. Fisch, MD, PhD[a], Alanna J. Church, MD[b],*

KEYWORDS

- Molecular diagnostics • Pediatric neoplasia • Next-generation sequencing
- Gene fusions • Pediatric cancer

KEY POINTS

- Pediatric neoplasms have different genetics, and fusions are particularly common.
- Small biopsies must be triaged to meet clinical demands.
- The care of children with benign and malignant neoplasms is increasingly supported by molecular diagnostics.

INTRODUCTION

Pediatric neoplasms are fundamentally different from adult neoplasms, with different diagnoses, tumor biology, tumor genomes, and treatment algorithms. Pediatric solid and brain tumors and hematologic malignances are relatively rare compared to their adult counterparts. Although the volume of cases may be low, the clinical impact of a correct diagnosis on the life of a child deserves special consideration, even within our cost-constrained health care systems.[1-3] An informed and inclusive molecular diagnostic program will include workflows, assays, and interpretation processes which accommodate young patients with cancer. Considerations for pediatric tumors begin with preanalytical factors, including tissue acquisition and handling, continue through analytical testing and interpretation of a given assay, and persist to include downstream implications for the patient, including clinical interpretation of genetic alterations, adjuvant and neoadjuvant treatment selection, and consideration of germline cancer predisposition. In this review, we focus on the unique elements of performing

[a] Massachusetts General Hospital, Harvard Medical School, 55 Fruit Street, Warren Building 225, Boston, MA 02114, USA; [b] Laboratory for Molecular Pediatric Pathology (LaMPP), Department of Pathology, Boston Children's Hospital, 300 Longwood Avenue, Boston, MA 02115, USA
* Corresponding author.
E-mail address: alanna.church@childrens.harvard.edu
Twitter: @AdamSFisch (A.S.F.); @AlannaChurch_MD (A.J.C.)

Clin Lab Med 42 (2022) 349–365
https://doi.org/10.1016/j.cll.2022.05.007
0272-2712/22/© 2022 Elsevier Inc. All rights reserved.

molecular diagnostics tailored to a predominantly pediatric patient population with benign and malignant neoplasms.

DISCUSSION
Small Biopsies and Tissue Allocation

Children and young adults presenting for diagnostic work-up of a suspected tumor have many unique clinical considerations. When considering the preanalytic factors for molecular diagnostics, we will focus on the challenges of sample size and assay design.

Owing to their small size and risk of procedure side effects, many surgeons and interventional radiologists prioritize less invasive procedures. Minimally invasive surgery, for instance, has progressed over the last 30 years from acquiring biopsies to tumor resections, and today is used for some complex cases[4]; imaging-guided percutaneous biopsy has been an even less invasive modality where applicable, with high sensitivity, specificity, and diagnostic accuracy.[5,6] Coupled with pediatric patients' relatively smaller overall size when compared to adults, biopsies taken for allocation to a variety of diagnostic modalities are often quite small, including core needle biopsies for mass lesions and minute bone marrows for hematolymphoid malignancies. Although pathologists working in clinical settings with a high proportion of pediatric patients are generally accustomed to the limited nature of tissue received, it is an important consideration both in histologic interpretation and molecular diagnostics. Specifically, smaller amounts of diagnostic tissue limit the number of ancillary histologic studies that can be performed (eg, immunohistochemistry, special stains) by a surgical pathologist, and require the pathologist to be even more aware of how much tissue remains in a block in case molecular testing is indicated. Careful management of the acquired tissue is necessary to properly triage tissues for necessary studies, including histologic work-up, various molecular tests, and additional techniques, including flow cytometry and electron microscopy. For some testing, it is imperative that fresh tissue be triaged appropriately into the necessary media for high-yield testing, including karyotyping and microarrays performed in the cytogenetics laboratory.[7] Last, as there continues to be a great need for more effective treatments for childhood cancers, consideration should be given to routine allocation of tissue to biorepositories for research.

Archival tissue is often the most readily available and widely used form of tissue for research purposes as FFPE tissue blocks are retained for long periods to meet clinical regulatory standards; fresh tissue is more difficult to acquire and less often procured as it often requires workflows that have been intentionally designed to include routine tissue allocation. Previous studies have shown the collaborative efforts necessary to establish such a system, and the benefits, in terms of broader study methods, that result from a streamlined process.[8] Within the molecular laboratory, smaller biopsies factor into the parameters used for clinical validation of a molecular assay, namely ensuring that the molecular assay's analytical sensitivity can meet the needs of routinely scant specimens, from a wide array of tissue types, with generally less viable tumor available for nucleic acid extraction.

Pediatric Cancer Genome

Many molecular targets are unique to childhood tumors, particularly those considered to have an embryonal histomorphology.[9,10] Pediatric neoplasms typically have a lower tumor mutational burden (TMB), but are also more likely to harbor structural rearrangements including gene fusions.[11-14]

Solid tumors, which are rare in adult populations, are seen more frequently in pediatric patients, particularly those of mesenchymal origin. Children and young adults diagnosed with soft tissue sarcomas tend to have a better prognosis than adults for a given tumor type in this category.[3,15,16] Within the family of mesenchymal tumors, which includes tumors of bone and soft tissue, the soft tissue sarcomas can be further subdivided into the more chemosensitive rhabdomyosarcomas (RMS), representing 40% of soft tissue sarcomas and 4% of pediatric tumors overall, and the less chemosensitive nonrhabdomyomatous soft tissue sarcomas that represent 3% of pediatric tumors and are bimodally seen in infants and young adults.[17–19] Many of the mesenchymal tumors seen in pediatrics, similar to adult soft tissue tumors, harbor characteristic gene fusions, including PAX3/PAX7::FOXO1 in alveolar RMS (ARMS), ETV6::NTRK3 in infantile fibrosarcoma, EWSR1::FLI1 in Ewing sarcoma, or fusions involving SS18 with SSX1, SSX2, or SSX4 in synovial sarcoma.[15] Some tumors have been shown to have recurrent SNVs, such as alterations in MYOD1 in spindle cell and sclerosing rhabdomyosarcoma,[19] whereas other tumors, such as osteosarcoma, have been shown to have more complex genetic findings, including recurrent inactivation of TP53 oftentimes due to structural rearrangements in the first intron.[15,16]

Pediatric tumors of the central nervous system (CNS) also harbor different molecular alterations than their adult counterparts. This group of tumors includes tumors of embryonal origin (rarely seen in adults) and mesenchymal origin. Gliomas represent a large proportion of CNS tumors in children but have unique molecular alterations which define the pediatric subtypes (Table 1).[20,21] The identification of sequence variants is important in children with CNS tumors, with the notable example of the diagnosis of diffuse midline glioma (previously known as diffuse intrinsic pontine glioma), characterized by hotspot variants in the H3 family of histone genes.[22] The identification of fusions is also important in this group of patients, as many entities are defined by unique fusions (see Table 1).[23]

Hematologic malignancies in children and adolescents have well-defined molecular pathways that drive molecular testing as part of the standard of care, much like diagnosis of hematolymphoid neoplasms in adults. Among leukemias, acute lymphoblastic leukemia (ALL) is the most common malignancy seen in the pediatric population, representing approximately a quarter of childhood cancers and divided into B-cell (B-ALL) and T-cell (T-ALL) lineages, respectively, accounting for 85% to 90% and 10% to 15% of ALL.[24,25] Tumor cells in B-ALL often have aneuploidy or harbor gene fusions, including BCR::ABL1, ETV6::RUNX1 (sometimes associated with intrachromosomal amplification of chromosome 21, iAMP21), TCF3::PBX1, IL3::IGH, or KMT2A rearrangements.[26–28] In patients with Philadelphia-like (Ph-like) B-ALL, a malignancy lacking the BCR::ABL1 fusion but similar in transcriptional profile to tumors with the fusion, over 90% of tumors have kinase-stimulating alterations, many of which are targetable with small molecular inhibitors.[29] More recent fusions have been identified in B-ALL, including TCF3::HLF or rearrangements involving MEF2D, DUX4, or ZNF384.[27] Generally, testing for chromosomal number, or ploidy, in B-ALL has predictive value for outcomes, namely hyperdiploid tumors (>50 chromosomes) often being driven by alterations in the Ras pathway with a better prognosis, whereas low-hypodiploid (31–39 chromosomes) and near-haploid (24–30 chromosomes) tumors have poor prognoses. Conversely, T-cell ALL (T-ALL) is more often associated with NOTCH1 or FBXW7 sequence variants; a small subset of T-ALL patients have tumors that are instead driven by translocations involving NOTCH1.[25] The frequency of genetic rearrangements necessitates the use of routine cytogenetics in the diagnosis of hematologic malignancies, including karyotype and FISH, and the involvement of fusion detection by next-generation sequencing when available.[27]

Table 1
Selected diagnostically significant alterations in pediatric extracranial solid tumors

Organ	Tumor	Alteration
Kidney	Clear cell sarcoma	BCOR-ITD
	Congenital mesoblastic nephroma	ETV6::NTRK3 fusion
	Translocation renal cell carcinoma	TFE3 or TFEB fusion
	Metanephric adenoma	BRAF p.V600E
	Rhabdoid tumor	SMARCB1 or SMARCA4 inactivation
	Cystic nephroma	DICER1 inactivation
Liver	Hepatoblastoma	CTNNB1 activation
	Fibrolamellar carcinoma	DNAJB1::PRKACA fusion
GI	Gastrointestinal stromal tumor	KIT or PDGFRA activation, or SDHB inactivation
Lung	Pleuropulmonary blastoma	DICER1 inactivation + RNaseIIb variant
Ovary	Juvenile granulosa cell tumor	AKT1 sequence variants
Peripheral nervous system	Paraganglioma	SDHA, SDHB, SDHC, or SDHD inactivation
Thyroid	PTC	BRAF p.V600E, RET fusions, NTRK fusions, or other kinase fusions
	PTC, cribriform morular variant	APC inactivation or CTNNB1 activation
	Follicular thyroid carcinoma	HRAS or NRAS activation, or PAX8::PPARG fusions, DICER1 variants, or PTEN inactivation
	NIFTP	HRAS or NRAS activation
	Multiple adenomas or adenomatous nodules	PTEN inactivation
	Medullary thyroid carcinoma	RET activation, HRAS or NRAS activation, or kinase fusions
Soft Tissue	Alveolar rhabdomyosarcoma	PAX3::FOXO1. PAX7::FOXO1 fusions
	Embryonal rhabdomyosarcoma	RAS pathway alterations, FGFR4 alterations
	Spindle cell rhabdomyosarcoma	MYOD1 p.L122R
	Solitary fibrous tumor	NAB2::STAT6
	Myofibroma	PDGFRB, NOTCH1, NOTCH3 variants
	Infantile fibrosarcoma	ETV6::NTRK3 fusion
	Desmoid fibromatosis	CTNNB1 activation
	Epithelioid hemangioendothelioma	WWTR1::CAMTA1, YAP1-TFE3
Bone & Cartilage	Aneurysmal bone cyst	USP6 fusion
	Giant cell tumor of bone	H3-3A p.G34W, p.G34L
	Mesenchymal chondrosarcoma	HEY1::NCOA2
	Chondroblastoma	H3-3A p.K36M

(continued on next page)

Table 1 (continued)		
Organ	Tumor	Alteration
Miscellaneous	Ewing sarcoma	EWSR1::FLI1, EWSR1::ERG
	CIC-rearranged sarcoma	CIC fusions
	BCOR-altered sarcoma	BCOR fusions and ITDs
	Desmoplastic small round cell tumor	EWSR1::WT1
	NUT midline carcinoma	BRD3::NUTM1, NRD4::NUTM1
	Epithelioid sarcoma	SMARCB1 or SMARCA4 inactivation

Abbreviations: NIFTP, noninvasive follicular thyroid neoplasm with papillary-like nuclear features; PTC, papillary thyroid carcinoma.
Data from Slack JC, Church AJ. Molecular Alterations in Pediatric Solid Tumors. Surg Pathol Clin. 2021;14(3):473-492. https://doi.org/10.1016/j.path.2021.05.010.

Assay Design

Given the unique molecular landscape of pediatric tumors, one must ensure a pediatric-centered approach to assay design in the early developmental stages of a molecular test. The inclusion of assays and targets that can identify diagnostically and therapeutically significant fusions is particularly important. The same principles seen for molecular diagnostics in the adult population apply, including the expected demand of the assay by clinician stakeholders, the ability to integrate the assay into the laboratory's current workflow, and the cost of on-boarding and maintaining the assay. Many of the off-the-shelf assay options have an adult-centric approach, such that custom assays are often needed to fully accommodate pediatric tumors.[30] Some programs may prefer to make use of reference laboratories or academic consultations for their youngest patients with cancer.

Clinical Interpretation of Alterations

Whether an assay is performed in-house or is outsourced, the clinical interpretation of any detected alterations should be undertaken with great care. As with adult neoplasms, clinical interpretation means evaluating evidence that an alteration has diagnostic, prognostic, or therapeutic impact.[15,31,32] Interpretation of variants in pediatric neoplasms is particularly challenging, given the rarity of these tumors; there is often not a large body of literature about the significance of any one alteration in these tumor types. We generally rely on inference from similar variants or evidence in other tumor types. Time and expertise are required to do a thorough analysis. Crowdsourcing efforts including the National Institutes of Health ClinGen working groups may provide important resources and alleviate some of the professional time required.[33]

With the advent of large-scale sequencing studies, even rare pediatric tumors are increasingly defined by their genotypes, thanks to characteristic alterations that can support a specific diagnosis.[34,35] Fusions are particularly relevant to the diagnosis of mesenchymal and hematopoietic origin. Key molecular alterations, which support a specific diagnosis in pediatric extracranial solid tumors and CNS tumors, are provided in **Tables 1** and **2**.

Molecularly informed risk stratification has become important for several pediatric brain, solid and hematologic neoplasms. Medulloblastomas are routinely subtyped into 4 molecularly defined groups which dictate therapeutic regimens (**Fig. 1**).[37]

Neuroblastoma patients are stratified according to their *MYCN* amplification status and may also make use of segmental copy number alterations for further stratification.[38] Pediatric hematologic malignancies rely heavily on molecular alterations for prognostication, including fusion status and *IKZF1* deletions.[39,40] Key molecular alterations with prognostic associations in B-ALL are summarized in **Table 3**. These risk stratification measures have had let to a significant improvement in survival for children with acute lymphoblastic leukemia, with an example provided in **Fig. 2**.[42] Prognostic associations in rare tumors are difficult to make because of the absence of large, stratified studies. It is the authors' opinions that prognostic associations without strong evidence should not be included in reports because of the stress and uncertainty that the patients and families may experience.[43]

The availability of targeted therapies has increased dramatically over the past decade, albeit more slowly for our young patients with cancer who may not be included in clinical trials, particularly those younger than 12 years.[44] Safety and efficacy studies may not have been completed, and issues of drug formulation may be relevant. Roughly half of all neoplasms in pediatric patients have a genetic alteration with a known targeted therapy.[11] Collaboration with pediatric oncologists who are familiar with the landscape of approved treatments and clinical trials is key to success and future development of targeted treatments available to children.[32] The age-agnostic global approval of NTRK inhibitors provides an important example of trials that include children and provide opportunities for precision medicine in pediatric cancers.[45] Other kinase inhibitors are increasingly available to children, with some dramatic clinical responses, as demonstrated in **Fig. 3**.

Germline Cancer Predisposition

Approximately 10% to 15% of pediatric patients with cancer have a germline genetic alteration with a known associated risk of developing cancer, most often in genes that code for repair proteins following DNA mismatch and double-stranded breaks.[47] The association of hematological malignancies is well-understood in the setting of certain constitutional syndromes. Patients with Down syndrome constitute approximately 1% to 5% of patients with acute myeloid leukemia, and also carry an increased risk for B-ALL (often with *CRLF2* rearrangements), whereas T-ALL is observed in patients with ataxia-telangiectasia or with germline variants in *RUNX1*.[25,48] Patients in families with general cancer predisposition syndromes are also at greater risk of developing ALL, particularly those harboring germline variants in *TP53*, *ETV6*, *PAX5*, and *IKZF1*, mirroring the same genes affected in the somatic genome in hematologic malignancies.[48]

Even when somatic testing is being performed, with tumor specimens being used, findings that lead to an indication of follow-up germline testing are seen in approximately 20% of cases.[30] Owing to the high pretest probability that a pediatric patient with cancer will have a germline cancer predisposition, it is advisable that the potential germline etiology of a variant identified by sequencing is considered. One approach to this important issue is to include molecular testing of separate, patient-matched, non-neoplastic tissues when testing tumor samples to provide a definitive source for each variant. This workflow can be complicated by the lack of availability of non-neoplastic tissues, particularly for patients with hematologic malignancies. Another approach is to provide a report that acknowledges the potential for germline disease associations and recommends follow-up with genetic counseling. Identification of germline cancer predisposition provides the patient and their family with options for screening and the prevention of future cancer risks.[47] Selected predisposition syndromes are summarized in **Table 4**.

Table 2
Selected diagnostically significant alterations in central nervous system tumors

Tumor Type	Tumors	Alterations
Pediatric-type diffuse low-grade gliomas	Diffuse astrocytoma, MYB- or MYBL1-altered	MYB, MYBL1
	Angiocentric glioma	MYB
	Polymorphous low-grade neuroepithelial tumor of the young	BRAF, FGFR family
	Diffuse low-grade glioma, MAPK pathway-altered	FGFR1, BRAF
Pediatric-type diffuse high-grade gliomas	Diffuse midline glioma, H3 K27-altered	H3 K27, TP53, ACVR1, PDGFRA, EGFR, EZHIP
	Diffuse hemispheric glioma, H3 G34-mutant	H3 G34, TP53, ATRX
	Diffuse pediatric-type high-grade glioma, H3-wildtype and IDH-wildtype	IDH-wildtype, H3-wildtype, PDGFRA, MYCN, EGFR
	Infant-type hemispheric glioma	NTRK family, ALK, ROS, MET
Astrocytic gliomas	Pilocytic astrocytoma	BRAF p.V600E or KIAA1549::BRAF fusion, NF1
	Astroblastoma, MN1-altered	MN1
Embryonal tumors	CNS tumor with BCOR internal tandem duplication	BCOR internal tandem duplication
	CNS embryonal tumor	
	Dysembryoplastic neuroepithelial tumor	FGFR1
	Medulloblastoma, WNT-activated	CTNNB1, APC
	Medulloblastoma, SHH-activated	TP53, PTCH1, SUFU, SMO, MYCN, GLI2
	Medulloblastoma, non-WNT/non-SHH	MYC, MYCN, PRDM6, KDM6A
	Atypical teratoid/rhabdoid tumor	SMARCB1, SMARCA4
	Embryonal tumor with multilayered rosettes	C19 MC, DICER1
	CNS neuroblastoma, FOXR2-activated	FOXR2
	CNS tumor with BCOR internal tandem duplication	BCOR
	Subependymal giant cell astrocytoma	TSC1, TSC2
Mesenchymal	Primary intracranial sarcoma, DICER1-mutant	DICER1
Ependymal	Supratentorial ependymomas	ZFTA, RELA, YAP1, MAML2
	Posterior fossa ependymomas	H3 K27me3, EZHIP (methylome)
	Spinal ependymomas	NF2, MYCN

Data from Louis DN, Perry A, Wesseling P, et al. The 2021 WHO Classification of Tumors of the Central Nervous System: a summary. Neuro-Oncol. 2021;23(8):1231-1251. https://doi.org/10.1093/neuonc/noab106.

Emerging Technologies

In pursuit of less invasive techniques for cancer diagnostics and disease monitoring, next-generation sequencing assays have recently been developed for the detection of relatively small amounts of circulating tumor DNA (ctDNA) in patient plasma.[68] Tumor ctDNA is derived from apoptotic or necrotic tumor cells, and abundance of ctDNA has been correlated with tumor type and disease burden, with some tumors generally having a higher propensity for releasing ctDNA, and patients with higher-stage

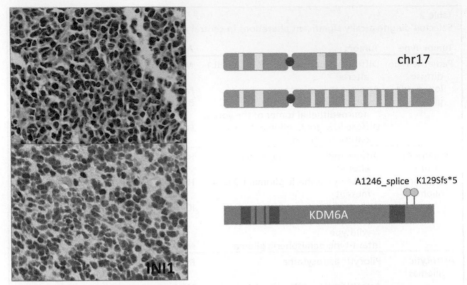

Fig. 1. Biopsy from a 9-year-old boy with a fourth ventricular mass. Histopathology shows a briskly mitotic "small blue cell tumor." The immunohistochemical profile is consistent with medulloblastoma (not pictured—abundant reactivity for synaptophysin, relatively fewer GFAP positive tumor cells, and no nuclear expression of beta-catenin). Nuclear retention of INI1 is important in excluding the diagnosis of atypical teratoid rhabdoid tumor (ATRT), which is histologically similar. Risk stratification for selection of treatment includes evaluation of both copy number alterations and sequence variants.[36] This case was evaluated by a large, targeted, DNA next-generation sequencing panel, which demonstrates loss of chr17p (consistent with the recurrent isodicentric chr17 alteration) and with 2 splice site variants in *KDM6A* (c.3736 + 1 G > C and c.3878_3878+6del, NM_021140.2). This combination of alterations assigns the patient to molecular group 4, the most common subtype in children, which is associated with an intermediate prognosis. (Images courtesy of Dr. Hart Lidov.)

malignancies generally having more readily detectable ctDNA.[69,70] These features have made ctDNA a promising tool for quantification of treatment response and, conversely, detection of disease recurrence as minimal residual disease (MRD).

There has been a significant investigation into the utility of ctDNA detection in pediatric brain tumors as they are among the most frequent pediatric neoplasms. In the setting of medulloblastoma, cerebrospinal fluid (CSF) has been shown to be a promising source of relatively abundant ctDNA to monitor for MRD and for longitudinal changes in tumor genetics following treatment and recurrence.[71] The characteristic alteration in H3K27M-mutant diffuse midline gliomas has also been successfully detected in ctDNA of CSF and plasma with sensitivity as high as 92%.[72,73] Although these assays mirror most current ctDNA sequencing assays targeting recurrent sequence variants, intended for an adult population, new methodologies have also emerged for detecting copy number alterations and translocations which constitute the majority of driver events in pediatric neoplasia. Low-pass whole genome sequencing in combination with hybrid capture assays have been developed to specifically target the copy number alterations and translocations that constitute the majority of driver events in pediatric neoplasia, particularly pediatric sarcomas.[74,75] As advancements are made in assay design and bioinformatics, many laboratories are

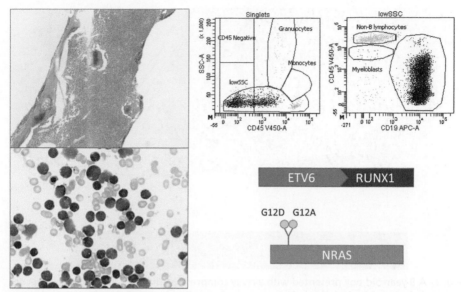

Fig. 2. Bone marrow biopsy from a 2-year-old girl, showing sheets of primitive lymphoid cells consistent with B-cell acute lymphoblastic leukemia (B-ALL). Risk stratification includes evaluation by multiple modalities. Flow cytometry was negative for other myeloid and T-lymphoid markers (CD15, CD117, CD3, CD5, CD7) with a DNA index of 1.0. Karyotype (not pictured) showed 46,XX,t(2;14)(p11.2;q32),add(12) (p12)[6]/47,sl,+10,del(15)(q11.2q15)[2]/48,sdl,+mar [7]/46,XX[7]. An *ETV6::RUNX1* fusion was identified by both FISH and by targeted RNA next-generation sequencing, which is associated with a better prognosis. DNA next-generation sequencing identified 2 *NRAS* variants (p.G12D and p.G12A, NM_002524.3) on different sequencing reads, which are recurrently identified in pediatric B-ALL.[41] (Images courtesy of Dr. Marian H. Harris.)

currently performing clinical sequencing on ctDNA for detection of disease recurrence, and are striving to further improve their assays' sensitivities to enable even earlier disease recurrence detection.[68]

Hypermutation, or a high TMB, is more common in adult malignancies than in pediatric cases, with approximately 14 times higher mutation frequencies.[12] When considering the clinical impact of TMB in pediatric tumors, it is important to identify hypermutated cases, and to think critically about the threshold used for the designation of "hypermutated." Tumors with ≥10 mutations per megabase (Mb) tested in pediatric patients are enriched for genetic alterations in genes coding for the mismatch repair pathway, including *MLH1*, *MSH2*, *PMS2*, *MSH6*, *POLE*, and *POLD1*; ultrahypermutated tumors in pediatric patients, with over 100 mutations per Mb, have been observed in hematolymphoid malignancies, colorectal cancers, and malignant gliomas.[11,12] These hypermutated tumors may be associated with cancer predisposition syndromes including Lynch syndrome or congenital mismatch repair deficiency, with significant implications in cancer risk for both the affected child and their family members.[43,47,49–52] TMB has also emerged as an important biomarker for predicting response to immuno-oncology therapies. Owing to the lower median and wide distribution of TMB in pediatric patients, careful consideration should be given to both assay design and to which thresholds are used to designate "hypermutant" status.[53] Additional ongoing studies may help to elucidate these details over the upcoming years.

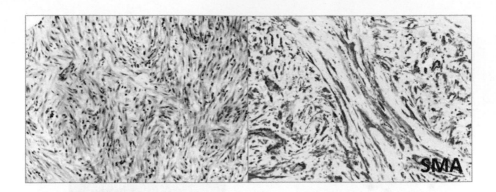

Fig. 3. A 9-year-old boy presented with airway compression due to a lung mass, along with perianal, leg, and brain lesions. A percutaneous needle biopsy of the chest wall shows a patternless arrangement of fibroblast-myofibroblast–like cells in a myxoid matrix with admixed inflammatory cells. Lesional cells show patchy positivity for SMA. A *TFG::ROS1* fusion was identified by targeted RNA next-generation sequencing, supporting a diagnosis of inflammatory myofibroblastic tumor. The patient responded favorably to targeted therapy with crizotinib followed by surgical resection of all masses, with additional details in press.46 (Images courtesy of Dr. Alyaa Al-Ibraheemi.)

Table 3
Common genetic alterations associated with prognosis in pediatric B-cell acute lymphoblastic leukemia

Prognostic Association	Alteration	Detection Method
Better prognosis	High hyperdiploidy	Karyotype
	ETV6::RUNX1	Karyotype, FISH, NGS
	NUTM1 rearrangement	Karyotype, FISH, NGS
Worse prognosis	Hypodiploidy	Karyotype
	KMT2A rearrangement	Karyotype, FISH, NGS
	BCR::ABL1 (Ph+)	Karyotype, FISH, NGS
	BCR::ABL1-like (Ph-like)	Karyotype, FISH, NGS
	IKZF1 intragenic deletion	MLPA, NGS
	TCF3::HLF	Karyotype, FISH, NGS
	MEF2D rearrangement	Karyotype, FISH, NGS
	Intrachromosomal amplification of chromosome 21 (iAMP21)	Karyotype, FISH, microarray
	BCL2 rearrangement	Karyotype, FISH, NGS
	MYC rearrangement	Karyotype, FISH, NGS

Data from Inaba H, Mullighan CG. Pediatric acute lymphoblastic leukemia. *Haematologica.* 2020;105(11):2524-2539. https://doi.org/10.3324/haematol.2020.247031 and Tran TH, Harris MH, Nguyen JV, et al. Prognostic impact of kinase-activating fusions and IKZF1 deletions in pediatric high-risk B-lineage acute lymphoblastic leukemia. *Blood Adv.* 2018;2(5):529-533. https://doi.org/10.1182/bloodadvances.2017014704.

Table 4
Selected genetic tumor predisposition syndromes associated with pediatric cancers

Syndrome	Genes	Associated Tumors
DICER1 Syndrome	DICER1	PPB
		Thyroid adenomas, multinodular goiter, and/or well-differentiated thyroid carcinoma
		Ovarian tumors including sex cord-stromal tumors
		Cystic nephroma
		Ciliary body medulloepithelioma
		Nasal chondromesenchymal hamartoma
		Embryonal rhabdomyosarcoma of the cervix or other sites
		Pituitary blastoma
		Pineoblastoma
		DICER1-associated CNS sarcoma
		ETMR-like (embryonal tumor with multilayer rosettes)
		Presacral malignant teratoid neoplasm of infancy
		Pleuropulmonary blastoma-like peritoneal sarcoma
Neurofibromatosis 1	NF1	Neurofibromas
		Plexiform neurofibromas
		Optic nerve and other central nervous system gliomas
		Malignant peripheral nerve sheath tumors
		JMML
		MDS/AML
Neurofibromatosis 2	NF2	Schwannomas
		Meningiomas
		Ependymomas
		Astrocytomas
Li Fraumeni	TP53	Adrenocortical carcinomas
		Breast cancer
		CNS tumors
		Osteosarcomas
		Soft-tissue sarcomas
		Others
Retinoblastoma	RB1	Retinoblastoma
		Osteosarcoma
Nevoid Basal Cell Carcinoma Syndrome	SUFU PTCH1	Jaw keratocysts
		Basal cell carcinomas
		Cardiac and ovarian fibromas
		Medulloblastoma
Constitutional Mismatch Repair Deficiency	MLH1 MSH2 MSH6 MS2	Colonic adenoma
		Colorectal carcinoma
		Carcinoma of the small intestine
		Hematologic
		Brain tumors

(continued on next page)

Table 4 (continued)		
Syndrome	**Genes**	**Associated Tumors**
Hereditary Paraganglioma-Pheochromocytoma Syndrome	MAX SDHA SDHAF2 SDHB SDHC SDHD TMEM127	Paragangliomas Pheochromocytomas GIST Pulmonary chondroma Renal cell carcinoma
Tuberous Sclerosis Complex	TSC1 TSC2	Facial angiofibromas Subependymal nodules Cortical dysplasias Subependymal giant cell astrocytomas Angiomyolipomas Kidney cysts Renal cell carcinomas Rhabdomyomas
Noonan syndrome	PTPN11	TMD JMML CMML
Shwachman-Diamond syndrome	SBDS	MDS/AML ALL
RUNX1 Familial Platelet Disorder with Associated Myeloid Malignancies	RUNX1	MDS/AML
ETV6 Thrombocytopenia and Predisposition to Leukemia	ETV6	ALL

Abbreviations: ALL, acute lymphoblastic leukemia; AML, acute myeloid leukemia; CMML, chronic myelomonocytic leukemia; JMML, juvenile myelomonocytic leukemia; MDS, myelodysplastic syndrome; PPB, pleuropulmonary blastoma; TMD, transient myeloproliferative disorder.
Data from Refs.[35,49–67]

SUMMARY

Molecular assays to support the care of children with tumors and hematologic neoplasia are evolving quickly. Pathology and oncology programs can support their youngest patients by designing assays that target actionable alterations for this patient population, and which can accommodate small biopsies. New and emerging technologies and the continued development of clinical associations for children with cancer will continue to evolve to support this important patient population.

CLINICS CARE POINTS

- Pediatric neoplasms have unique molecular signatures, different from their adult counterparts
- Fusions and copy number alterations are particularly common, and clinically relevant, in pediatric tumors
- Designing a suite of molecular assays, which include children with cancer, may require addition of unique targets
- Tissue allocation can be challenging due to small biopsies

- Diagnostic, prognostic, and therapeutic associations with strong evidence are available for children with cancer

---

DISCLOSURE

A.J. Church Medical Advisory Board for Bayer Oncology.

REFERENCES

1. Dixon SB, Chen Y, Yasui Y, et al. Reduced morbidity and mortality in survivors of childhood acute lymphoblastic leukemia: a report from the childhood cancer survivor study. J Clin Oncol 2020;38(29):3418–29.
2. Armstrong GT, Liu Q, Yasui Y, et al. Late mortality among 5-year survivors of childhood cancer: a summary from the Childhood Cancer Survivor Study. J Clin Oncol 2009;27(14):2328–38.
3. Siegel DA, Richardson LC, Henley SJ, et al. Pediatric cancer mortality and survival in the United States, 2001-2016. Cancer 2020;126(19):4379–89.
4. Fuchs J. The role of minimally invasive surgery in pediatric solid tumors. Pediatr Surg Int 2015;31(3):213–28.
5. Ilivitzki A, Abugazala M, Arkovitz M, et al. Ultrasound-guided core biopsy as the primary tool for tissue diagnosis in pediatric oncology. J Pediatr Hematol Oncol 2014;36(5):333–6.
6. Garrett KM, Fuller CE, Santana VM, et al. Percutaneous biopsy of pediatric solid tumors. Cancer 2005;104(3):644–52.
7. Cooley LD, Morton CC, Sanger WG, et al. Section E6.5-6.8 of the ACMG technical standards and guidelines: chromosome studies of lymph node and solid tumor-acquired chromosomal abnormalities. Genet Med 2016;18(6):643–8.
8. Pinches RS, Clinton CM, Ward A, et al. Making the most of small samples: optimization of tissue allocation of pediatric solid tumors for clinical and research use. Pediatr Blood Cancer 2020;67(9). https://doi.org/10.1002/pbc.28326.
9. Kram DE, Henderson JJ, Baig M, et al. Embryonal tumors of the central nervous system in children: the era of targeted therapeutics. Bioeng Basel Switz 2018; 5(4):E78.
10. Gadd S, Huff V, Walz AL, et al. A Children's Oncology Group and TARGET initiative exploring the genetic landscape of Wilms tumor. Nat Genet 2017;49(10): 1487–94.
11. PedBrain-Seq Project ICGC, MMML-Seq Project ICGC, Gröbner SN, et al. The landscape of genomic alterations across childhood cancers. Nature 2018; 555(7696):321–7.
12. Campbell BB, Light N, Fabrizio D, et al. Comprehensive analysis of hypermutation in human cancer. Cell 2017;171(5):1042–56.e10.
13. Dupain C, Harttrampf AC, Urbinati G, et al. Relevance of fusion genes in pediatric cancers: toward precision medicine. Mol Ther Nucleic Acids 2017;6:315–26.
14. Sweet-Cordero EA, Biegel JA. The genomic landscape of pediatric cancers: implications for diagnosis and treatment. Science 2019;363(6432):1170–5.
15. Slack JC, Church AJ. Molecular alterations in pediatric solid tumors. Surg Pathol Clin 2021;14(3):473–92.
16. Hingorani P, Janeway K, Crompton BD, et al. Current state of pediatric sarcoma biology and opportunities for future discovery: a report from the sarcoma translational research workshop. Cancer Genet 2016;209(5):182–94.

17. Lautz TB, Hayes-Jordan A. Recent progress in pediatric soft tissue sarcoma therapy. Semin Pediatr Surg 2019;28(6):150862.

18. Ingley KM, Cohen-Gogo S, Gupta AA. Systemic therapy in pediatric-type soft-tissue sarcoma. Curr Oncol 2020;27(11):6–16.

19. Agaram NP, LaQuaglia MP, Alaggio R, et al. MYOD1-mutant spindle cell and sclerosing rhabdomyosarcoma: an aggressive subtype irrespective of age. A reappraisal for molecular classification and risk stratification. Mod Pathol 2019; 32(1):27–36.

20. Nobre L, Zapotocky M, Ramaswamy V, et al. Outcomes of BRAF V600E pediatric gliomas treated with targeted BRAF inhibition. JCO Precis Oncol 2020;4. PO.19.00298.

21. Ryall S, Zapotocky M, Fukuoka K, et al. Integrated molecular and clinical analysis of 1,000 pediatric low-grade gliomas. Cancer Cell 2020;37(4):569–83.e5.

22. Johnson A, Severson E, Gay L, et al. Comprehensive genomic profiling of 282 pediatric low- and high-grade gliomas reveals genomic drivers, tumor mutational burden, and hypermutation signatures. Oncologist 2017;22(12):1478–90.

23. Fangusaro J, Bandopadhayay P. Advances in the classification and treatment of pediatric brain tumors. Curr Opin Pediatr 2021;33(1):26–32.

24. Ward E, DeSantis C, Robbins A, et al. Childhood and adolescent cancer statistics, 2014. CA Cancer J Clin 2014;64(2):83–103.

25. Harris MH, Czuchlewski DR, Arber DA, et al. Genetic testing in the diagnosis and biology of acute leukemia. Am J Clin Pathol 2019;152(3):322–46.

26. Swerdlow SH, Campo E, Harris NL, et al. WHO classification of tumours of haematopoietic and lymphoid tissues 2011;117(19):5019–32.

27. Harris MH. Gene rearrangement detection in pediatric leukemia. Clin Lab Med 2021;41(3):551–61.

28. National Comprehensive Cancer Network. Acute lymphoblastic leukemia (Version 2.2021). Available at: https://www.nccn.org/professionals/physician_gls/pdf/all. pdf. Accessed October 1, 2021.

29. Roberts KG, Li Y, Payne-Turner D, et al. Targetable kinase-activating lesions in Ph-like acute lymphoblastic leukemia. N Engl J Med 2014;371(11):1005–15.

30. Surrey LF, MacFarland SP, Chang F, et al. Clinical utility of custom-designed NGS panel testing in pediatric tumors. Genome Med 2019;11(1):32.

31. Cheng L, Pandya PH, Liu E, et al. Integration of genomic copy number variations and chemotherapy-response biomarkers in pediatric sarcoma. BMC Med Genomics 2019;12(S1):23.

32. Oberg JA, Glade Bender JL, Sulis ML, et al. Implementation of next generation sequencing into pediatric hematology-oncology practice: moving beyond actionable alterations. Genome Med 2016;8(1):133.

33. Ritter DI, Rao S, Kulkarni S, et al. A case for expert curation: an overview of cancer curation in the Clinical Genome Resource (ClinGen). Cold Spring Harb Mol Case Stud 2019;5(5):a004739.

34. Kallen ME, Hornick JL. The 2020 WHO classification: what's new in soft tissue tumor Pathology? Am J Surg Pathol 2021;45(1):e1–23.

35. Louis DN, Perry A, Wesseling P, et al. The 2021 WHO classification of tumors of the central nervous system: a summary. Neuro-Oncol 2021;23(8):1231–51. Available at: https://Publications.Iarc.Fr/Book-And-Report-Series/Who-Classification-Of-Tumours/WHO-Classification-Of-Tumours-Of-Haematopoietic-And-Lymphoid-Tissues-2017.

36. Schwalbe EC, Lindsey JC, Nakjang S, et al. Novel molecular subgroups for clinical classification and outcome prediction in childhood medulloblastoma: a cohort study. Lancet Oncol 2017;18(7):958–71.
37. Ramaswamy V, Remke M, Bouffet E, et al. Risk stratification of childhood medulloblastoma in the molecular era: the current consensus. Acta Neuropathol (Berl) 2016;131(6):821–31.
38. Pinto NR, Applebaum MA, Volchenboum SL, et al. Advances in risk classification and treatment Strategies for Neuroblastoma. J Clin Oncol 2015;33(27):3008–17.
39. Vrooman LM, Blonquist TM, Harris MH, et al. Refining risk classification in childhood B acute lymphoblastic leukemia: results of DFCI ALL Consortium Protocol 05-001. Blood Adv 2018;2(12):1449–58.
40. Burns MA, Place AE, Stevenson KE, et al. Identification of prognostic factors in childhood T-cell acute lymphoblastic leukemia: results from DFCI ALL Consortium Protocols 05-001 and 11-001. Pediatr Blood Cancer 2021;68(1):e28719.
41. Messina M, Chiaretti S, Wang J, et al. Prognostic and therapeutic role of targetable lesions in B-lineage acute lymphoblastic leukemia without recurrent fusion genes. Oncotarget 2016;7(12):13886–901.
42. Pui C-H, Yang JJ, Hunger SP, et al. Childhood acute lymphoblastic leukemia: progress through collaboration. J Clin Oncol 2015;33(27):2938–48.
43. Robinson JO, Wynn J, Biesecker B, et al. Psychological outcomes related to exome and genome sequencing result disclosure: a meta-analysis of seven Clinical Sequencing Exploratory Research (CSER) Consortium studies. Genet Med 2019;21(12):2781–90.
44. Langenberg KPS, Looze EJ, Molenaar JJ. The landscape of pediatric precision oncology: program design, actionable alterations, and clinical trial development. Cancers 2021;13(17):4324.
45. Scott LJ. Larotrectinib: first global approval. Drugs 2019;79(2):201–6.
46. Wachter F, Al-Ibraheemi A, Trissal M, et al. Molecular characterization of inflammatory tumors facilitates initiation of effective therapy. Pediatrics 2021;148(6). e2021050990.
47. Fiala EM, Jayakumaran G, Mauguen A, et al. Prospective pan-cancer germline testing using MSK-IMPACT informs clinical translation in 751 patients with pediatric solid tumors. Nat Cancer 2021;2(3):357–65.
48. Inaba H, Mullighan CG. Pediatric acute lymphoblastic leukemia. Haematologica 2020;105(11):2524–39.
49. Yuan H, Ji J, Shi M, et al. Characteristics of pan-cancer patients with ultrahigh tumor mutation burden. Front Oncol 2021;11:682017.
50. Waterfall JJ, Meltzer PS. Avalanching mutations in biallelic mismatch repair deficiency syndrome. Nat Genet 2015;47(3):194–6.
51. Sinicrope FA. Lynch syndrome-associated colorectal cancer. N Engl J Med 2018; 379(8):764–73.
52. Durno C, Ercan AB, Bianchi V, et al. Survival benefit for individuals with constitutional mismatch repair deficiency undergoing Surveillance. J Clin Oncol 2021; 39(25):2779–90.
53. Noskova H, Kyr M, Pal K, et al. Assessment of tumor mutational burden in pediatric tumors by real-life whole-exome sequencing and in Silico Simulation of targeted gene panels: how the choice of method could affect the clinical decision? Cancers 2020;12(1):E230.
54. Tran TH, Harris MH, Nguyen JV, et al. Prognostic impact of kinase-activating fusions and IKZF1 deletions in pediatric high-risk B-lineage acute lymphoblastic leukemia. Blood Adv 2018;2(5):529–33.

55. Schultz KAP, Stewart DR, Kamihara J, et al. DICER1 tumor predisposition. In: Adam MP, Ardinger HH, Pagon RA, et al, editors. GeneReviews® [Internet]. Seattle (WA): University of Washington, Seattle; 2020. p. 1993–2022. Available at: https://www.ncbi.nlm.nih.gov/books/NBK196157/.

56. Friedman JM. Neurofibromatosis 1. In: Adam MP, Ardinger HH, Pagon RA, et al, editors. GeneReviews® [Internet]. Seattle (WA): University of Washington, Seattle; 2022. p. 1993–2022. Available at: https://www.ncbi.nlm.nih.gov/books/NBK1109/.

57. Evans DG. Neurofibromatosis 2. In: Adam MP, Ardinger HH, Pagon RA, et al, editors. GeneReviews® [Internet]. Seattle (WA): University of Washington, Seattle; 2018. p. 1993–2022. Available at: https://www.ncbi.nlm.nih.gov/books/NBK1201/.

58. Schneider K, Zelley K, Nichols KE, et al. Li-fraumeni syndrome. In: Adam MP, Ardinger HH, Pagon RA, et al, editors. GeneReviews® [Internet]. Seattle (WA): University of Washington, Seattle; 2019. p. 1993–2022. Available at: https://www.ncbi.nlm.nih.gov/books/NBK1311/.

59. Lohmann DR, Gallie BL. Retinoblastoma. In: Adam MP, Ardinger HH, Pagon RA, et al, editors. GeneReviews® [Internet]. Seattle (WA): University of Washington, Seattle; 2018. p. 1993–2022. Available at: https://www.ncbi.nlm.nih.gov/books/NBK1452/.

60. Evans DG, Farndon PA. Nevoid Basal cell carcinoma syndrome. In: Adam MP, Ardinger HH, Pagon RA, et al, editors. GeneReviews® [Internet]. Seattle (WA): University of Washington, Seattle; 2018. p. 1993–2022. Available at: https://www.ncbi.nlm.nih.gov/books/NBK1151/.

61. Idos G, Valle L. Lynch syndrome. In: Adam MP, Ardinger HH, Pagon RA, et al, editors. GeneReviews® [Internet]. Seattle (WA): University of Washington, Seattle; 2021. p. 1993–2022. Available at: https://www.ncbi.nlm.nih.gov/books/NBK1211/.

62. Else T, Greenberg S, Fishbein L. Hereditary Paraganglioma-Pheochromocytoma syndromes. In: Adam MP, Ardinger HH, Pagon RA, et al, editors. GeneReviews® [Internet]. Seattle (WA): University of Washington, Seattle; 2018. p. 1993–2022. Available at: https://www.ncbi.nlm.nih.gov/books/NBK1548/.

63. Northrup H, Koenig MK, Pearson DA, et al. Tuberous Sclerosis complex. In: Adam MP, Ardinger HH, Pagon RA, et al, editors. GeneReviews® [Internet]. Seattle (WA): University of Washington, Seattle; 2021. p. 1993–2022. Available at: https://www.ncbi.nlm.nih.gov/books/NBK1220/.

64. Allanson JE, Roberts AE. Noonan syndrome. In: Adam MP, Ardinger HH, Pagon RA, et al, editors. GeneReviews® [Internet]. Seattle (WA): University of Washington, Seattle; 2022. p. 1993–2022. Available at: https://www.ncbi.nlm.nih.gov/books/NBK1124/.

65. Nelson A, Myers K. Shwachman-diamond syndrome. In: Adam MP, Ardinger HH, Pagon RA, et al, editors. GeneReviews® [Internet]. Seattle (WA): University of Washington, Seattle; 2018. p. 1993–2022. Available at: https://www.ncbi.nlm.nih.gov/books/NBK1756/.

66. Deuitch N, Broadbridge E, Cunningham L, et al. RUNX1 familial Platelet disorder with associated myeloid malignancies. In: Adam MP, Ardinger HH, Pagon RA, et al, editors. GeneReviews® [Internet]. Seattle (WA): University of Washington, Seattle; 2021. p. 1993–2021. Available at: https://www.ncbi.nlm.nih.gov/books/NBK568319/.

67. Porter CC, Di Paola J, Pencheva B. ETV6 thrombocytopenia and predisposition to leukemia. In: Adam MP, Ardinger HH, Pagon RA, et al, editors. GeneReviews®

[Internet]. Seattle (WA): University of Washington, Seattle; 2020. p. 1993–2021. Available at: https://www.ncbi.nlm.nih.gov/books/NBK564234/.
68. Alix-Panabières C, Pantel K. Clinical applications of circulating tumor cells and circulating tumor DNA as liquid biopsy. Cancer Discov 2016;6(5):479–91.
69. Diaz LA, Bardelli A. Liquid biopsies: genotyping circulating tumor DNA. J Clin Oncol 2014;32(6):579–86.
70. Bettegowda C, Sausen M, Leary RJ, et al. Detection of circulating tumor DNA in early- and late-stage human malignancies. Sci Transl Med 2014;6(224):224ra24.
71. Escudero L, Llort A, Arias A, et al. Circulating tumour DNA from the cerebrospinal fluid allows the characterisation and monitoring of medulloblastoma. Nat Commun 2020;11(1):5376.
72. Mueller S, Jain P, Liang WS, et al. A pilot precision medicine trial for children with diffuse intrinsic pontine glioma-PNOC003: a report from the Pacific Pediatric Neuro-Oncology Consortium. Int J Cancer 2019;145(7):1889–901.
73. Panditharatna E, Kilburn LB, Aboian MS, et al. Clinically relevant and minimally invasive tumor Surveillance of pediatric diffuse midline gliomas using patient-derived liquid biopsy. Clin Cancer Res 2018;24(23):5850–9.
74. Shah AT, Azad TD, Breese MR, et al. A comprehensive circulating tumor DNA assay for detection of translocation and copy-number changes in pediatric sarcomas. Mol Cancer Ther 2021;1535–7163. https://doi.org/10.1158/1535-7163. MCT-20-0987. MCT-20-0987.
75. Klega K, Imamovic-Tuco A, Ha G, et al. Detection of somatic structural variants enables quantification and characterization of circulating tumor DNA in children with solid tumors. JCO Precis Oncol 2018;(2):1–13.

FURTHER READING

Church AJ, Corson LB, Kao P-C, et al. Molecular profiling identifies targeted therapy opportunities in pediatric solid cancer. Nature Medicine 2022. https://doi.org/10.1038/s41591-022-01856-6. In press.

Specimen Considerations in Molecular Oncology Testing

Qiong Gan, MD, PhD, Sinchita Roy-Chowdhuri, MD, PhD*

KEYWORDS

- Specimen • Tissue journey • Molecular testing • Targeted therapy

KEY POINTS

- Pathologists play a pivotal role in molecular oncology testing by providing oversight through the entire tissue journey.
- Concurrently acquired core biopsy and fine-needle aspiration specimens are frequently complementary for both diagnosis and oncology testing, especially when paired with a rapid on-site evaluation.
- Different types of specimens, including histology, cytology, and liquid biopsy, provide a wide variety of options to maximize the chance of testing success.
- The main types of molecular oncology testing fall into three major categories: DNA-based, RNA-based, and protein-based assays.

INTRODUCTION

Advances in our understanding of the molecular basis of cancer have led to the development of targeted therapies that are able to target specific alterations in the oncogenic pathway and can yield significant benefits to the patient's overall and/or progression-free survival. Appropriate management of patients with solid organ and hematologic malignancies is frequently directed by molecular signatures that have necessitated molecular testing as part of the standard of care for these patients. Evaluation of the tumor biomarker profile through assessing nucleic acids and proteins can provide a detailed genomic map to guide precise individual treatment decisions. Molecular testing provides not only predictive, prognostic, and therapeutic information but also a snapshot of the genomic landscape of the tumor, allowing for monitoring the patient for tumor evolution, development of therapeutic resistance mechanisms, and detection of minimal residual disease.

Molecular oncology testing comes with several specific requirements for specimen collection, handling, and processing. The molecular oncology testing field is rapidly

Conflict of Interest: The authors have nothing to disclose.
Department of Anatomic Pathology, The University of Texas MD, Anderson Cancer Center, 1515 Holcombe Boulevard, Houston, TX 77030, USA
* Corresponding author.
E-mail address: sroy2@mdanderson.org

Clin Lab Med 42 (2022) 367–383
https://doi.org/10.1016/j.cll.2022.04.002
0272-2712/22/© 2022 Elsevier Inc. All rights reserved.
labmed.theclinics.com

evolving with a growing number of clinically relevant biomarkers, shifting the focus from disease-specific single gene testing to broad panel-based tests that are capable of identifying alterations in myriad genes or their products. Being aware that different sample types possess specific advantages and limitations, the preanalytical variables due to sampling techniques, specimen preparation and processing methods, tumor heterogeneity and the advantages, and limitations of various testing methodologies can help the pathologist develop optimal strategies to maximize the utilization of valuable tissue specimens. Therefore, in this review, we summarize the strengths and weaknesses of different specimen types that are widely used in the clinical practice of molecular oncology testing. We hope to provide valuable information to laboratories in choosing optimal clinical specimens to achieve comprehensive molecular testing that formulates individually tailored treatment plans for patients with cancer.

TISSUE ACQUISITION AND PROCESSING

Targeted therapy starts with the acquisition of adequate and appropriate tissue because the accuracy of molecular oncology testing is affected by both the quality and the quantity of tumor tissue obtained.

The Role of the Pathologist in the Era of Molecular Oncology Testing

Pathologists are at the forefront of managing patient specimens for diagnostically relevant tests as well as potential downstream biomarker tests stemming from the diagnosis. Therefore, it is important that they have a good understanding of sample requirements for different test platforms, along with the strengths and limitations of the testing platforms. Given the importance of collecting adequate tumor tissue for a variety of biomarkers that guide patient care, the pathologist should play a central role in providing oversight of the entire tumor tissue journey, optimizing the use of resources and tumor tissue sampling and processing in a personalized workflow for patients with cancer. Indeed, pathologists should oversee and manage the tumor tissue's handling and processing while communicating with the key personnel involved and consulting on diagnostic assay outputs. Therefore, it is essential that pathologists stay up-to-date with molecular testing requirements to better triage specimens, serve as patient advocates, and advise clinicians about testing options. These involve optimizing and ensuring sample adequacy and integrating and streamlining downstream testing. The era of precision medicine in the oncology setting has brought new responsibilities and challenges to pathologists, given the rapid and constant evolution of molecular pathology and the wide range of molecular tests currently used in clinical medicine.

The Collection of Specimens

At the time of tissue acquisition, the variability in tumor sampling procedures can affect diagnosis as well as the execution and accuracy of downstream testing. After the identification of the biomarker and the tissue source from which the biomarker will be assayed, the most important consideration is how the sample will be collected and preserved in the clinical setting. Three key guiding principles related to specimen collection include: (a) the collection method should use the least invasive or minimally invasive technique, if possible; (b) the amount of specimen should be sufficient for diagnosis and possible downstream ancillary testing; and (c) the collection and preservation method should be technically and logistically feasible in a clinical setting.

The tumor sampling procedures include surgical resection, excisional biopsy, core needle biopsy (CNB), fine-needle aspiration (FNA), and exfoliative specimens, including cerebrospinal fluid, urine, washings/brushings/lavages, and serous cavity body fluid specimens. The decision for sampling modality is based on the clinical stage of disease and the selection of the most suitable procedure to obtain sufficient tissue to fit assay requirements, whether it is from a primary or metastatic site, facilitating both morphologic diagnosis and downstream biomarker testing. During tumor sampling, the proceduralists aim to obtain an appropriate amount of diagnostic material while minimizing the risk of complications. Open biopsy has a reported high diagnostic accuracy; however, it carries a high risk of complications and may not be cost-effective.[1] FNA techniques were developed as a less invasive alternative to open biopsy, which is cost-effective and can be performed in an outpatient setting with little equipment requirement and minimal adverse events. Nonetheless, the diagnostic accuracy depends on the location and size of the tumor, the experience of the proceduralist, and the diagnostic interpretation skills of the pathologist. In general, FNA specimens provide a higher tumor fraction for molecular testing than concurrently acquired CNB samples due to lower amounts of stromal tissue that are aspirated in the process (**Fig. 1**).[2] In contrast, CNB provides a cylindrical core of tissue, allowing for the evaluation of tissue architecture, unlike FNA samples.[3,4] It offers a satisfactory tissue specimen, with standardized and rapid sample preparation, with a better turnaround time of diagnosis compared with open biopsy. Specimens concurrently acquired from CNB and FNA procedures are frequently complementary not only for diagnostic purposes[5] and are used in conjunction for biomarker testing in many scenarios (see **Fig. 1**).[2,6,7] Studies have shown that next-generation sequencing (NGS) success rates were similar across various types of solid tumors sampled by various techniques after adjusting for input DNA.[8,9]

The Importance of Rapid on-Site Evaluation

Rapid on-site evaluation (ROSE) is a clinical service to provide adequacy assessment of an FNA biopsy or touch imprints of a CNB in real-time, although the procedure is ongoing. The primary benefit of ROSE is the ability to direct the proceduralist on the adequacy of the sample procured, the need for additional material, and to triage the collected specimen material for the appropriate ancillary testing. During ROSE,

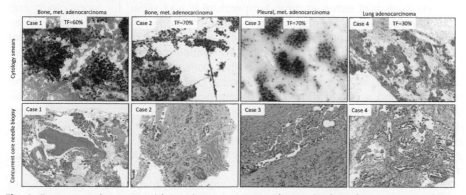

Fig. 1. Representative cases with specimens concurrently acquired cytology smears and core needle biopsy that were frequently complementary not only for diagnostic purposes and were used in conjunction for biomarker testing in many scenarios. For all these cases, cytology smears were selected for next-generation sequencing (NGS) due to the suboptimal tumor fraction (TF) in the current core biopsy (TF<20%). The TF values of these cytology cases were obtained from the final NGS results.

pathologists can proactively communicate with the proceduralist about the adequacy of the specimen collected, the preliminary diagnosis, and coordinate any special handing for downstream testing. This applies not only for diagnostic adequacy, but ROSE can also assess other crucial factors, such as tumor viability, necrosis, and tumor cellularity, especially in cases where specimen procurement is performed primarily for molecular testing. Thus, ROSE can decrease the incidence of insufficient tumor samples, mitigate the need for resampling, and in turn, reduce delays in the turnaround time of the test. ROSE has been reported to improve specimen adequacy, diagnostic yield, and turnaround times and support optimal specimen triage across different procedures, including the setting of endobronchial ultrasound-guided transbronchial needle aspiration (EBUS-TBNA) of mediastinal lymph nodes[10] and endoscopic ultrasound (EUS)-FNA of solid gastrointestinal lesions.[11–14] Despite the advantages of using ROSE, providing this service is not without challenges that often limit its widespread use in clinical practice. The primary concerns are the personnel staffing, cost-effectiveness and the resource and infrastructure impediments to performROSE.[15,16] In specific situations, telepathology using high-resolution digital imaging technologies may be used to provide ROSE service as an effective and potential time-efficient solution.[17–20]

SPECIMEN PROCESSING AND PRE-ANALYTIC VARIABLES INFLUENCING SPECIMENS

Following tissue sample acquisition, a number of additional pre-analytic variables should be considered. These include the type of preservation (fixation vs freezing), type of fixative, ischemic time, fixation conditions, decalcification reagents, storage time, and condition. All of these pre-analytical factors impact the quality of nucleic acids and proteins present within the tissue sample and can play a major role in the success of biomarker testing. Tissue procured via biopsy and surgery could be processed fresh frozen, but for clinical purposes are routinely processed through formalin fixation after gross examination and tissue sectioning, if needed for larger specimens. Fresh frozen tissue at ultra-low temperature is associated with better quality nucleic acid and is more favorable to the analysis of long DNA segments, whereas the lack of morphologic evaluation as well as the demand for more specialized handling and storage makes it more amenable for use in a research setting than a clinical laboratory. Formalin fixation of tissue at room temperature is well-suited for morphologic and other pathologic assessments, making it preferable for use in clinical practice. However, formalin fixation has certain limitations, such as DNA fragmentation, chemical cross-linking, artifactual mutations, and slow fixation (penetration rate of 1 mm per hour), which are well recognized.[21,22] Another fixative commonly used in cytology is alcohol-based fixatives because of their rapid action, ability to clear mucous and obscuring blood, and overall improved morphology. Specimen with alcohol-based fixation has been reported to yield even superior quantity and quality of genomic material, although alcohol-based fixative might give variable results for immunostaining.[23–25] Thus, awareness of these pre-analytical variables and standardized specimen management and processing is a prerequisite for reliable and accurate molecular testing.

Besides standardizing specimen processing, some proactive approaches during specimen processing could help minimize the loss of tissue due to refacing of the block. These include:

a. Preparation of extra unstained sections upfront for requested or anticipated ancillary testing is particularly useful for timely, efficient triage of small specimens for appropriate molecular tests once the diagnosis has been rendered.

b. Separate embedding of tissue core fragments if necessary. For example, placing each core in separated cassette, if >5 cores, place 2 cores in each cassette. This approach enables each core to be assessed independently and allows tissue samples to be reserved for molecular testing or additional testing. The pathologist could determine the optimal tissue block, such as a block only for molecular testing[26] for downstream processing, depending on tissue availability and testing requirements (discussed in the next section).

c. Guiding tissue grossing by pathologists, such as the biopsy of bone lesions. Since decalcification agents that use harsh acids are detrimental to the tissue for biomarker testing, a biopsy taken from a bone lesion involved by metastatic carcinoma (eg, lung, breast) could be split into softer tissue fragments to avoid decalcification, which could be prioritized for molecular testing if sufficient, and harder tissue fragments for decalcification using agents such as ethylenediaminetetraacetic acid to allow for efficient sectioning which could be used for immunostaining and molecular testing.

PRE-ANALYTIC EVALUATION AND TRIAGE OF SPECIMEN

Pre-analytic evaluation of all available pathology specimens plays an important role in the success of subsequent molecular oncology testing. The proper selection of tumor samples for downstream molecular testing is critical to generate accurate results and guide therapeutic management.

Which Specimen to Choose and What Type of Specimen Could Be Used for Molecular Oncology Testing?

The treating physician may sometimes specify which sample and what type of test to perform to guide precise and individualized treatment decisions. In general, if there are multiple specimens or tumor blocks and/or cytologic specimens available for biomarker testing, the most recent specimen from the metastasis or recurrence is usually recommended for testing as tumor heterogeneity has been reported in primary versus metastatic lesions and the metastatic site is thought to best represent the tumor evolution.[27–30] If the designated specimen is unsuitable, alternatives including archival material could be queried within the context of the requested tests. In case there are concurrently acquired core biopsy and FNA specimens or touch-prep smears, these specimens could be combined for molecular testing as long as they were obtained from the same site during the same procedure.[2,7] The relevant specimen with adequate cellularity and the highest tumor fraction is usually chosen for testing to maximize the chances of testing success. Overall, the specimen type and clinical context will determine how specimens and slide preparations are prioritized for pathologic evaluation and ancillary molecular testing (**Table 1**).

Histologic tissue specimen

Histologic tissue specimens were the first specimen preparation that was optimized for molecular oncology tests and remains the cornerstone of biomarker testing. Depending on the techniques used for sampling, the specimen ranges from small CNB to large surgical resection. These tissues provide relatively larger specimen volume; however, they may also contain abundant non-tumor components such as fibroconnective tissue and surrounding inflammation. Therefore, pathologic evaluation of tissue specimen and demarcation of appropriate areas of tumor cells are important to guarantee adequate tumor fraction for downstream testing.

Table 1
Clinical specimens used for biomarker testing

Specimen Type	Resection or Biopsy	Cytology • Cell Block	Cytology • Touch Imprint • Direct Smears	Cytology • Cytospins • Liquid Based Cytology	Blood-Based Liquid Biopsy
ROSE for adequacy assessment	No[a]	No	Yes	No	No
Fixation	Formalin[b]	Formalin[c]	Variable[d]	Variable[d]	None
Processing	Paraffin	Paraffin	Variable[e]	Variable[e]	None
Biomarker testing (Yes/No)					
DNA/RNA-based assays	Yes	Yes	Yes[f]	Yes[f]	Yes[f]
FISH	Yes	Yes	Yes[f]	Yes[f]	No
Gene expression	Yes	Yes	Yes[f]	Yes[f]	No
IHC	Yes	Yes	Yes[g]	Yes[f]	No

Abbreviations: CSF, cerebrospinal fluid; Fish, fluorescence in situ hybridization; FNA, fine needle aspiration; IHC, immunohistochemistry/immunocytochemistry; LBC, liquid-based cytology; ROSE, rapid on-site evaluation.

[a] Except in cases with touch imprint.
[b] 10% neutral buffered formalin, recommended.
[c] CB preparations are often prefixed in other fixatives such as ethanol or methanol before formalin fixation.
[d] Variety of fixatives such as ethanol, Carnoys, CytoLyt.
[e] Variety of processing techniques and staining such as Papanicolaou, Diff-Quik; residual LBC nucleic acid extraction can be performed without additional processing/staining/cover slipping.
[f] With appropriate assay validation for the specimen preparation.
[g] With appropriate assay validation; however, the number of TP/smear slides available for potential IHC may be limited.

Cytology specimen

Until recently, the utility of cytology specimens in molecular testing has been underutilized and even excluded from molecular testing due to a lack of familiarity with cytologic preparations, pre-analytical variables, and the tedious process of additional validation. The variety and versatility of cytology specimen preparations provide a few advantages in terms of molecular testing and are considered equivalent or superior to some surgical specimens for testing. Cytology specimens include cell block (CB) preparation, direct smear, cytospin preparations, liquid-based cytology (LBC), and "liquid biopsy" options, such as supernatants and residual specimens. CBs could be considered "hybrid" versions of cytologic and histologic samples. The usefulness of CBs has been widely demonstrated.[31] Most CB preparations use formalin fixation for processing, similar to histologic specimen processing. Therefore, a major benefit of using CBs instead of other cytologic preparations is the ability to perform ancillary studies, including molecular testing, without the need for additional validation. However, while choosing among different types of cyto preparations, it should be taken into consideration that the formalin fixation used for CB preparations may give rise to confounding artifacts and loss of nucleic acid yield, similar to their histologic counterparts.

Direct smears have been demonstrated to be suitable for molecular testing, including NGS analysis.[32–34] DNA extracted from smears and subjected to NGS yielded higher rates of mutation than did DNA extracted from CBs.[35] Besides being suitable for DNA-based NGS analysis, direct smears are also appropriate for RNA-based NGS testing.[36] In the appropriate clinical and molecular testing settings, suitable smears may be used in cytology laboratories as the primary source for NGS analysis and thus spare CB slides for diagnostic analyses and immune-based prognostic testing [eg, immunohistochemistry (IHC)-based biomarker testing] as well as fluorescence in-situ hybridization assays.

LBC offers the ability to use scraped material from LBC slides for molecular testing as well as retrieve nucleic acids from residual material.[37] Its overall ease in terms of specimen collection, transportation, and a well-preserved sample with minimal background blood and debris makes it an attractive preparation for molecular testing.[38] Another major advantage of this approach is that LBC samples can be used to build quality controls for different NGS platforms to standardize molecular procedures on cytologic specimens.[39]

Discarded supernatant fluids and residual LBC specimens of FNA and exfoliative specimens after centrifugation and cell pelleting may be a valuable source of high-quality nucleic acids for molecular purposes due to their ability to extract nucleic acids directly without the impact of pre-analytical variables such as preservatives, fixatives, and stains.[40] Especially in situations where the cellular material is limited, such as EUS-guided FNA of pancreas[41]and thyroid,[42–44]EBUS-TBNA of lung cancer,[45] the success of using residual LBC preparation and/or supernatant of cytology specimens to detect clinically relevant mutations provides an exciting new paradigm for the use of cytopathology samples inpatient care. Using the residual or supernatant specimen for molecular testing by the NGS platform has been incorporated into the clinical workflow, thus improving the turnaround time and reducing costs associated with specimen processing.[37] Despite the success of using supernatants for molecular testing, the lack of morphologic evaluation in the specimen limits the interpretation of mutation-negative results. The fact that most of the DNA retrieved from supernatants is high molecular weight DNA that suggests that the DNA is largely from cellular components instead of tumor-derived cell-free DNA (cfDNA).[40] Hence, the cellularity of the FNA smears may be used as a surrogate for correlation when interpreting a negative mutational result.

Liquid biopsy
Liquid biopsy, while most commonly performed using plasma samples, can be performed from any body fluids, such as urine, cerebrospinal fluid, saliva, effusions, washings, and aspirates, to analyze different types of biomolecules including circulating tumor DNA (ctDNA), circulating tumor cells, and exosomes.[46] It provides an option for an alternative to tissue biopsy or cytology when the latter is absent or unavailable or inadequate for biomarker testing. As mentioned, the most widely used liquid biopsy involves testing of plasma-derived ctDNA obtained via a simple blood draw. ctDNA is cfDNA that is shed from tumor cells into the circulatory system by apoptosis, necrosis, or secretion.[47] In the case of solid malignancies, ctDNA makes up only a small fraction of cfDNA. The major advantages of liquid biopsy include the rapid turnaround time, especially in the setting of an insufficient tissue sample, thus allowing clinically relevant therapeutic decisions without delay or a need for re-biopsy.[48] For example, FDA has expanded the approval of using blood-based liquid biopsy test for all patients with advanced non-small-cell lung carcinoma (NSCLC), ovarian cancer, breast cancer, and prostate cancer.[49] Liquid biopsy can be considered at the time of initial diagnosis in all patients who need tumor molecular profiling, particularly when tumor tissue is scarce, unavailable, or for patients in whom invasive procedures may be risky or contraindicated. In addition, liquid biopsy is minimally invasive, can be repeated easily, and ctDNA can potentially provide a more comprehensive and representative molecular profile on the genetic landscapes of tumors and

thus overcome tumor heterogeneity compared with single site-specific sampling.[50] The contributing fraction of ctDNA to the total cfDNA increases with increasing tumor burden and, as such, it could be used to dynamically monitor tumor burden.[51] These advantages make liquid biopsies an attractive testing substrate in patients with advanced-stage cancer with dynamic monitoring of therapy response, early detection of resistance and new driver mutations, and knowledge of tumor recurrence even months before clinical relapse.[52,53] While compared with tissue biopsy, liquid biopsy has the advantages of being minimally invasive, having a shorter turnaround time and potentially lower overall health care costs; however, the testing success of liquid biopsy assays depends on the tumor burden in the patient. Hence, suboptimal sensitivity limits its use as a complete replacement for tissue-based testing. Negative liquid biopsy results should be considered noncontributory and followed-up with tissue sampling and tissue-based molecular testing. Further, as liquid biopsy is limited primarily to molecular characterization, the need to confirm the tissue of origin and perform tissue-based testing such as IHC biomarkers will limit its complete replacement of tumor biopsy. Several analytical methods are available for ctDNA analysis. Mutant enriched-polymerase chain reaction (PCR), Scorpion Amplified Refractory Mutation System, and peptide nucleic acid clamping provide greater sensitivity compared with traditional sequencing methods.[54] Digital droplet PCR, BEAMing (beads, emulsions, amplification, and magnetics), and NGS also demonstrate greater sensitivity and are now routinely used.[55–57]

What Are the Important Parameters Evaluated During Pre-analytic Specimen Evaluation?

For both histology and cytology specimens, important parameters that are evaluated include overall cellularity, tumor fraction, tumor viability, and background material such as mucin and blood (see **Fig. 1**). The overall cellularity plays an important role in molecular testing since it is directly corresponding to the DNA/RNA input, a critical quality control step of achieving a high success rate for NGS mutational analysis.[36,58] Based on the calculation that a single nucleated cell yields approximately 6–7 pg of DNA[59] it will need about 1500 whole cells to obtain 10 ng DNA, assuming an extraction efficiency of 100%. The number of unstained slides needed from the formalin-fixed paraffin-embedded (FFPE) block depends on the size of the tumor area. Hypocellular specimens require a greater number of unstained sections to ensure adequate cellularity for nucleic acid extraction and vice versa. In a large tumor excision sample, a single unstained section with a tumor-rich area might be adequate to yield adequate NA. The tumor fraction requirement for the molecular test depends on the analytical sensitivity of the platform.[60] For NGS testing, the approximate limit of detection is ranging from 5% to 10%, depending on the depth of sequencing coverage.[8] As somatic mutations usually affect one of two alleles in oncogenes, the minimum tumor fraction is ~10 to 20% for conventional NGS platforms, such as the Ion Torrent platform. In small specimens, tumor enrichment is a key component of molecular testing to meet the minimum threshold of tumor fraction for the platform, and such a strategy is routinely used when sections do not meet the tumor cellularity requirement. The most commonly used strategies are manual microdissection and laser-capture microdissection.

Tumor necrosis is an interesting variable to evaluate. Tumor death could be caused by either necrosis or apoptosis. Necrosis typically leads to autolysis of cellular components, which is incompatible with PCR-based sequencing tests. In contrast, apoptosis associated with nuclear and DNA fragmentation is presumed to be compatible with PCR-based testing. Necrotic tumor in post-chemotherapy treatment can yield fragmented DNA suitable for molecular testing. Consequently, samples with an insufficient viable tumor but abundant tumor necrosis may be adequate for NGS testing.[61,62] For cytology specimen, the parameters for evaluation need to be expanded to include types of preparation, fixative, stains, and slides.

What Method to Choose?

Molecular oncology testing and issues related to methodology

Many different testing methods ranging from simple to complex are used to detect molecular alterations that are diagnostic, prognostic, or predictive for patients with cancer. The main types of molecular oncology tests largely fall into three major categories: tests analyzing DNA, tests analyzing mRNA, and those analyzing protein expressions.[63] These approaches are often complementary but depending on the quantity and quality of the available material, the access to technical platforms, the turnaround time, and the expertise of the team. Given the different nature of the assays used to assess the status of genes and biomarkers, this has implications for specimen processing and triage procedures. There are methodology-related issues that may also closely relate to specimen feasibility. Adopting a more sensitive method is very important to identify molecular targets accurately and also provides another way to preserve tissue due to the decrease in the minimum requirement of testing materials. A variety of methods might be needed as the number of biomarkers, to be tested, is increasing due to the increment in the available matched targeted therapy. The quantity and quality requirements for a molecular test will be assay and specimen specific. The success of these biomarker assays depends on the quality of the nucleic acid and protein in the tested sample and correlates with several pre-analytic factors related to specimen collection and processing that have been discussed above.[9,64–66] It should be kept in mind that the results of the same factors detected by different method might have different implications. For example, in lung cancer, epidermal growth factor receptor (EGFR) DNA mutations but not EGFR protein levels by IHC predict sensitivity to EGFR tyrosine kinase inhibitors.[67]

The types of gene alteration occurring in cancers and their detection

DNA-based alterations: The four main types of alterations are single nucleotide variants, also known as point mutations; small duplications of consecutive nucleotides, insertions or deletions involving one or a few nucleotides, or more complex mutations involving simultaneous deletions and insertions of one or a few bases (indels); exon or gene copy number changes; and structural variants such as translocations or inversions often resulting in gene fusions. With the number of druggable gene aberrations and predictive biomarkers growing in oncology, NGS technologies have increasingly substituted for conventional techniques in routine molecular pathology in a more efficient, cost-saving and tissue-saving manner.[68]

RNA-based alterations: RNA-based alterations include actionable gene fusions, such as ALK, ROS1, RET, NTRK, and so forth. Also, splice variants arising out of alternative splicing points that can lead to different biological properties, such as MET splicing variant in patients with cancer, are frequently interrogated by RNA-based assays.[69] Generally, as mRNAs are less stable compared with DNA, they are often too degraded for analysis in clinical samples; thus, it is easier to use DNA to detect alterations, although RNA-based testing for fusion detection is known to be superior to DNA-based testing.[70] The RNA quality and quantity are strongly impacted by a number of pre-analytic variables, including specimen preparation type, the volume of tissue available, the specimen processing (eg, fixation), and storage conditions.[36] Fixatives containing formaldehyde can cause RNA degradation and modification by cross-linking of cytosine residues.[21]

To overcome the limitation that RNA recovered from routine specimens is often unsuitable for RNA-based gene array methodology and to encourage the implementation of gene expression analysis assays in clinical practice, new platforms based on innovative technologies have emerged in clinical practice.[71,72] In particular, multiplex digital color-coded barcode technology represents a fascinating option to evaluate both gene expression and fusion/translocation detection.[73] This assay is suitable in a clinical setting as the RNA can be extracted from FFPE samples as well as a variety of cytology specimen preparations without any significant difference in generating results. In contrast to NGS, this platform is a viable option for a single tube assay to evaluate multiple gene fusions even when the extracted RNA is of poor quality and target capture amplification fails. Although the literature investigating the feasibility of such systems to analyze RNA from cytologic smears is very limited, the application of these assays is feasible in cytology.[74,75] The implementation of new-generation technologies, such as NGS and multiplex digital color-coded barcode technology, allows maximizing the yield of molecular tests on small routine biopsy or cytology samples through integrated analysis of DNA and RNA for better diagnostic and therapeutic strategies.

Protein-based alterations: In the clinical practice of precision medicine, protein-based alterations of several predictive biomarkers are evaluated primarily by IHC. The IHC can be used to detect changes at the protein level that results not only from gene aberrations, most commonly gene amplifications, but also from specific DNA rearrangements or point mutation (such as *EML4::ALK* inversion in NSCLC and *IDH1/2* mutations in glioma).[76] The use of IHC has extended to biomarkers of response to immune-therapy agents, including programmed death-ligand 1 (PD-L1) expression[77,78] or mismatch repair status,[79,80] which determines the eligibility for therapies that are based on anti-PD-1/PD-L1 agents in certain tumor types. The FFPE tissue from surgical resection and CNB are the main material used clinically for biomarker testing due to well-characterized validation protocols and has been extended to cytology-garnered material such as cytology CB. Because of the great variation in the preparation steps of cytology specimens in terms of the types of fixative, length of fixation, and CB preparation method, FFPE-optimized IHC protocols require validation and additional optimization before use in cytology specimens. Validation and comparison to the results obtained with tissue biopsies should be performed preferably on the same patient. Studies evaluating IHC-based predictive markers have shown high concordance between cytology CB and histology specimens.[81–84] When cytology smears are the only available material, immunocytochemical staining (ICC) may be used. However, cytology specimens without fixation, fixation other than with formalin, and so forth make standardization of ICC approaches difficult. Of particular importance, alcohol fixation of cytologic specimen gives variable results for ICC depending on the antibody and the epitope.[23,24] Buonocore and colleagues have reported that the fixation method in head and neck cytology CB preparation has a significant impact on p16 staining in head and neck squamous cell carcinoma in that formalin-fixed CB outperformed CytoLyt-fixed CB.[85] The type of fixative can cause decreased antigenicity of certain antibodies have been reported, including mindbomb E3 ubiquitin protein ligase 1, estrogen receptor, and S100.[23,24,85,86] It is thus particularly important to know the impact of pre-analytic factors when the interpretation and report of IHC staining results are quantitative such as in many of these biomarkers.

Few caveats related to the specimen should be kept in mind when IHC or ICC is performed. CBs or material with adequate number of tumor cells but not necessarily an adequate tumor fraction for molecular tests could be triaged for IHC or ICC tests.

Some predictive markers have a minimum requirement of viable tumor cells, such as PD-L1 evaluation requires a minimum number of 100 tumor cells for assessment. If not, a deeper level of the block or another potential block could be considered. The other major issue for small biopsy or cytology samples is potential spatial heterogeneous expression of some markers and temporal heterogeneity expression (ie, altered expression in primary vs metastatic tumors) as reported in PD-L1expression.[81,87] Some of the other limitations associated with cytology specimens include challenging interpretation of membranous staining on non-CB cytology specimen in which the cell membranes are intact and not cut, and thus the membranous staining may mimic cytoplasmic staining instead, overinterpretation of staining due to edge or crush artifact, nonspecific staining of non-tumor cells especially in effusion samples and high background staining interfering with evaluation of these predictive biomarkers.[88,89] In addition, other than in NSCLC using tumor percentage score (TPS) which counts only tumor cells to report PD-L1 result, evaluation and reporting of PD-L1 combined positive score (CPS) that takes into account staining of tumor cells as well as infiltrating immune cells in cytology sample is not well established in other organ tumors due to challenges in identifying tumor-infiltrating inflammatory cells or even differentiating tumor cells from immune cells. Therefore, in a limited small specimen, assessing PD-L1 CPS should be evaluated only in the context of sufficient and intact tissue fragments or with cautious use of TPS, which, as reported, could be used interchangeably with a TPS of 50% to determine the PD-L1 status.[90]

SUMMARY

The molecular oncology testing in precision medicine of patients with cancer remains in constant evolution as newer biomarkers are added to the oncologists treating armamentarium. As the number of druggable gene aberrations and predictive biomarkers grows in oncology, implementation of systems to maximize tissue usage, such as the establishment and utilization of precise workflow and optimized standard operating procedures, is likely to provide patient benefits in the form of reduced requirements for repeated procedures, reduced turnaround time of testing result report, and reduced overall medical cost. Therefore, individual institutions need to have their own standard operating procedures related to tissue acquisition, specimen processing and handling, specimen selection, molecular test interpretation, reporting the tests results, and making treatment decisions with well-documented and standardized protocols.

CLINICS CARE POINTS

- Individual institutions should have their own standard operating procedures in place related to molecular oncology testing.
- Results of the same analytes detected by different methods might have different implications.
- Different types of cytology specimens as well as liquid biopsy are great alternatives to histologic specimens for molecular oncology testing.

REFERENCES

1. Kasraeian S, Allison DC, Ahlmann ER, et al. A comparison of fine-needle aspiration, core biopsy, and surgical biopsy in the diagnosis of extremity soft tissue masses. ClinOrthopRelat Res 2010;468(11):2992–3002.

2. Roy-Chowdhuri S, Chen H, Singh RR, et al. Concurrent fine needle aspirations and core needle biopsies: a comparative study of substrates for next-generation sequencing in solid organ malignancies. Mod Pathol 2017;30(4): 499–508.

3. Klein A, Fell T, Birkenmaier C, et al. Relative sensitivity of core-needle biopsy and incisional biopsy in the diagnosis of musculoskeletal sarcomas. Cancers (Basel) 2021;13(6):1393.

4. Birgin E, Yang C, Hetjens S, et al. Core needle biopsy versus incisional biopsy for differentiation of soft-tissue sarcomas: a systematic review and meta-analysis. Cancer 2020;126(9):1917–28.

5. Joudeh AA, Shareef SQ, Al-Abbadi MA. Fine-needle aspiration followed by core-needle biopsy in the same setting: modifying our approach. ActaCytol 2016; 60(1):1–13.

6. VanderLaan PA. Fine-needle aspiration and core needle biopsy: an update on 2 common minimally invasive tissue sampling modalities. Cancer Cytopathol 2016; 124(12):862–70.

7. Chen L, Jing H, Gong Y, et al. Diagnostic efficacy and molecular testing by combined fine needle aspiration and core needle biopsy in patients with a lung nodule. Cancer Cytopathol 2020;128(3):201–6.

8. Goswami RS, Luthra R, Singh RR, et al. Identification of factors affecting the success of next-generation sequencing testing in solid tumors. Am J ClinPathol 2016;145(2):222–37.

9. Roy-Chowdhuri S, Stewart J. Preanalytic variables in cytology: lessons learned from next-generation sequencing-the MD Anderson experience. Arch Pathol Lab Med 2016;140(11):1191–9.

10. Sehgal IS, Dhooria S, Aggarwal AN, et al. Impact of rapid on-site cytological evaluation (ROSE) on the diagnostic yield of transbronchial needle aspiration during mediastinal lymph node sampling: systematic review and meta-analysis. Chest 2018;153(4):929–38.

11. Collins BT, Murad FM, Wang JF, et al. Rapid on-site evaluation for endoscopic ultrasound-guided fine-needle biopsy of the pancreas decreases the incidence of repeat biopsy procedures. Cancer Cytopathol 2013;121(9):518–24.

12. Ishizawa T, Makino N, Matsuda A, et al. Usefulness of rapid on-site evaluation specimens from endoscopic ultrasound-guided fine-needle aspiration for cancer gene panel testing: a retrospective study. PLoS One 2020;15(1):e0228565.

13. Sandoh K, Ishida M, Okano K, et al. Utility of endoscopic ultrasound-guided fine-needle aspiration cytology in rapid on-site evaluation for the diagnosis of gastric submucosal tumors: retrospective analysis of a single-center experience. DiagnCytopathol 2019;47(9):869–75.

14. Tamura T, Yamashita Y, Ueda K, et al. Rapid on-site evaluation by endosonographers during endoscopic ultrasonography-guided fine-needle aspiration for diagnosis of gastrointestinal stromal tumors. ClinEndosc 2017;50(4):372–8.

15. Sauter JL, Chen Y, Alex D, et al. Results from the 2019 American Society of Cytopathology survey on rapid onsite evaluation (ROSE)-part 2: subjective views among the cytopathology community. J Am SocCytopathol 2020;9(6):570–8.

16. VanderLaan PA, Chen Y, Alex D, et al. Results from the 2019 American Society of Cytopathology survey on rapid on-site evaluation-Part 1: objective practice patterns. J Am SocCytopathol 2019;8(6):333–41.

17. Pantanowitz L, Sinard JH, Henricks WH, et al. Validating whole slide imaging for diagnostic purposes in pathology: guideline from the College of American

Pathologists Pathology and Laboratory Quality Center. Arch Pathol Lab Med 2013;137(12):1710–22.

18. Lin O. Telecytology for rapid on-site evaluation: current status. J Am SocCytopathol 2018;7(1):1–6.

19. Lin O, Rudomina D, Feratovic R, et al. Rapid on-site evaluation using telecytology: a major cancer center experience. DiagnCytopathol 2019;47(1):15–9.

20. Sirintrapun SJ, Rudomina D, Mazzella A, et al. Robotic telecytology for remote cytologic evaluation without an on-site cytotechnologist or cytopathologist: an active quality assessment and experience of over 400 cases. J Pathol Inform 2017;8:35.

21. Srinivasan M, Sedmak D, Jewell S. Effect of fixatives and tissue processing on the content and integrity of nucleic acids. Am J Pathol 2002;161(6):1961–71.

22. Williams C, Ponten F, Moberg C, et al. A high frequency of sequence alterations is due to formalin fixation of archival specimens. Am J Pathol 1999;155(5):1467–71.

23. Buonocore DJ, Konno F, Jungbluth AA, et al. CytoLyt fixation significantly inhibits MIB1immunoreactivity whereas alternative Ki-67 clone 30-9 is not susceptible to the inhibition: critical diagnostic implications. Cancer Cytopathology 2019; 127(10):643–9.

24. Gruchy JR, Barnes PJ, Dakin Hache KA. CytoLyt(R) fixation and decalcification pretreatments alter antigenicity in normal tissues compared with standard formalin fixation. ApplImmunohistochemMolMorphol 2015;23(4):297–302.

25. Panzacchi S, Gnudi F, Mandrioli D, et al. Effects of short and long-term alcohol-based fixation on Sprague-Dawley rat tissue morphology, protein and nucleic acid preservation. ActaHistochem 2019;121(6):750–60.

26. Aisner DL, Rumery MD, Merrick DT, et al. Do more with less: tips and techniques for maximizing small biopsy and cytology specimens for molecular and ancillary testing: the university of Colorado experience. Arch Pathol Lab Med 2016; 140(11):1206–20.

27. Gomes-Lima CJ, Shobab L, Wu D, et al. Do molecular profiles of primary versus metastatic radioiodine refractory differentiated thyroid cancer differ? Front Endocrinol 2021;12:623182.

28. Lee CC, Soon YY, Lum JHY, et al. Frequency of discordance in programmed death-ligand 1 (PD-L1) expression between primary tumors and paired distant metastases in advanced cancers: a systematic review and meta-analysis. ActaOncol 2020;59(6):696–704.

29. Manson QF, Schrijver W, TerHoeve ND, et al. Frequent discordance in PD-1 and PD-L1 expression between primary breast tumors and their matched distant metastases. ClinExpMetastasis 2019;36(1):29–37.

30. Naso JR, Banyi N, Al-Hashami Z, et al. Discordance in PD-L1 scores on repeat testing of non-small cell lung carcinomas. Cancer Treat Res Commun 2021;27: 100353.

31. Nambirajan A, Jain D. Cell blocks in cytopathology: an update. Cytopathology 2018;29(6):505–24.

32. Kanagal-Shamanna R, Portier BP, Singh RR, et al. Next-generation sequencing-based multi-gene mutation profiling of solid tumors using fine needle aspiration samples: promises and challenges for routine clinical diagnostics. Mod Pathol 2014;27(2):314–27.

33. Khode R, Larsen DA, Culbreath BC, et al. Comparative study of epidermal growth factor receptor mutation analysis on cytology smears and surgical pathology specimens from primary and metastatic lung carcinomas. Cancer Cytopathol 2013;121(7):361–9.

34. Velizheva NP, Rechsteiner MP, Wong CE, et al. Cytology smears as excellent starting material for next-generation sequencing-based molecular testing of patients with adenocarcinoma of the lung. Cancer Cytopathol 2017;125(1):30–40.

35. Fielding D, Dalley AJ, Bashirzadeh F, et al. Diff-quik cytology smears from endobronchial ultrasound transbronchial needle aspiration lymph node specimens as a source of DNA for next-generation sequencing instead of cell blocks. Respiration 2019;97(6):525–39.

36. Ramani NS, Chen H, Broaddus RR, et al. Utilization of cytology smears improves success rates of RNA-based next-generation sequencing gene fusion assays for clinically relevant predictive biomarkers. Cancer Cytopathol 2021;129(5):374–82.

37. Doxtader EE, Cheng YW, Zhang Y. Molecular testing of non-small cell lung carcinoma diagnosed by endobronchial ultrasound-guided transbronchial fine-needle aspiration: the cleveland clinic experience. Arch Pathol Lab Med 2019;143(6): 670–6.

38. Bellevicine C, Malapelle U, Vigliar E, et al. Epidermal growth factor receptor test performed on liquid-based cytology lung samples: experience of an academic referral center. ActaCytol 2014;58(6):589–94.

39. Malapelle U, Mayo-de-Las-Casas C, Molina-Vila MA, et al. Consistency and reproducibility of next-generation sequencing and other multigene mutational assays: a worldwide ring trial study on quantitative cytological molecular reference specimens. Cancer Cytopathol 2017;125(8):615–26.

40. Roy-Chowdhuri S, Mehrotra M, Bolivar AM, et al. Salvaging the supernatant: next generation cytopathology for solid tumor mutation profiling. Mod Pathol 2018; 31(7):1036–45.

41. Finkelstein SD, Bibbo M, Kowalski TE, et al. Mutational analysis of cytocentrifugation supernatant fluid from pancreatic solid mass lesions. DiagnCytopathol 2014; 42(8):719–25.

42. Krane JF, Cibas ES, Alexander EK, et al. Molecular analysis of residual ThinPrep material from thyroid FNAs increases diagnostic sensitivity. Cancer Cytopathol 2015;123(6):356–61.

43. Kwon H, Kim WG, Eszlinger M, et al. Molecular diagnosis using residual liquid-based cytology materials for patients with nondiagnostic or indeterminate thyroid nodules. EndocrinolMetab(Seoul) 2016;31(4):586–91.

44. Ye W, Hannigan B, Zalles S, et al. Centrifuged supernatants from FNA provide a liquid biopsy option for clinical next-generation sequencing of thyroid nodules. Cancer Cytopathol 2019;127(3):146–60.

45. Guibert N, Tsukada H, Hwang DH, et al. Liquid biopsy of fine-needle aspiration supernatant for lung cancer genotyping. Lung Cancer 2018;122:72–5.

46. Michela B. Liquid biopsy: a family of possible diagnostic tools. Diagnostics (Basel) 2021;11(8):1391.

47. Schwarzenbach H, Hoon DSB, Pantel K. Cell-free nucleic acids as biomarkers in cancer patients. Nat Rev Cancer 2011;11(6):426–37.

48. Rolfo C, Mack PC, Scagliotti GV, et al. Liquid biopsy for advanced non-small cell lung cancer (NSCLC): a statement paper from the IASLC. J ThoracOncol 2018; 13(9):1248–68.

49. Ignatiadis M, Sledge GW, Jeffrey SS. Liquid biopsy enters the clinic - implementation issues and future challenges. Nat Rev ClinOncol 2021;18(5):297–312.

50. Russano M, Napolitano A, Ribelli G, et al. Liquid biopsy and tumor heterogeneity in metastatic solid tumors: the potentiality of blood samples. J ExpClinCancer Res 2020;39(1):95.

51. Diehl F, Schmidt K, Choti MA, et al. Circulating mutant DNA to assess tumor dynamics. Nat Med 2008;14(9):985–90.
52. Sorensen BS, Wu L, Wei W, et al. Monitoring of epidermal growth factor receptor tyrosine kinase inhibitor-sensitizing and resistance mutations in the plasma DNA of patients with advanced non-small cell lung cancer during treatment with erlotinib. Cancer 2014;120(24):3896–901.
53. Diaz LA Jr, Williams RT, Wu J, et al. The molecular evolution of acquired resistance to targeted EGFR blockade in colorectal cancers. Nature 2012; 486(7404):537–40.
54. Lin CC, Huang WL, Wei F, et al. Emerging platforms using liquid biopsy to detect EGFR mutations in lung cancer. Expert Rev MolDiagn 2015;15(11):1427–40.
55. Hindson CM, Chevillet JR, Briggs HA, et al. Absolute quantification by droplet digital PCR versus analog real-time PCR. Nat Methods 2013;10(10):1003–5.
56. Chen M, Zhao H. Next-generation sequencing in liquid biopsy: cancer screening and early detection. Hum Genomics 2019;13(1):34.
57. Garcia-Foncillas J, Alba E, Aranda E, et al. Incorporating BEAMing technology as a liquid biopsy into clinical practice for the management of colorectal cancer patients: an expert taskforce review. Ann Oncol 2017;28(12):2943–9.
58. Roy-Chowdhuri S, Goswami RS, Chen H, et al. Factors affecting the success of next-generation sequencing in cytology specimens. Cancer Cytopathol 2015; 123(11):659–68.
59. Ranek L. Cytophotometric studies of the DNA, nucleic acid and protein content of human liver cell nuclei. ActaCytol 1976;20(2):151–7.
60. Jennings LJ, Arcila ME, Corless C, et al. Guidelines for validation of next-generation sequencing-based oncology panels: a Joint consensus recommendation of the association for molecular pathology and college of American pathologists. J MolDiagn 2017;19(3):341–65.
61. Chen H, Luthra R, Goswami RS, et al. Analysis of pre-analytic factors affecting the success of clinical next-generation sequencing of solid organ malignancies. Cancers (Basel) 2015;7(3):1699–715.
62. Jabbar K, Routbort M, Singh C, et al. Impact of tumor necrosis on success of clinical next generation sequencing. Mod Pathol 2015;28:501a.
63. El-Deiry WS, Goldberg RM, Lenz HJ, et al. The current state of molecular testing in the treatment of patients with solid tumors, 2019. CACancer J Clin 2019;69(4): 305–43.
64. Bass BP, Engel KB, Greytak SR, et al. A review of preanalytical factors affecting molecular, protein, and morphological analysis of formalin-fixed, paraffin-embedded (FFPE) tissue: how well do you know your FFPE specimen? Arch Pathol Lab Med 2014;138(11):1520–30.
65. da Cunha Santos G, Saieg MA. Preanalytic specimen triage: smears, cell blocks, cytospin preparations, transport media, and cytobanking. Cancer Cytopathol 2017;125(S6):455–64.
66. Padmanabhan V, Steinmetz HB, Rizzo EJ, et al. Improving adequacy of small biopsy and fine-needle aspiration specimens for molecular testing by next-generation sequencing in patients with lung cancer: a quality improvement study at Dartmouth-Hitchcock medical center. Arch Pathol Lab Med 2017;141(3): 402–9.
67. Sholl LM, Xiao Y, Joshi V, et al. EGFR mutation is a better predictor of response to tyrosine kinase inhibitors in non-small cell lung carcinoma than FISH, CISH, and immunohistochemistry. Am J ClinPathol 2010;133(6):922–34.

68. Hinrichs JW, van Blokland WT, Moons MJ, et al. Comparison of next-generation sequencing and mutation-specific platforms in clinical practice. Am J ClinPathol 2015;143(4):573–8.

69. Majeed U, Manochakian R, Zhao Y, et al. Targeted therapy in advanced non-small cell lung cancer: current advances and future trends. J HematolOncol 2021; 14(1):108.

70. Davies KD, Lomboy A, Lawrence CA, et al. DNA-based versus RNA-based detection of MET exon 14 skipping events in lung cancer. J ThoracOncol 2019; 14(4):737–41.

71. Byron SA, Van Keuren-Jensen KR, Engelthaler DM, et al. Translating RNA sequencing into clinical diagnostics: opportunities and challenges. Nat Rev Genet 2016;17(5):257–71.

72. Kirchner M, Neumann O, Volckmar AL, et al. RNA-based detection of gene fusions in formalin-fixed and paraffin-embedded solid cancer samples. Cancers (Basel) 2019;11(9):1309.

73. Goytain A, Ng T. NanoStringnCounter technology: high-throughput RNA validation. MethodsMol Biol 2020;2079:125–39.

74. Aguado C, Gimenez-Capitan A, Roman R, et al. RNA-based multiplexing assay for routine testing of fusion and splicing variants in cytological samples of NSCLC patients. Diagnostics (Basel) 2020;11(1):15.

75. Gentien D, Piqueret-Stephan L, Henry E, et al. Digital multiplexed gene expression analysis of mRNA and miRNA from routinely processed and stained cytological smears: a proof-of-principle study. ActaCytol 2021;65(1):88–98.

76. Reuss DE, Sahm F, Schrimpf D, et al. ATRX and IDH1-R132H immunohistochemistry with subsequent copy number analysis and IDH sequencing as a basis for an "integrated" diagnostic approach for adult astrocytoma, oligodendroglioma and glioblastoma. ActaNeuropathol 2015;129(1):133–46.

77. Ancevski Hunter K, Socinski MA, Villaruz LC. PD-L1 testing in guiding patient selection for PD-1/PD-L1 inhibitor therapy in lung cancer. MolDiagnTher 2018; 22(1):1–10.

78. Cheung CC, Barnes P, Bigras G, et al. Fit-for-purpose PD-L1 biomarker testing for patient selection in immuno-oncology: Guidelines for clinical laboratories from the Canadian association of pathologists-Association canadienneDes pathologistes (CAP-ACP). ApplImmunohistochemMolMorphol 2019;27(10):699–714.

79. Asaoka Y, Ijichi H, Koike K. PD-1 blockade in tumors with mismatch-repair deficiency. N Engl J Med 2015;373(20):1979.

80. Le DT, Durham JN, Smith KN, et al. Mismatch repair deficiency predicts response of solid tumors to PD-1 blockade. Science 2017;357(6349):409–13.

81. Heymann JJ, Bulman WA, Swinarski D, et al. PD-L1 expression in non-small cell lung carcinoma: comparison among cytology, small biopsy, and surgical resection specimens. Cancer Cytopathol 2017;125(12):896–907.

82. Jacobi EM, Landon G, Broaddus RR, et al. Evaluating mismatch repair/microsatellite instability status using cytology effusion specimens to determine eligibility for immunotherapy. Arch Pathol Lab Med 2020;145(1):46–54.

83. Lozano MD, Abengozar-Muela M, Echeveste JI, et al. Programmed death-ligand 1 expression on direct Pap-stained cytology smears from non-small cell lung cancer: comparison with cell blocks and surgical resection specimens. Cancer Cytopathol 2019;127(7):470–80.

84. Pisapia P, Lozano MD, Vigliar E, et al. ALK and ROS1 testing on lung cancer cytologic samples: Perspectives. Cancer Cytopathol 2017;125(11):817–30.

85. Buonocore DJ, Fowle E, Lin O, et al. Cytologic evaluation of p16 staining in head and neck squamous cell carcinoma in CytoLyt versus formalin-fixed material. Cancer Cytopathol 2019;127(12):750–6.
86. Gong Y, Symmans WF, Krishnamurthy S, et al. Optimal fixation conditions for immunocytochemical analysis of estrogen receptor in cytologic specimens of breast carcinoma. Cancer 2004;102(1):34–40.
87. Wang H, Agulnik J, Kasymjanova G, et al. Cytology cell blocks are suitable for immunohistochemical testing for PD-L1 in lung cancer. Ann Oncol 2018;29(6): 1417–22.
88. Noll B, Wang WL, Gong Y, et al. Programmed death ligand 1 testing in non-small cell lung carcinoma cytology cell block and aspirate smear preparations. Cancer Cytopathol 2018;126(5):342–52.
89. Skov BG, Skov T. Paired comparison of PD-L1 expression on cytologic and histologic specimens from malignancies in the lung assessed with PD-L1IHC 28-8pharmDx and PD-L1IHC22C3pharmDx. ApplImmunohistochemMolMorphol 2017;25(7):453–9.
90. Emancipator K, Huang L, Aurora-Garg D, et al. Comparing programmed death ligand 1 scores for predicting pembrolizumab efficacy in head and neck cancer. Mod Pathol 2021;34(3):532–41.

Utility of Single-Gene Testing in Cancer Specimens

Mehenaz Hanbazazh, MD[a,b], Diana Morlote, MD[b],
Alexander C. Mackinnon, MD, PhD[b], Shuko Harada, MD[b,*]

KEYWORDS

• Molecular • Single-gene testing • NGS • Sanger • PCR • Automated assay

KEY POINTS

- Choosing between single-gene testing and NGS depends on several clinical, analytical, and economic factors.
- Communication with the ordering clinician, knowing the main purpose for the required molecular testing, and understanding the laboratory potentialities, help in determining the appropriate and most suitable technique.
- Each methodology has its own advantages and disadvantages.

INTRODUCTION

The implementation of molecular profiling enhanced the field of oncology and precision medicine. Twenty-four years after the discovery of DNA by Watson and Crick in 1953, Fredrick Sanger developed the dideoxy sequencing method in 1977 to sequence the first full genome.[1] This was followed by the introduction of the polymerase chain reaction (PCR) in 1983 allowing the analysis of small amounts of DNA and RNA.[2] PCR revolutionized molecular diagnostics and led to an explosion in the number of new single-gene assays, which are tests that identify disease-associated genetic variants in a single target. PCR-based molecular testing frequently used capillary electrophoresis and hybridization with sequence-specific probes, and single-gene testing remained an excellent and dominant option for the next 3 decades. In 2005, next-generation sequencing (NGS) technology was developed and provided the ability to sequence multiple genes simultaneously using one sample.[3] Later, the US Food and Drug Administration (FDA) approved NGS for clinical applications, leading to the introduction of competing platforms and a dramatic drop in the cost of DNA and RNA sequencing.[4]

[a] Department of Pathology, Faculty of Medicine, University of Jeddah, Jeddah, Saudi Arabia;
[b] Division of Genomic Diagnostics & Bioinformatics, Department of Pathology, University of Alabama at Birmingham, 619 19th Street South, Birmingham, AL 35249-7331, USA
* Corresponding author.
E-mail address: sharada@uabmc.edu

Clin Lab Med 42 (2022) 385–394
https://doi.org/10.1016/j.cll.2022.05.001
0272-2712/22/© 2022 Elsevier Inc. All rights reserved.

During this genomic era, characterized by a wide variety of molecular technologies and extensive demand for mutation profiling, there remains significant uncertainty about the most practical and cost-effective approaches for a laboratory to adopt. Several considerations may be taken into account when deciding which molecular diagnostic tools to implement. In this review, we evaluate several single-gene testing options with regard to clinical indications, utilities, advantages, and limitations.

SINGLE-GENE TESTING METHODOLOGY
Sanger Sequencing

Sanger sequencing, also known as "dideoxy sequencing" or "sequencing by termination," uses dideoxynucleotides (ddNTPs) to randomly terminate a growing DNA strand. Each of the 4 ddNTPs is labeled with a different fluorescent dye. This creates DNA fragments of different lengths and different fluorescent labels, which are then resolved by capillary electrophoresis. Sanger sequencing, which was used to sequence the first human genomes, generates long sequencing reads and is considered the gold standard for DNA sequencing. It has been used to identify many clinically significant variants such as *EGFR* in nonsmall cell lung cancer (NSCLC), *KRAS* in colorectal cancer, and *BRAF* in melanoma.[5] It can detect changes in DNA sequence up to 1000 bp including base pair substitutions, insertions, and deletions. However, it is limited in detecting gene copy number variants (CNV) and large chromosomal abnormalities.[6,7] Sanger sequencing can be performed using small amounts of input DNA (5–10 ng) per amplicon, but this comes at the cost of sensitivity, which requires 15% to 20% variant allele fraction or 30% to 40% tumor nuclei in the sample, for reliable variant detection.[8,9] Other limitations include extensive hands-on time, long turnaround time (TAT), and difficulty with precise determination of variant allele fraction.[7,9] Sanger method is relatively expensive and becomes cost-prohibitive for projects analyzing large numbers of genes or samples.[6]

Allele-Specific Polymerase Chain Reaction

A few years after the discovery of PCR, Newton and coworkers established allele-specific PCR in 1989.[10] Allele-specific PCR, also known as amplification refractory mutation system (ARMS), uses unique combinations of DNA primers designed to specifically target and amplify both the variant and wild type alleles, which can then be distinguished and quantified using real-time PCR or other downstream methodologies.[7,10,11] A single PCR product will be generated in samples that are homozygous for either the mutant or wild type allele, whereas 2 PCR products will be generated in heterozygous samples-one PCR product derived from the mutant allele and the other from the wild type allele.[12] Allele-specific real-time PCR has numerous advantages over Sanger method including fast TAT, low cost, and high sensitivity (1%–5%), making it particularly useful in small biopsies with low tumor content. Some of the FDA-approved assays use this methodology because of these advantages. Nevertheless, this technique is limited through its design to identify known single nucleotide variant (SNV) that are commonly mutated in cancer, such as *KRAS* in colon cancer and *BRAF* in melanoma.[5,6]

Melt Curve Analysis

Melting curve analysis is a post-PCR method based on the detection of differences in the melting temperature (Tm) of DNA as it denatures and transitions from double-stranded DNA (dsDNA) to single-stranded DNA (ssDNA). DNA is mixed with dyes that intercalate and fluoresce when the DNA is double stranded. Fluorescence is detected continuously as the temperature rises. As the rising temperature passes the Tm, the DNA melts into single strands causing the intercalated dyes to dissociate and no longer fluoresce. Tm depends on numerous factors, such as the DNA length, sequence, and guanine-cytosine (GC) content.[13] Consequently, PCR products corresponding to the different alleles have different Tm, and this can be quantified using melting curve analysis.[5,9] Although melting curve analysis is considered a simple, rapid, highly sensitive, and inexpensive tool for mutation screening, melting curve is limited by the fact that it is qualitative and cannot determine the sequence of the variant; subsequent sequencing methods are needed for this.[5,9]

Fragment Analysis and Restriction Fragment Length Polymorphism Analysis

Fragment analysis method is based on distinguishing the size of DNA fragments and is most often used for detecting insertions, deletions, or polymorphic alleles. The DNA fragments are labeled with fluorescent dye during PCR. PCR products are separated by capillary electrophoresis and analyzed according to their size. Due to its high sensitivity, simplicity, and speed, fragment analysis is used in a wide range of applications including genotyping, loss of heterozygosity, and microsatellite instability. As it is based on size, peak intensity measurement can be used for relative quantification, and prior sequence knowledge is not required.[14] Most notably, fragment analysis compliments the limitation of NGS for detecting large indels. Combining fragment analysis with NGS improves the sensitivity and accuracy of the detection of FLT3-ITD (internal tandem duplication) and MET exon 14 splice site deletion in acute myeloid leukemia (AML) and NSCLC, respectively.[15–17] Furthermore, restriction fragment length polymorphism (RFLP) analysis combines restriction enzyme digestion—which digests PCR products based on the presence of restriction site sequences—with fragment analysis to differentiate mutated products from wild type.

Automated System

One of the most notable technological advances in single-gene testing is the introduction of fully automated assay systems. The main advantages are minimal hands-on time, rapid TAT, and integrated interpretation and reporting-all of which help reduce the risk of contamination and human error. Additionally, it is considered one of the easiest and fastest molecular assays to validate making it an attractive molecular diagnostics platform for most laboratories, including laboratories that do not have experience with complex molecular protocols. In regards to cost, the higher cost of automated test systems can be offset by reduced labor and informatics costs.[18]

The Idylla platform (Biocartis, Mechelen, Belgium) is a real-time PCR-based automated assay that uses closed, fully integrated cartridges for multiplex interrogation of hotspots involving BRAF, KRAS, NRAS, and EGFR oncogenes. Idylla also supports the detection of fusion genes and MSI analysis.[19] Idylla combines the advantages of limited hands-on-time (2 minutes), short TAT (85–180 minutes), sample versatility (solid and liquid biopsy), multiplexing capability, and ease of use. In a recent comparative analysis, the Idylla BRAF, EGFR, and KRAS mutation tests showed a very high overall agreement with NGS (100%, 94%, and 94%, respectively).[20–22] Although it is limited by the range of mutations that can be detected, Idylla is a robust, practical option-especially for small samples and for laboratories with limited resources.

The GeneXpert BCR-ABL (Cepheid, Sunnyvale, CA) is another automated test for quantifying BCR::ABL1 transcripts in chronic myeloid leukemia (CML) through quantitative reverse-transcriptase (RT)-PCR. The test was approved by the FDA in 2019. An updated version of the assay, Xpert BCR-ABL Ultra, has improved the limit of detection going as low as 0.0030%.[23] The cartridges are disposable, closed, and include all of the reagents needed for RT-PCR. The test provides fast TAT (less than 3 hours), which significantly reduces the time for diagnosis, initial management, and shortens the length of hospital stays.[24]

PROS AND CONS OF SINGLE-GENE TESTING

In the current era of molecular diagnostics for cancer—with constant development and introduction of new techniques and platforms—it can be very challenging to choose the appropriate test for a particular patient or clinical scenario. Multiple factors need to be addressed to select the best approach, including clinical history, sample assessment, indication for molecular testing, TAT, and cost of the test.[25,26] NGS attracts huge attention due to the continuous advancement in the technology, sequencing platforms, multiplexing, and an expansion of the range of genetic alterations that can be detected. NGS is characterized by high sensitivity to detect low-fraction variants and comprehensive coverage. The ability to sequence whole exomes and whole genomes rather than mutational hotspots or targeted, disease-focused gene panels adds additional value-particularly in the context of clinical trials as NGS can find therapeutically targetable mutations in unexpected genes.[27,28] Because of these advantages, many studies propose using NGS methods for routine clinical practice. Furthermore, emerging NGS technologies providing short hands-on time, and rapid TAT challenge the value and practicality of single-gene testing platforms and assays. Nevertheless, NGS is associated with high capital and operational costs, long TAT, laborious processes, complex bioinformatics, lack of standardized guidelines, and challenging interpretations—including the detection and annotation of variants of uncertain significance (VUS). These barriers can make it difficult to implement NGS as the laboratories only testing platform.[9,29] With all being said, it is predictable for NGS to overcome most of these challenges in the near future, especially with the continuous growth, advancement, and improvement in its technology and data interpretation.[5,30–32]

On the other hand, single-gene tests are easier to develop, simple to validate, and direct to perform using relatively inexpensive equipment. The interpretation is straightforward with no need for sophisticated bioinformatics support. Because of the low cost and relatively short TAT, single-gene assays are a practical consideration. The main limitation of single-gene assays is the subsequent additional testing required when initial results are negative or inconclusive due to the narrow coverage of single-gene testing. Additionally, some single-gene assays, such as Sanger sequencing, are unable to identify low-fraction genetic variants present in subclonal populations of cells (**Table 1**). Some laboratories use a sequential testing approach by initially testing for the most common mutations followed by additional testing for less common variants.[33] However, this strategy has disadvantages—it is slower, consumes large amounts of resources, requires large tumor size, and ultimately can be more expensive than a single, upfront NGS test.[34] For straightforward clinical scenarios, limited specimens, small numbers of targets, monitoring a particular alteration, low budget situations, or the urgent need for results, single-gene assays are a reasonable choice for testing (**Fig. 1**).[35,36]

CLINICAL UTILITY

The implementation of molecular profiling contributed to the field of oncology by increasing our understanding of the molecular mechanisms of tumors, confirming the diagnosis, predicting prognosis, and guiding therapy. While the demand for molecular testing is increasing as it becomes a fundamental part of the routine pathology workup, the amount of diagnostic tissue submitted for molecular analysis is actually

Table 1
Pros and cons of different single-gene testing assays and NGS

Assay	Pros	Cons
Sanger sequencing	"Gold standard"; ability to detect most sequence variants	Low sensitivity Need 30%–40% tumor Labor intensive Low throughput
Melt Curve Analysis	Fast TAT Less labor	Dose not provide exact sequence
Allele-specific PCR/ARMS	Fast TAT High sensitivity	Only detect the mutations targeted by primers
Fragment analysis and RFLP	Inexpensive Prior sequence knowledge is not required	Long hands-on time Time-consuming
Automated system	Fast TAT Easy to validate Minimal hands-on time Integrated interpretation and reporting	Limited to specific variants
Next-Generation Sequencing	More comprehensive High throughput High sensitivity Sample multiplexing Better picture for tumor heterogeneity	May have longer turnaround time Labor intensive Complex workflow Large DNA/RNA input Need informatics pipeline and storage Challenging interpretation

decreasing. This is due in large part to the predominant use of minimally invasive procedures such as fine-needle aspiration (FNA) or the extensive use of Immunohistochemistry (IHC) and special stains before molecular testing, which exhaust small tissue samples.[37] As a result, molecular laboratories oftentimes face challenges when performing NGS on minimal samples with scant lesional tissue. In such scenarios, single-gene testing represents an alternative solution.[21] This is particularly important in lung cancer, whereby many patients are diagnosed with advanced stage disease by small biopsies and baseline IHC and molecular testing for *EGFR, ALK, MET,* and *ROS1* are required to initiate optimal therapy.[38–41] Consequently, strategies and methods to improve the adequacy of biopsies and maximize the utility of small samples should always be considered. For example, many cancer centers use rapid on-site assessment for the adequacy of cytology specimen for molecular testing. Other ways to fully use small tissue samples include macro- and micro-dissection for tumor cell enrichment and application of emerging NGS technologies.[37,38]

Another example of the beneficial role of single-gene testing is its use for the identification of specific, known variants commonly mutated in cancer-related genes in rapid TAT. This provides a feasible, fast, sensitive, and cost-effective approach for diagnostic molecular profiling. *BRAF* codon 600 mutations in exon 15 in melanoma represent a good example of using single-gene testing. The FDA and the European Medicines Agency (EMA) approved Vemurafenib and Dabrafenib as selective inhibitors of *BRAF* codon 600 mutations for the treatment of unresectable or metastatic melanoma. Targeted therapy dramatically improved the prognosis of metastatic melanoma and therefore necessitated the need for rapid *BRAF* V600 analysis.[42] Several single-gene methods exist to evaluate *BRAF V600* mutations, including Sanger

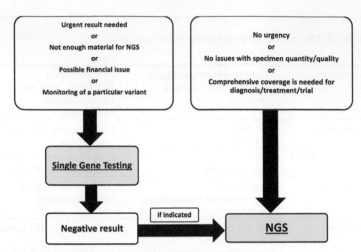

Fig. 1. Suggested scheme for single-gene testing and NGS.

sequencing, allele-specific reverse transcriptase PCR, high-resolution melting curve analysis, and the rapid automated Idylla system. It is worth noting that the FDA has approved the Cobas *BRAF* V600 Mutation test by Roche (Indianapolis, IN), which detects approximately 80% of melanoma mutations. The assay uses formalin-fixed paraffin-embedded tumor samples and has a sensitivity of greater than 99% and limit of detection of < 4–5% variant allele fraction.[7]

Isocitrate dehydrogenase enzyme isoform 1 and 2 (*IDH1/2*) mutation testing is another example of the utility of single-gene testing. Mutations in *IDH1/2* play an important role in the diagnosis and prognosis of a large proportion of WHO grade II and III diffuse gliomas. In cases of oligodendroglioma, the presence of *IDH 1/2* mutation and 1p/19q deletion is a defining feature. *IDH1/2* mutated-gliomas are associated with younger age, better prognosis, and increased overall survival.[43] *IDH1/2* mutations are also observed in a subset of hematopoietic diseases, such as AML and provide prognostic value as well as target therapy options. However, in contrast to CNS tumors, *IDH1/2* mutations in hematologic disorders are associated with worse prognosis and shorter overall survival.[44] The most common *IDH* mutation affects *IDH1* codon 132 (R132H is the most frequent), followed by mutations involving *IDH2* codon R140 and R172. The fact that most of the *IDH1/2* gene mutations occur in specific hotspots makes it relatively simple to target them by different assays. A common and very practical approach is to start with testing for these common variants. However, *IDH1/2* negative tumors need additional testing by more comprehensive methods to detect less common variants.[45] Different highly sensitive assays have been developed to tests for *IDH1/2* mutations.[46,47] Testing can be part of a gene panel or as gene-specific tests, including PCR-based methods, high resolution melting curve analysis, Sanger sequencing, pyrosequencing, and NGS. Abbott Real-Time *IDH1*, which is a quantitative PCR-based assay, is FDA-approved for the detection of *IDH1* p.R132 mutations (R132C, R132H, R132G, R132S, and R132L) in AML cases.

It is also worth mentioning that screening for *IDH1* R132H, *BRAF* V600E, *ALK,* and *ROS1* gene rearrangement can be performed by IHC as a routine histopathological examination.

CML requires prompt molecular analysis for the *BCR::ABL1* fusion for initial diagnosis and regular molecular monitoring to determine molecular response to the therapy and minimal residual disease (MRD). Karyotyping, fluorescence in situ hybridization (FISH), and PCR are available techniques for CML diagnosis and monitoring.[24] Quantitative reverse transcriptase PCR of *BCR::ABL1* mRNA is one of the most sensitive methods for monitoring CML and is considered the standard clinical practice for follow-up.[48,49] GeneXpert *BCR-ABL*, an automated, FDA approved, real-time reverse transcription PCR test, is used for quantifying *BCR::ABL1* transcript in peripheral blood for patients with CML. It provides excellent sensitivity, specificity, and fast TAT making it a good cost-effective option. The systems use GeneXpert cartridges, which include reagents needed to detect *BCR::ABL1* fusion genes resulting from 2 major p210 breakpoints—translocation e13a2/b2a2 and e14a2/b3a2. However, it does not differentiate between the 2 fusion transcripts and does not monitor other rare fusion transcripts.[18,48]

SUMMARY

Despite the explosive growth of NGS, single-gene testing remains a beneficial and complimentary testing option in certain situations. Each method has its own benefits and limitations. Communication with the ordering clinician, understanding the intended reason for the molecular test, and recognizing the capabilities of the laboratory help in determining the most appropriate and suitable single-gene assay to use.

CLINICS CARE POINTS

- Single-gene testing is a practical approach to identify common variants in small samples and with rapid turnaround time.

- Inconclusive or negative results by single-gene testing assays might require additional testing for more comprehensive coverage.

- Genexpert BCR-ABL, Cobas BRAF V600 mutation test by Roche, and Abbott real-time IDH1 are examples of FDA-approved single-gene testing assays.

DISCLOSURE

The authors have nothing to disclose.

REFERENCES

1. Kumar R, Jorben J, Yadav RR, et al. Genomics and its application in crop improvement. J Pharmacognosy Phytochemistry 2020;9(1):547–52.
2. Hongbao M. Development application polymerase chain reaction (PCR). J Am Sci 2005;1(3):1–15.
3. Van Dijk EL, Auger H, Jaszczyszyn Y, et al. Ten years of next-generation sequencing technology. Trends Genetics 2014;30(9):418–26.
4. Karlovich CA, Williams PM. Clinical applications of next-generation sequencing in precision oncology. Cancer J 2019;25(4):264–71.
5. Ross JS, Cronin M. Whole cancer genome sequencing by next-generation methods. Am J Clin Pathol 2011;136(4):527–39.
6. Tafe LJ, Arcila ME. Genomic medicine: a practical guide. New York: Springer; 2019.
7. Curry JL, Torres-Cabala CA, Tetzlaff MT, et al. Molecular platforms utilized to detect BRAF V600E mutation in melanoma 2012;31(4):267–73.

ɔ. Calvayrac O, Pradines A, Pons E, et al. Molecular biomarkers for lung adenocarcinoma. Eur Respir J 2017;49(4). https://doi.org/10.1183/13993003.01734-2016.

9. Khoo C, Rogers TM, Fellowes A, et al. Molecular methods for somatic mutation testing in lung adenocarcinoma: EGFR and beyond. Transplant Lung Cancer Res 2015;4(2):126–41.

10. Newton C, Graham A, Heptinstall L, et al. Analysis of any point mutation in DNA. the amplification refractory mutation system (ARMS). Nucleic Acids Res 1989; 17(7):2503–16.

11. Darawi MN, Ai-Vyrn C, Ramasamy K, et al. Allele-specific polymerase chain reaction for the detection of alzheimer's disease-related single nucleotide polymorphisms. BMC Med Genet 2013;14(1):1–8.

12. Goswami RS, Harada S. An overview of molecular genetic diagnosis techniques. Curr Protoc Hum Genet 2020;105(1):e97.

13. Farrar JS, Wittwer C. High-resolution melting curve analysis for molecular diagnostics. In: Patrinos GP, editor. Molecular diagnostics. Philadelphia: Elsevier; 2017. p. 79–102.

14. Scientific TF. DNA fragment analysis by capillary electrophoresis. Carlsbad: Thermo FIsher Sicentific. Inc 2014.

15. Sakaguchi M, Nakajima N, Yamaguchi H, et al. The sensitivity of the FLT3-ITD detection method is an important consideration when diagnosing acute myeloid leukemia. Leuk Res Rep 2020;13:100198.

16. Loyaux R, Blons H, Garinet S, et al. 4MO MET exon 14 screening strategy: how not to miss large deletions. Ann Oncol 2020;31:S1218.

17. Kim Y, Lee G, Park J, et al. Quantitative fragment analysis of FLT3-ITD efficiently identifying poor prognostic group with high mutant allele burden or long ITD length. Blood Cancer J 2015;5(8):e336.

18. López-Jorge C, Gómez-Casares M, Jiménez-Velasco A, et al. Comparative study of BCR-ABL1 quantification: xpert assay, a feasible solution to standardization concerns. Ann Hematol 2012;91(8):1245–50.

19. Harada S, Morlote D. Molecular pathology of colorectal cancer. Adv Anat Pathol 2020;27(1):20–6.

20. Van Haele M, Vander Borght S, Ceulemans A, et al. Rapid clinical mutational testing of KRAS, BRAF and EGFR: a prospective comparative analysis of the idylla technique with high-throughput next-generation sequencing. J Clin Pathol 2020;73(1):35–41.

21. Huang H, Springborn S, Haug K, et al. Evaluation, validation, and implementation of the idylla system as rapid molecular testing for precision medicine. J Mol Diagn 2019;21(5):862–72.

22. Tsongalis GJ, Al Turkmani MR, Suriawinata M, et al. Comparison of tissue molecular biomarker testing turnaround times and concordance between standard of care and the biocartis idylla platform in patients with colorectal cancer. Am J Clin Pathol 2020;154(2):266–76.

23. Dominy KM, Simon IM, Sorouri-Khorashad J. Evaluation of xpert® BCR-ABL ultra for the confirmation of BCR-ABL1 international scale conversion factors for the molecular monitoring of chronic myeloid leukaemia. Int J Lab Hematol 2021; 43(1):e31–4.

24. Jobbagy Z, van Atta R, Murphy KM, et al. Evaluation of the cepheid GeneXpert BCR-ABL assay. J Mol Diagn 2007;9(2):220–7.

25. Pruneri G, De Braud F, Sapino A, et al. Next-generation sequencing in clinical practice: is it a cost-saving alternative to a single-gene testing approach? PharmacoEconomics-Open 2021;5(2):285–98.

26. Lynce F, Isaacs C. How far do we go with genetic evaluation? gene, panel, and tumor testing. Am Soc Clin Oncol Educ Book 2016;36:e72–8.
27. Hiemenz MC, Kadauke S, Lieberman DB, et al. Building a robust tumor profiling program: synergy between next-generation sequencing and targeted single-gene testing. PloS one 2016;11(4):e0152851.
28. Colomer R, Mondejar R, Romero-Laorden N, et al. When should we order a next generation sequencing test in a patient with cancer? EClinicalMedicine 2020;25:100487.
29. Park E, Shim HS. Detection of targetable genetic alterations in Korean lung cancer patients: a comparison study of single-gene assays and targeted next-generation sequencing. Cancer Res Treat 2020;52(2):543–51.
30. Dalal AA, Guerin A, Mutebi A, et al. Economic analysis of BRAF gene mutation testing in real world practice using claims data: costs of single gene versus panel tests in patients with lung cancer. J Med Econ 2018;21(7):649–55.
31. Altimari A, de Biase D, De Maglio G, et al. 454 next generation-sequencing outperforms allele-specific PCR, sanger sequencing, and pyrosequencing for routine KRAS mutation analysis of formalin-fixed, paraffin-embedded samples. Onco Targets Ther 2013;6:1057–64.
32. de Biase D, Acquaviva G, Visani M, et al. Molecular diagnostic of solid tumor using a next generation sequencing custom-designed multi-gene panel. Diagnostics 2020;10(4):250.
33. Momeni-Boroujeni A, Salazar P, Zheng T, et al. Rapid EGFR mutation detection using the idylla platform: single-institution experience of 1200 cases analyzed by an in-house developed pipeline and comparison with concurrent next-generation sequencing results. J Mol Diagn 2021;23(3):310–22.
34. Pennell NA, Mutebi A, Zhou Z, et al. Economic impact of next-generation sequencing versus single-gene testing to detect genomic alterations in metastatic non–small-cell lung cancer using a decision analytic model. JCO Precision Oncol 2019;3:1–9.
35. Tan AC, Lai GG, San Tan G, et al. Utility of incorporating next-generation sequencing (NGS) in an asian non-small cell lung cancer (NSCLC) population: incremental yield of actionable alterations and cost-effectiveness analysis. Lung Cancer 2020;139:207–15.
36. Kuo FC, Mar BG, Lindsley RC, et al. The relative utilities of genome-wide, gene panel, and individual gene sequencing in clinical practice. Blood J Am Soc Hematol 2017;130(4):433–9.
37. Aisner DL, Rumery MD, Merrick DT, et al. Do more with less: Tips and techniques for maximizing small biopsy and cytology specimens for molecular and ancillary testing: the university of Colorado experience. Arch Pathol Lab Med 2016;140(11):1206–20.
38. Lozano MD, Echeveste JI, Abengozar M, et al. Cytology smears in the era of molecular biomarkers in non–small cell lung cancer: doing more with less. Arch Pathol Lab Med 2018;142(3):291–8.
39. Canberk S, Engels M. Cytology samples and molecular biomarker testing in lung cancer—advantages and challenges. Virchows Archiv 2021;1–13.
40. Sigel CS, Moreira AL, Travis WD, et al. Subtyping of non-small cell lung carcinoma: a comparison of small biopsy and cytology specimens. J Thorac Oncol 2011;6(11):1849–56.
41. Roy-Chowdhuri S, Aisner DL, Allen TC, et al. Biomarker testing in lung carcinoma cytology specimens: a perspective from members of the pulmonary pathology society. Arch Pathol Lab Med 2016;140(11):1267–72.

42. Barbano R, Pasculli B, Coco M, et al. Competitive allele-specific TaqMan PCR (cast-PCR) is a sensitive, specific and fast method for BRAF V600 mutation detection in melanoma patients. Sci Rep 2015;5(1):1–11.

43. Ichimura K. Molecular pathogenesis of IDH mutations in gliomas. Brain Tumor Pathol 2012;29(3):131–9.

44. Dang L, Jin S, Su SM. IDH mutations in glioma and acute myeloid leukemia. Trends Mol Med 2010;16(9):387–97.

45. Wongsurawat T, Jenjaroenpun P, De Loose A, et al. A novel Cas9-targeted long-read assay for simultaneous detection of IDH1/2 mutations and clinically relevant MGMT methylation in fresh biopsies of diffuse glioma. Acta Neuropathol Commun 2020;8(1):1–13.

46. Catteau A, Girardi H, Monville F, et al. A new sensitive PCR assay for one-step detection of 12 IDH1/2 mutations in glioma. Acta neuropathologica Commun 2014;2(1):1–12.

47. Patel KP, Barkoh BA, Chen Z, et al. Diagnostic testing for IDH1 and IDH2 variants in acute myeloid leukemia: an algorithmic approach using high-resolution melting curve analysis. J Mol Diagn 2011;13(6):678–86.

48. Enjeti A, Granter N, Ashraf A, et al. A longitudinal evaluation of performance of automated BCR-ABL1 quantitation using cartridge-based detection system. Pathology 2015;47(6):570–4.

49. Radich J, Yeung C, Wu D. New approaches to molecular monitoring in CML (and other diseases). Blood 2019;134(19):1578–84.

Analytical Principles of Cancer Next Generation Sequencing

Tatyana Gindin, MD, PhD[a], Susan J. Hsiao, MD, PhD[b],*

KEYWORDS

- Cancer • Oncology • Molecular diagnostics • Next generation sequencing
- Analytical

KEY POINTS

- Molecular profiling of tumor samples by next generation sequencing may be challenging as tumor samples may be small or compromised due to storage and fixation issues, and frequently have admixed normal.
- During the assay design process, steps may be taken during sample processing, library preparation, and bioinformatics analysis steps to address the unique challenges and clinical questions for somatic molecular testing.
- Control samples and quality control metrics should be monitored to assess the performance of the assay to detect somatic variants.

INTRODUCTION

Molecular profiling and biomarker detection in tumor samples by next generation sequencing (NGS) provide key information that may be used to guide patient management and therapy selection that allows the delivery of personalized medicine. NGS or "massively parallel" sequencing are the terms used to refer collectively to a range of sequencing technologies that involve analysis of large numbers of different DNA sequences in parallel (ie, in a single reaction). The past decade has seen an exponential increase in novel methodologies in template generation and sequencing that were developed to address a range of questions in clinical practice and cancer research. As an example, tumor mutation burden (TMB), defined as the number of mutations per megabase of sequence, predicts response to immune checkpoint inhibitor therapy.[1–4] TMB is readily detectable using large NGS-based cancer panels or cancer whole exome sequencing (WES) studies. Other biomarkers detectable by NGS include

[a] Department of Pathology, NYU Grossman School of Medicine, 240 East 38th Street, 22-66, New York, NY 10016, USA; [b] Department of Pathology & Cell Biology, Columbia University Medical Center, 630 West 168th Street, P&S 16-409A, New York, NY 10032, USA
* Corresponding author.
E-mail address: sjh2155@cumc.columbia.edu

Clin Lab Med 42 (2022) 395–408
https://doi.org/10.1016/j.cll.2022.04.003
0272-2712/22/© 2022 Elsevier Inc. All rights reserved.

point mutations, insertion/deletion mutations, copy number alterations, and gene fusions. These biomarkers can support the diagnosis of malignancy, inform prognosis, and identify therapeutic targets.

Optimization and validation of the performance characteristics of a cancer NGS assay is critical for the accurate detection of biomarkers. The analytical phase of NGS testing typically encompasses steps including DNA fragmentation, end repair, adapter ligation, library enrichment, sequencing, and bioinformatics analysis. DNA fragmentation is, generally, done by mechanical shearing (eg, sonication or nebulization) or enzymatic digestion. This step produces fragments of a size compatible with short read sequencing lengths. The end repair step is required following fragmentation if the fragmentation method does not produce blunt ends. The end repair step fills in 5′ overhangs, trims 3′ overhangs, and phosphorylates the 5′ nucleotide to provide a blunt end to which adapters can ligate. The end repair step is generally not required if polymerase chain reaction (PCR) amplification is used for library enrichment of target sequences. As part of library preparation, the enrichment step can enhance the coverage of specific genetic regions such as cancer-specific genes or all coding exons in the case of WES. For whole genome sequencing (WGS), the complete genomic DNA is sequenced and hence no enrichment step is required. Following preparation of libraries and addition of patient-specific barcodes, the libraries are pooled and loaded onto the sequencer. Sequence data is bioinformatically processed with steps including demultiplexing to assign reads to patient samples, alignment to a reference genome, variant calling, and annotation.

There are specific considerations for the analysis of tumor samples, due to the nature of tumor samples, the frequent presence of admixed normal, and the clinical context and clinical utilization of the assay at each step in the analytical phase of cancer NGS testing (**Fig 1**). The analytical principles for cancer NGS will be the main focus of this article.

TUMOR NGS SPECIMEN PROCESSING CONSIDERATIONS

Tumor samples routinely submitted for cancer NGS testing include blood, bone marrow, cytologic preparations (cell blocks, smears), and formalin fixed, paraffin embedded tissue (FFPE). Tumor samples can be challenging samples to sequence for several reasons, including: 1) low input from limited tissue obtained from minimally invasive biopsies, 2) low tumor fraction from samples with inflammatory infiltrate or a highly cellular background, or 3) poor DNA quality, primarily for FFPE samples where the formalin fixation and storage can result in DNA–protein or DNA–DNA crosslinks, cytosine deamination, DNA fragmentation, oxidized bases, or apurinic sites.[5–9] The preanalytical specimen considerations around specimen collection, transport, and storage are discussed in detail in another article in this series (see Qiong Gan and Sinchita Roy-Chowdhuri's article, "Specimen Considerations in Molecular Oncology Testing," in this issue). We discuss here strategies that may be used during specimen processing.

Deamination of cytosine to uracil occurs frequently in FFPEs.[5–8] If unrepaired, cytosine deamination results in C>T or G>A transitions. Particularly in tumor samples with limited input, PCR amplification from a limited number of genomic equivalents followed by sequencing may result in artifactual calls that are above calling thresholds. Indeed, multiple studies have found a significant proportion of variant calls from tumor FFPE samples to arise from deamination events.[6,10,11] In cells, spontaneous deamination is repaired by uracil-DNA glycosylases (UDGs), a family of enzymes in which uracil-N-glycosylase (UNG) is a member. UDG catalyzes hydrolysis in the N-glycosylic

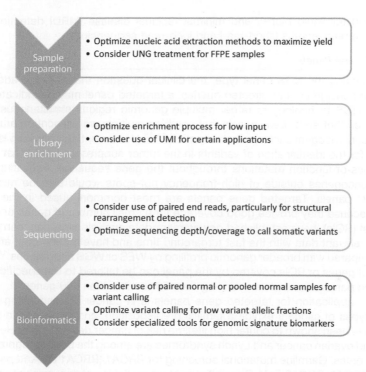

Sample preparation
- Optimize nucleic acid extraction methods to maximize yield
- Consider UNG treatment for FFPE samples

Library enrichment
- Optimize enrichment process for low input
- Consider use of UMI for certain applications

Sequencing
- Consider use of paired end reads, particularly for structural rearrangement detection
- Optimize sequencing depth/coverage to call somatic variants

Bioinformatics
- Consider use of paired normal or pooled normal samples for variant calling
- Optimize variant calling for low variant allelic fractions
- Consider specialized tools for genomic signature biomarkers

Fig. 1. Assay design considerations for cancer testing at each step of the NGS testing process.

bond, resulting in an abasic site that can then be repaired by the base excision repair (BER) pathway. Studies have examined the use of UNG treatment to reduce deamination artifact and have found UNG treatment to reduce C>T and G>A transition mutations.[6,11,12] Incorporation of a UNG treatment step may be considered for assays using FFPE specimens.

In addition to cytosine deamination, another DNA lesion that may occur is oxidation of guanine caused by hydroxy radicals, generating 8-oxoguanine, which pairs with adenine and results in G>T and C>A transversions. This lesion may be repaired by 8-oxoguanine DNA glycosylase and the BER pathway.[9,13] Other DNA damage seen in FFPE includes nicks and blocked 3′ ends. Multiple commercial products are available to repair these types of FFPE-associated DNA damage events. Although the components of commercial FFPE repair kits are proprietary, they generally contain DNA glycosylase to remove the damaged base, apurinic/apyrimidinic endonuclease to cut the backbone, end processing with polynucleotide kinase, DNA polymerase for gap filling, and ligase for nick ligation.

TUMOR NEXT GENERATION SEQUENCING ASSAY DESIGN CONSIDERATIONS

NGS methodologies can be subdivided into several different ways, by the type of the nucleic acid source (DNA vs RNA), the resolution (single cell vs bulk sequencing), the amount of genome sequenced ("hot-spot" gene panels vs WES and WGS/transcriptome sequencing), the library-enrichment approach (hybrid capture vs amplicon based), the sensitivity or read depth (low pass whole genome sequencing vs ultradeep sequencing for liquid biopsy and minimal residual disease [MRD] detection), and sequencing read lengths (short-read and long-read sequencing).

Targeted Gene Panels

When selecting the NGS panel type, the clinical question that is being addressed should be considered. For directed queries, a targeted panel may be indicated. The ability of NGS technology to target multiple genomic regions simultaneously gave rise to small "hot-spot" gene panels that combine multiple well-described mutational hot-spots in oncogenes into a single reaction.[14,15] However, this approach is not as effective for the identification of variants in the tumor suppressor genes that tend to exhibit loss-of-function mutations throughout the gene sequence. Activating mutations in oncogenes outside of high-frequency hot-spots would also be missed by "hot-spot" panels. Targeted gene panels are most commonly used in the clinical setting because they provide good coverage for a small number of genes or regions of interest (ROIs), have established downstream data analysis pipelines, can provide clinically relevant data with the fast turnaround time and have greater cost efficiency when compared with broader genomic profiling by WES or WGS approaches.[16–18] The number of genes or ROIs covered by the panel can be tailored to the specific cancer type or be pan cancer and vary ranging from 50 to more than 500 genes.

Another application for targeted gene panels is in cancer predisposition testing. Several types of cancers exhibit a familial predisposition, and mutations in specific genes have been shown to confer high lifetime risk of cancer development. Hereditary breast and ovarian cancer and Lynch syndromes are among the best-recognized cancer syndromes. Germline mutational screening for *BRCA1* (BRCA1 DNA Repair Associated), *BRCA2* (BRCA2 DNA Repair Associated), and mismatch repair genes (*MLH1* [MutL Homolog 1], *MSH2*, *MSH6*, or *PMS2* [PMS1 Homolog 2, Mismatch Repair System Component]) has had a major impact on genetic counseling with effects of numerous additional genes involved in homologous recombination and mismatch repair pathways being discovered. Gene-panel testing offers a fast and reliable approach to genetic diagnostics of hereditable cancer syndromes and allows design of personalized preventive measures with diagnostic yield greatly increased compared with singe gene testing.[19,20]

Whole Exome Sequencing and Whole Genome Sequencing

Depending on the cancer type and the panel size, recent studies showed that between 50% and 70% of patients remain mutation-negative after gene-panel testing with less than 30% of patients displaying actionable mutations.[16,21] Expanding the panel testing to WES is attractive for clinical use because expanding of the ROIs to all exonic regions of the genome allows identification of additional disease-causing and actionable mutations. However, there are several tradeoffs to covering more of the genome space including the loss of sequencing depth that decreases sensitivity of testing by not allowing to confidently call the variants with low allele fraction, particularly for subclonal somatic variants or tumors that show heterogeneity. In addition, WES typically requires paired germline sequencing to allow identification of true somatic mutations, which can increase the cost of sequencing and complexity of bioinformatics analysis.

WGS has multiple advantages over the panel-based sequencing methods. It enables simultaneous detection of single nucleotide, copy number, and structural variants (gene fusions) and, hence, can result in a substantial increase in actionable findings. Several recent studies demonstrated that ~60% of patients with advanced metastatic cancer had actionable variants identified using WGS.[22,23] In addition, library preparation for WGS does not need to include the enrichment step and, thus, the genomic ROIs are covered more uniformly without the introduction of PCR errors and other biases associated with library preparation steps. However, the increase in the number of covered bases (~3 billion for WGS) compared with WES (WES targets approximately 3% of the whole genome) results in significant increase in sequencing costs that are still a barrier for incorporation of WGS into routine clinical practice. In addition, lower coverage, as with WES, can make detection of variants at low variant allelic fractions difficult. Another application of WGS is low-pass (low-coverage) WGS. Low-pass WGS has been used as a low-cost high-throughput alternative to genotyping arrays and pharmacogenomics. Recent advances in bioinformatics analysis allowed the use of low-pass WGS for accurate detection of copy number variants and large chromosomal rearrangements at a fraction of a cost of WGS deep sequencing methods.[24–26]

Amplicon versus Hybrid Capture

When considering library enrichment, 2 approaches are generally available: amplicon sequencing and hybrid capture.[27–29] For amplicon-based sequencing, the ROIs are amplified by PCR using the set of specific primers before sequencing. The advantages of amplicon-based methods are low DNA input, fast turnaround time, and the ease of bioinformatics analysis. However, the PCR amplification can introduce bias, affecting predicted variant allele frequencies and copy number changes, as well as propagate amplification errors.

In hybrid capture, relevant DNA sequences are hybridized to probes and biotin—streptavidin system is used to pull down the hybridized sequences as the nonbound DNA is washed away. This method introduces less error due to fewer PCR amplification cycles when compared with the amplicon-based methods. Hybrid capture is more reliable for copy number detection and is able to identify fusion events because at least one partner will be pulled down by the baited DNA. However, this method requires higher input DNA concentration and more advanced bioinformatics analysis pipelines. Coverage may be lower in regions that are difficult to capture, and off target reads can add cost to the sequencing reaction.

Long Read Sequencing

All abovementioned NGS methods use short-read sequencing—the most commonly used technology in the clinical setting because of the lower cost and relatively high accuracy. However, long-read sequencing is starting to gain traction because it has unique advantages in improving the read alignments (eg, for de novo genome assembly) and simplifying bioinformatics pipelines. In clinical practice, most long-read sequencing efforts have centered predominantly on structural DNA variants and RNA sequencing and are focused on the discovery of novel fusion and splicing isoforms that are relevant to tumor progression or treatment resistance.[30–32] Currently, the error rates for long-read technologies are too high to be used in clinical practice for reproducible somatic variant detection.

RNA Sequencing

RNA sequencing has many advantages over DNA-based methods for several clinical applications including enhanced ability to detect gene fusions, splicing variants, noncoding RNA species, and define cancer-specific gene expression signatures among others.[33] RNA sequencing allows precise identification of all the genes that are transcribed from DNA in specific tumor sample (termed "transcriptome") as well as defines relative abundance of different gene transcripts (gene expression levels). Transcribed sequences also include untranslated (nonprotein-coding) RNA species such as microRNAs that have been recently implicated in tumorigenesis.[34,35] Because RNA sequencing data only provides information on genes that are expressed in the sample, it enriches for functionally relevant mutations that otherwise might have been of too low abundance to be detected by DNA-based methods.

RNA-based methods are particularly useful when interrogating fusion events and splice variants.[36] By assessing RNA transcripts directly, large intronic sequences are removed allowing for more efficient sequencing and ability to ascertain the in-frame status of the resultant transcript. RNA-based methods also allow detection of novel fusion products with previously uncharacterized fusion partners. Most human genes exist as different isoforms due to alternative splicing. Mutations in splicing machinery in cancer can result in change in relative abundance of gene transcripts and formation of novel isoforms, some with novel or opposite functional consequences. RNA-based sequencing can precisely measure the levels of different isoforms and determine whether the pathogenic splicing event has occurred.[37]

Another key clinical application of RNAseq is based on measurement of differential expression of target genes using whole transcriptome analysis. This methodology has been successfully used to discover novel gene expression-based biomarkers. Gene expression signatures have been developed for several cancer types and are being widely used for diagnosis, risk stratification, as well as prediction of treatment responses.[38,39] Molecular classification has been developed and validated for a range of cancer types including large B-cell lymphomas, thyroid, breast, and pediatric brain cancer among others.[40–42]

Single cell RNA sequencing (scRNA-seq) is currently primarily used in the research setting but clinical applications are emerging. In scRNA-seq, single cells are isolated, RNA is reverse transcribed, barcoded, and library is generated and sequenced. Bioinformatics analysis of the resulting data, with transcript quantification and clustering analysis, allows the identification of cell types in a heterogeneous tumor and a view of the regulatory networks.[43–45] Clinical applications of scRNA-seq include prediction of prognosis and drug resistance.

APPLICATION-SPECIFIC ASSAY DESIGN CONSIDERATIONS

In addition to some of the more general considerations described above, specific cancer applications have unique design considerations, both from the library/sequencing aspects and from the bioinformatics analysis aspects. Laboratories considering these clinical applications may be able to adopt existing assays and bioinformatics pipelines to detect these biomarkers or may need to design specific assays to meet the requirements for detection (**Table 1**).

Genetic Signatures (MSI/tumor mutation burden/homologous recombination deficiency)

Computational analysis of NGS sequencing data from large patient cohorts resulted in identification of different patterns of somatic mutations and led to discovery of specific mutational signatures related to underlying mechanisms of mutagenesis.[46] Examples of mutational signatures are deamination of cytosines in cancer associated with aging, excess of G to T transversions from exposure to polycyclic aromatic hydrocarbons in tobacco smoke, and dimerization of adjacent pyrimidine nucleic acids by ultraviolet radiation.[47] In recent years, several mutational signatures have been successfully used the in clinical setting as predictors of response to several therapy modalities. For instance, it has been shown that a subset of colorectal and endometrial cancers with inactivation of mismatch repair proteins (*MLH1*, *MSH2*, *MSH6*, or *PMS2*) display a characteristic

Table 1 Cancer applications and their respective NGS analytical considerations		
Cancer Application	**NGS Analytical Considerations**	**References**
Targeted panel sequencing/hotspot panel	High sequencing depths Amplicon-based libraries Hybrid capture libraries	14–18
ctDNA or MRD detection	UMI High sequencing depth	60–64,67
Structural variant detection (RNA)	Anchored multiplex PCR RNA sequencing	33,36
Structural variant detection (DNA)	Long reads	30
TMB/microsatellite instability	Large panel or whole exome or whole genome Paired normal; if tumor only, use bioinformatics approaches to identify somatic variants	48,49 57–59
Mutation signatures (eg, HRD)	Large panel or whole exome or whole genome Bioinformatics approaches	55,56
Copy number variant detection	Paired normal; if tumor only, use bioinformatics approaches for normalization Copy number backbone	16–18
Tumor microenvironment	Single cell RNASeq	43–45
Gene expression	Transcriptome	38,39

pattern of insertions and deletions in the regions of repetitive DNA tracts (microsatellites). Germline mutations in mismatch repair proteins are associated with Lynch syndrome conferring increased risk for the development of several cancers, most commonly colorectal and endometrial but also of ovarian, urinary tract, and gastrointestinal tract origins. NGS provides the opportunity to interrogate large numbers of microsatellite loci without the need for additional testing concurrently with identification of other genomic variants.[48,49] Presence of microsatellite instability (MSI) was shown to be associated with the response to immune checkpoint inhibitor therapy across tumor types.[50–52]

Another independent biomarker of response to immunotherapy is tumor mutational burden (TMB). Some mutational processes generate large number of somatic mutations in the course of cancer development. It has been hypothesized that large number of mutations in tumor DNA can result in presentation of novel peptides (neoantigens) to the immune system and subsequently elicit host response. TMB is calculated as the total number of somatic mutations per coding area of a sequenced tumor genome, and high TMB has been associated with favorable response to immune checkpoint inhibitor regardless of cancer type.[53,54]

Another emerging mutational signature-based biomarker is homologous recombination deficiency (HRD). HRD is most commonly associated with BRCA1 or BRCA2 loss-of-function mutations but it has been recognized that the homologous recombination pathway is composed of several genes with mutational profiles that have not been fully characterized. Mutational patterns of nucleotide substitutions, deletions, and copy number losses have been aggregated into the scoring system that has been shown to predict the improved response to Poly(ADP-Ribose) Polymerase inhibitors and platinum chemotherapy even in the absence of *BRCA1* or *BRCA2* loss-of-function alterations. HRD scoring system has been successfully applied to gynecologic cancers including those of ovarian and endometrial origins.[55,56]

Detection of these signatures requires the use of WES, WGS, or targeted panels large enough to provide representative sampling of the cancer genome. For TMB assessment, for example, studies have examined the effect of panel size on the accuracy of TMB, and a panel covering at least 1 Mb of sequence is recommended.[57–59] Other considerations include use of a paired normal specimen to exclude germline variants from TMB calculation. If tumor only sequencing is performed, the use of population databases, pooled normal samples, and other approaches can be considered.

Circulating Tumor DNA

Another significant advance in the application of NGS testing in clinical setting is liquid biopsy—a technique for analyzing circulating tumor DNA (ctDNA) for clinically significant point mutations, copy number alterations, and structural rearrangements. Several advantages of evaluating ctDNA over tissue DNA include being minimally invasive, providing a comprehensive view of tumor genetics from multiple metastatic sites in a single test, and ability to follow the dynamic changes in ctDNA during therapy for the development of resistance mutations, other targetable variants, and assessing tumor burden of the disease to identify early signs of progression.[60–64] Generally, the concentration of ctDNA in peripheral blood of cancer patients can vary from less than 5 to more than 1000 ng/mL. Hence, analyzing ctDNA requires a great increase in sequencing depth when compared with the panel-based methods. The error rates of amplicon-based or hybrid capture methods are too high to be able to differentiate the low variant fraction changes from technical artifacts. The use of additional barcoding with unique molecular identifiers (UMIs) allows significant error reduction.[65,66] UMIs involve barcoding of individual DNA template molecules during NGS library preparation with subsequent ability to trace all sequencing reads back to a single original DNA template. Aligning the reads with the same barcode and treating them as a single read by generating the consensus sequence, enables one to differentiate the true low-frequency variants from PCR and sequencing errors. The same technology has been recently implemented for MRD testing in hematologic malignancies where presence of MRD and early molecular relapse has been used to inform clinical decisions.[67]

CONTROL SAMPLES

Inclusion of control samples allows for detection of unexpected errors that may occur at any point throughout the testing process. No template control (NTC) samples allow one to assess for potential contamination, which can occur at any step in the process but particularly during steps in which PCR amplification of the library occurs. NTC samples may be assessed following library preparation for the presence of measurable nucleic acids. Some laboratories may choose to process the NTC sample past the library preparation step through sequencing and analysis steps. Sequencing NTC samples can help identify potential issues around index hopping or barcode contamination.

Positive control samples are ideally processed with clinical samples through all phases of testing, including nucleic acid extraction, library preparation, sequencing, and bioinformatics analysis steps. Sources for positive control samples include patient samples, well-characterized cell lines, and engineered (eg, oligonucleotide or plasmid) control samples. The positive control sample should demonstrate the ability of the assay to detect variants at the assay's validated limit of detection. In practice, this can be achieved readily through the use of mixtures of cell lines to generate a variety of variant types at a range of variant allelic fractions. Cell lines are available from cell line repositories such as Coriell or American Type Culture Collection. Sequence data from HapMap samples are available through the Genome in a Bottle consortium and sequence data from cancer cell lines are available through the Cancer Cell Line Encyclopedia project.[68–71] Patient samples or cell lines may not be available for less common alterations, such as rare mutations, uncommon fusion genes, large deletions/duplications, copy number alterations, or specific genomic signatures. Engineered positive control materials are a good resource to confirm the ability to detect rare cancer genomic alterations.

Another consideration for cancer sequencing is the inclusion of normal controls in the assay to aid in the detection of somatic variants. Some laboratories may choose to run paired normal samples to improve the ability to call somatic variants, copy number alterations, microsatellite instability, TMB, or gene expression changes, as well as evaluate sample identity. Other laboratories use a panel or pool of normal samples, which can also allow for normalization and recognition of artifactual calls.

QUALITY CONTROL AND QUALITY ASSURANCE

Monitoring quality control parameters and ongoing quality assurance procedures helps ensure the cancer NGS assay is performing as designed and unexpected errors did not occur. Specific quality control metrics may vary depending on the analytes being detected as well as the performance characteristics established during validation. In general, laboratories should consider monitoring the nucleic acid quantity and quality (particularly for RNA or nucleic acids extracted from FFPE), the library preparation process, the sequencing metrics, and the bioinformatics process.

Multiple options are available for each of these quality control markers. To evaluate nucleic acid quantity spectrophotometric or fluorometric measurements can be taken, and electrophoresis can be used to analyze the integrity and fragment size of nucleic acids. Additional metrics following bioinformatics analysis can also inform of potential issues with nucleic acid input. For example, a higher than expected duplication rate may indicate less than expected amplifiable DNA present in the sample that resulted in a low-complexity library. The library preparation process can be evaluated by quantifying the amount of library generated, as well as by electrophoresis to ensure the library products are of the expected size (and minimal-to-no adapter or primer dimers present). Following sequencing, analysis of metrics such as the percentage of on-target reads, the depth of coverage, and uniformity of coverage may highlight errors that may have occurred during library preparation. Sequencing quality control metrics may vary depending on the sequencing platform used. In general, the percentage of reads and bases at or above quality score thresholds should meet the cutoffs established by the manufacturer. Quality metrics for bioinformatics processes examine features such as the number and quality of variants identified, variant allelic fraction, read depth, transition/transversion and heterozygous/homozygous ratio, and strand bias (see Somak Roy's article, "Principles and Validation of Bioinformatics Pipeline for Cancer Next Generation Sequencing," in this issue on Bioinformatics for further detailed information).

Ongoing quality assurance measures should be used by the laboratory as part of the quality management system. As an example of a quality assurance measure, a laboratory should have a policy for confirmatory testing of detected variants by orthogonal methods such as Sanger sequencing, digital droplet PCR, fluorescence in situ hybridization, microarray, or other methods. Proficiency testing is another important mechanism to assess assay performance and unexpected errors. Formal proficiency testing surveys such as those offered by the College of American Pathologists, alternative assessments using blinded or interlaboratory samples, or in silico mutagenized files for bioinformatics analyses, are all examples of proficiency testing that laboratories can participate in.

SUMMARY

The analysis of cancer specimens by NGS presents unique challenges but the genomics data obtained provides information crucial for therapeutic management. Tumor samples are increasingly being profiled not just for a small subset of hotspot mutations but also for a variety of alterations including copy number, structural variants, and genomic signatures. Common challenges to most cancer NGS assays include fixation-related artifacts for DNA extracted from FFPE, low input, and low tumor fraction, which necessitate higher sequencing depths. Assay design requires consideration of these factors as well as the technical limitations of sequencing and bioinformatics pipelines, all in the context of the biomarkers desired to be assessed. General design principles as well as application-specific considerations were highlighted here to guide other laboratories. Another key component of clinical cancer NGS testing is the selection and inclusion of control samples, during the optimization and familiarization, and validation stages, and also as a part of quality control and an ongoing quality assurance program.

CLINICS CARE POINTS

- Consider UNG treatment of FFPEs, particularly for samples that have been stored for longer periods of time.
- Amplicon-based libraries are helpful to achieve high depths from low-input samples. Use of UMIs can enhance sensitivity and are important for applications such as ctDNA or MRD.
- Genomic region covered and sequencing depth should be optimized for the biomarkers and analytes detected.
- Specialized bioinformatics approaches are necessary for detection of genomic signatures such as TMB or MSI or for specific applications such as liquid biopsy.

DISCLOSURE

S.J. Hsiao has received honoraria from Illumina, Loxo Oncology, Opentrons Labworks and Medscape and institutional research funding from Bristol Myers Squibb.

REFERENCES

1. Hellmann MD, Paz-Ares L, Bernabe Caro R, et al. Nivolumab plus ipilimumab in advanced non-small-cell lung cancer. N Engl J Med 2019;381(21):2020–31.
2. Hellmann MD, Ciuleanu TE, Pluzanski A, et al. Nivolumab plus ipilimumab in lung cancer with a high tumor mutational burden. N Engl J Med 2018;378(22): 2093–104.
3. Snyder A, Makarov V, Merghoub T, et al. Genetic basis for clinical response to CTLA-4 blockade in melanoma. N Engl J Med 2014;371(23):2189–99.

4. Samstein RM, Lee CH, Shoushtari AN, et al. Tumor mutational load predicts survival after immunotherapy across multiple cancer types. Nat Genet 2019;51(2): 202–6.
5. Ferruelo A, El-Assar M, Lorente JA, et al. Transcriptional profiling and genotyping of degraded nucleic acids from autopsy tissue samples after prolonged formalin fixation times. Int J Clin Exp Pathol 2011;4(2):156–61.
6. Do H, Dobrovic A. Sequence artifacts in DNA from formalin-fixed tissues: causes and strategies for minimization. Clin Chem 2015;61(1):64–71.
7. Rait VK, Zhang Q, Fabris D, et al. Conversions of formaldehyde-modified 2'-deoxyadenosine 5'-monophosphate in conditions modeling formalin-fixed tissue dehydration. J Histochem Cytochem 2006;54(3):301–10.
8. Jackson DP, Lewis FA, Taylor GR, et al. Tissue extraction of DNA and RNA and analysis by the polymerase chain reaction. J Clin Pathol 1990;43(6):499–504.
9. Lindahl T. Instability and decay of the primary structure of DNA. Nature 1993; 362(6422):709–15.
10. Robbe P, Popitsch N, Knight SJL, et al. Clinical whole-genome sequencing from routine formalin-fixed, paraffin-embedded specimens: pilot study for the 100,000 Genomes Project. Genet Med 2018;20(10):1196–205.
11. Berra CM, Torrezan GT, de Paula CA, et al. Use of uracil-DNA glycosylase enzyme to reduce DNA-related artifacts from formalin-fixed and paraffin-embedded tissues in diagnostic routine. Appl Cancer Res 2019;39(1):7.
12. Prentice LM, Miller RR, Knaggs J, et al. Formalin fixation increases deamination mutation signature but should not lead to false positive mutations in clinical practice. PLoS One 2018;13(4):e0196434.
13. David SS, O'Shea VL, Kundu S. Base-excision repair of oxidative DNA damage. Nature 2007;447(7147):941–50.
14. de Leng WW, Gadellaa-van Hooijdonk CG, Barendregt-Smouter FA, et al. Targeted next generation sequencing as a reliable diagnostic assay for the detection of somatic mutations in tumours using minimal DNA amounts from formalin fixed paraffin embedded material. PLoS One 2016;11(2):e0149405.
15. Prendergast EN, Elvin JA. Genomic profiling of gynecologic cancers and implications for clinical practice. Curr Opin Obstet Gynecol 2017;29(1):18–25.
16. Zehir A, Benayed R, Shah RH, et al. Mutational landscape of metastatic cancer revealed from prospective clinical sequencing of 10,000 patients. Nat Med 2017;23(6):703–13.
17. Frampton GM, Fichtenholtz A, Otto GA, et al. Development and validation of a clinical cancer genomic profiling test based on massively parallel DNA sequencing. Nat Biotechnol 2013;31(11):1023–31.
18. Williams HL, Walsh K, Diamond A, et al. Validation of the Oncomine focus panel for next-generation sequencing of clinical tumour samples. Virchows Arch 2018; 473(4):489–503.
19. Aloraifi F, McDevitt T, Martiniano R, et al. Detection of novel germline mutations for breast cancer in non-BRCA1/2 families. FEBS J 2015;282(17):3424–37.
20. Farmer H, McCabe N, Lord CJ, et al. Targeting the DNA repair defect in BRCA mutant cells as a therapeutic strategy. Nature 2005;434(7035):917–21.
21. Sholl LM, Do K, Shivdasani P, et al. Institutional implementation of clinical tumor profiling on an unselected cancer population. JCI Insight 2016;1(19):e87062.
22. Priestley P, Baber J, Lolkema MP, et al. Pan-cancer whole-genome analyses of metastatic solid tumours. Nature 2019;575(7781):210–6.
23. Chrystoja CC, Diamandis EP. Whole genome sequencing as a diagnostic test: challenges and opportunities. Clin Chem 2014;60(5):724–33.

24. Chen X, Chang CW, Spoerke JM, et al. Low-pass whole-genome sequencing of circulating cell-free DNA demonstrates dynamic changes in genomic copy number in a squamous lung cancer clinical cohort. Clin Cancer Res 2019;25(7): 2254–63.

25. Ruhen O, Mirzai B, Clark ME, et al. Comparison of circulating tumour DNA and extracellular vesicle DNA by low-pass whole-genome sequencing reveals molecular drivers of disease in a breast cancer patient. Biomedicines 2020;9(1):14.

26. Smyth EC, Vlachogiannis G, Hedayat S, et al. EGFR amplification and outcome in a randomised phase III trial of chemotherapy alone or chemotherapy plus panitumumab for advanced gastro-oesophageal cancers. Gut 2021;70(9):1632–41.

27. Samorodnitsky E, Jewell BM, Hagopian R, et al. Evaluation of hybridization capture versus amplicon-based methods for whole-exome sequencing. Hum Mutat 2015;36(9):903–14.

28. Mardis ER. Next-generation sequencing platforms. Annu Rev Anal Chem (Palo Alto Calif) 2013;6:287–303.

29. Kadri S, Long BC, Mujacic I, et al. Clinical validation of a next-generation sequencing genomic Oncology panel via cross-platform benchmarking against established amplicon sequencing assays. J Mol Diagn 2017;19(1):43–56.

30. Sakamoto Y, Zaha S, Suzuki Y, et al. Application of long-read sequencing to the detection of structural variants in human cancer genomes. Comput Struct Biotechnol J 2021;19:4207–16.

31. Leung SK, Jeffries AR, Castanho I, et al. Full-length transcript sequencing of human and mouse cerebral cortex identifies widespread isoform diversity and alternative splicing. Cell Rep 2021;37(7):110022.

32. De Paoli-Iseppi R, Gleeson J, Clark MB. Isoform age - splice isoform profiling using long-read technologies. Front Mol Biosci 2021;8:711733.

33. Wang Y, Mashock M, Tong Z, et al. Changing technologies of RNA sequencing and Their applications in clinical Oncology. Front Oncol 2020;10:447.

34. Anastasiadou E, Jacob LS, Slack FJ. Non-coding RNA networks in cancer. Nat Rev Cancer 2018;18(1):5–18.

35. Huarte M, Rinn JL. Large non-coding RNAs: missing links in cancer? Hum Mol Genet 2010;19(R2):R152–61.

36. Park HJ, Baek I, Cheang G, et al. Comparison of RNA-based next-generation sequencing assays for the detection of NTRK gene fusions. J Mol Diagn 2021; 23(11):1443–51.

37. Davies KD, Lomboy A, Lawrence CA, et al. DNA-based versus RNA-based detection of MET exon 14 skipping events in lung cancer. J Thorac Oncol 2019;14(4):737–41.

38. Varnier R, Sajous C, de Talhouet S, et al. Using breast cancer gene expression signatures in clinical practice: unsolved issues, ongoing trials and future perspectives. Cancers (Basel) 2021;13(19):4840.

39. Jensen MB, Laenkholm AV, Balslev E, et al. The Prosigna 50-gene profile and responsiveness to adjuvant anthracycline-based chemotherapy in high-risk breast cancer patients. NPJ Breast Cancer 2020;6:7.

40. Roschewski M, Phelan JD, Wilson WH. Molecular classification and treatment of diffuse large B-cell lymphoma and primary Mediastinal B-cell lymphoma. Cancer J 2020;26(3):195–205.

41. Cacciotti C, Fleming A, Ramaswamy V. Advances in the molecular classification of pediatric brain tumors: a guide to the galaxy. J Pathol 2020;251(3):249–61.

42. Guerreiro Stucklin AS, Ramaswamy V, Daniels C, et al. Review of molecular classification and treatment implications of pediatric brain tumors. Curr Opin Pediatr 2018;30(1):3–9.
43. Rosati D, Giordano A. Single-cell RNA sequencing and bioinformatics as tools to decipher cancer heterogenicity and mechanisms of drug resistance. Biochem Pharmacol 2021;195:114811.
44. Tang F, Barbacioru C, Wang Y, et al. mRNA-Seq whole-transcriptome analysis of a single cell. Nat Methods 2009;6(5):377–82.
45. Andrews TS, Kiselev VY, McCarthy D, et al. Tutorial: guidelines for the computational analysis of single-cell RNA sequencing data. Nat Protoc 2021;16(1):1–9.
46. Alexandrov LB, Nik-Zainal S, Wedge DC, et al. Signatures of mutational processes in human cancer. Nature 2013;500(7463):415–21.
47. Seo KY, Jelinsky SA, Loechler EL. Factors that influence the mutagenic patterns of DNA adducts from chemical carcinogens. Mutat Res 2000;463(3):215–46.
48. Pang J, Gindin T, Mansukhani M, et al. Microsatellite instability detection using a large next-generation sequencing cancer panel across diverse tumour types. J Clin Pathol 2020;73(2):83–9.
49. Bonneville R, Krook MA, Chen HZ, et al. Detection of microsatellite instability biomarkers via next-generation sequencing. Methods Mol Biol 2020;2055:119–32.
50. Hause RJ, Pritchard CC, Shendure J, et al. Classification and characterization of microsatellite instability across 18 cancer types. Nat Med 2016;22(11):1342–50.
51. Sahin IH, Akce M, Alese O, et al. Immune checkpoint inhibitors for the treatment of MSI-H/MMR-D colorectal cancer and a perspective on resistance mechanisms. Br J Cancer 2019;121(10):809–18.
52. Andre T, Shiu KK, Kim TW, et al. Pembrolizumab in microsatellite-instability-high advanced colorectal cancer. N Engl J Med 2020;383(23):2207–18.
53. Hellmann MD, Nathanson T, Rizvi H, et al. Genomic features of response to combination immunotherapy in patients with advanced non-small-cell lung cancer. Cancer Cell 2018;33(5):843–52.e4.
54. Van Allen EM, Miao D, Schilling B, et al. Genomic correlates of response to CTLA-4 blockade in metastatic melanoma. Science 2015;350(6257):207–11.
55. Konstantinopoulos PA, Ceccaldi R, Shapiro GI, et al. Homologous recombination deficiency: exploiting the fundamental vulnerability of ovarian cancer. Cancer Discov 2015;5(11):1137–54.
56. Pennington KP, Walsh T, Harrell MI, et al. Germline and somatic mutations in homologous recombination genes predict platinum response and survival in ovarian, fallopian tube, and peritoneal carcinomas. Clin Cancer Res 2014; 20(3):764–75.
57. Vega DM, Yee LM, McShane LM, et al. Aligning tumor mutational burden (TMB) quantification across diagnostic platforms: phase II of the Friends of Cancer Research TMB Harmonization Project. Ann Oncol 2021;32(12):1626–36.
58. Stenzinger A, Endris V, Budczies J, et al. Harmonization and standardization of panel-based tumor mutational burden measurement: real-world results and recommendations of the quality in pathology study. J Thorac Oncol 2020;15(7): 1177–89.
59. Buchhalter I, Rempel E, Endris V, et al. Size matters: dissecting key parameters for panel-based tumor mutational burden analysis. Int J Cancer 2019;144(4): 848–58.
60. Zill OA, Banks KC, Fairclough SR, et al. The landscape of actionable genomic alterations in cell-free circulating tumor DNA from 21,807 advanced cancer patients. Clin Cancer Res 2018;24(15):3528–38.

61. Jensen TJ, Goodman AM, Kato S, et al. Genome-wide sequencing of cell-free DNA identifies copy-number alterations that can Be used for monitoring response to immunotherapy in cancer patients. Mol Cancer Ther 2019;18(2):448–58.
62. Chae YK, Oh MS. Detection of minimal residual disease using ctDNA in lung cancer: current evidence and future directions. J Thorac Oncol 2019;14(1):16–24.
63. Khagi Y, Goodman AM, Daniels GA, et al. Hypermutated circulating tumor DNA: correlation with response to checkpoint inhibitor-based immunotherapy. Clin Cancer Res 2017;23(19):5729–36.
64. Gandara DR, Paul SM, Kowanetz M, et al. Blood-based tumor mutational burden as a predictor of clinical benefit in non-small-cell lung cancer patients treated with atezolizumab. Nat Med 2018;24(9):1441–8.
65. Schmitt MW, Kennedy SR, Salk JJ, et al. Detection of ultra-rare mutations by next-generation sequencing. Proc Natl Acad Sci U S A 2012;109(36):14508–13.
66. Young AL, Wong TN, Hughes AE, et al. Quantifying ultra-rare pre-leukemic clones via targeted error-corrected sequencing. Leukemia 2015;29(7):1608–11.
67. Chen X, Cherian S. Role of minimal residual disease testing in acute Myeloid leukemia. Clin Lab Med 2021;41(3):467–83.
68. Ball MP, Thakuria JV, Zaranek AW, et al. A public resource facilitating clinical use of genomes. Proc Natl Acad Sci U S A 2012;109(30):11920–7.
69. Barretina J, Caponigro G, Stransky N, et al. The Cancer Cell Line Encyclopedia enables predictive modelling of anticancer drug sensitivity. Nature 2012; 483(7391):603–7.
70. Zook JM, Catoe D, McDaniel J, et al. Extensive sequencing of seven human genomes to characterize benchmark reference materials. Sci Data 2016;3:160025.
71. Zook JM, McDaniel J, Olson ND, et al. An open resource for accurately benchmarking small variant and reference calls. Nat Biotechnol 2019;37(5):561–6.

Principles and Validation of Bioinformatics Pipeline for Cancer Next-Generation Sequencing

Somak Roy, MD

KEYWORDS

- Cancer • Sequencing • High throughput • Bioinformatics • Pipeline • Validation
- Containers • Automation

KEY POINTS

- Clinical bioinformatics plays a key role in the implementation of clinical NGS testing infrastructure.
- NGS bioinformatics pipeline needs to be validated as part of an end-to-end NGS assay validation before clinical use.
- The validation cohort should be representative of the types of samples, types of variants, lower limits of detection of the assay, as well as sequence context of the panel.
- Software containers and modern software automation tools can allow building of a scalable and reliable clinical bioinformatics infrastructure.

INTRODUCTION

Next-generation sequencing (NGS)-based molecular tests have revolutionized the practice of medicine with the ability to personalize diagnosis, risk assessment, and treatment of patients with cancer. In the setting of cancer predisposition, especially in the pediatric age group, NGS-based testing is increasingly playing an important role in improving overall patient care. Given the vast amounts of quantitative and complex sequencing data generated by high-throughput sequencers, resource-intensive data processing pipelines are imperative to analyze the data and identify genetic alterations of clinical relevance. Bioinformatics, specifically in the context of genomics and molecular pathology, is a field of science that uses computational, mathematical, and statistical tools to collect, organize, and analyze large and complex genetic sequencing data and related biological data. A set of bioinformatics algorithms, when executed in a predefined sequence to process NGS data, is collectively referred

Department of Pathology, Cincinnati Children's Hospital Medical Center, R.2040 240 Albert Sabin Way, Cincinnati, OH 45229, USA
E-mail address: somak.roy@cchmc.org

Clin Lab Med 42 (2022) 409–421
https://doi.org/10.1016/j.cll.2022.05.006
0272-2712/22/© 2022 Elsevier Inc. All rights reserved.

labmed.theclinics.com

to as a bioinformatics pipeline.[1] Clinical molecular laboratories performing NGS-based tests may implement one or more bioinformatics pipelines that are either custom-developed by the laboratory or provided by the sequencing platform or a third-party vendor or a combination of both. A bioinformatics pipeline typically depends on the availability of several resources, including adequate storage, compute units, network connectivity, and an appropriate software execution environment. Provisioning such resources consistently and on-demand can present several challenges in a clinical laboratory environment during the implementation of an NGS-based assay. This article will discuss some important practical considerations for laboratory directors and bioinformatics personnel when developing, validating, and managing NGS bioinformatics resources for a clinical laboratory. This article is not a comprehensive guide for all aspects of bioinformatics resource development. The readers are suggested to follow the references below for additional details.

BACKGROUND

Clinical bioinformatics is an emerging subspecialty in laboratory medicine that is focused on the application of bioinformatics principles, methods, and software tools to analyze, integrate, and understand biological and health care data in a clinical setting.[2] Clinical bioinformatics has several applications in a clinical molecular laboratory offering NGS-based tumor (somatic) testing. NGS technology enables the generation of several million to billion short reads of DNA and RNA sequences isolated from a tumor sample. In contrast to traditional Sanger Sequencing technology with a read lengths of 500 to 900 bp, short reads of NGS range in size from 75 to 300 bp depending on the application and sequencing chemistry. Newer NGS technologies (PacBio, Nanopore, 10x Genomics) enable longer read sequences in excess of 10 kilobases[3] Converting RNA to cDNA molecule using Reverse-transcriptase polymerase chain reaction (RT-PCR) enables oncogenic fusion detection by NGS testing. Unlike Sanger sequencing, the high-throughput nature of NGS provides quantitative information (depth of coverage) due to the high level of sequence redundancy at a given locus. This nature of the NGS data enables the identification of a vast repertoire of cancer-related genetic alterations from a single NGS run using different bioinformatics algorithms[4] (**Fig. 1**).

The bioinformatics pipeline for DNA sequencing using NGS involves the alignment of the raw sequence reads from a FASTQ or an unaligned BAM (uBAM) file against the human reference genome. The FASTQ and uBAM file formats store short sequences as plain text with metadata information about each short sequence such as base quality score (Q-score) and read identifiers (**Fig. 2**). The sequence alignment process assigns a positional context to the short reads in the reference genome and generates several metadata fields, including alignment characteristics (matches, mismatches, and gaps) in CIGAR (Concise Idiosyncratic Gapped Alignment Report) format and mate-pair information. The aligned sequences and the related metadata are stored in a Sequence Alignment Mapping (SAM/BAM; https://samtools.github.io/hts-specs/SAMv1.pdf; see **Fig. 3**) or CRAM[5] file format. The BAM file is consumed by downstream algorithms to identify a range of different genetic alterations, including single-nucleotide variants (SNV), Insertion and Deletions (Indels), and tumor mutational burden (TMB).[4,6] One of the common ways of estimating copy number alterations (CNA) from aligned sequencing reads is using the depth of coverage approach. More extensive and specific DNA sequencing strategies can also enable the identification of large structural variants (SV), including gene fusions, and microsatellite instability (MSI).[6,7] The split-read alignment strategy can identify gene fusions

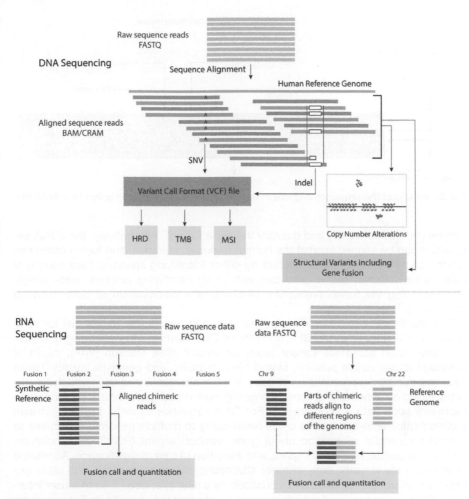

Fig. 1. Summarizes the high-level workflow of an NGS bioinformatics pipeline for DNA and RNA sequencing.

from genomic DNA sequencing.[7] For RNA-based gene fusion detection using NGS, one of the bioinformatics approaches involves the alignment of the cDNA sequences to an artificially constructed genome containing a list of known fusion sequences. The total number of reads from the sample that align to one of the known fusion sequences

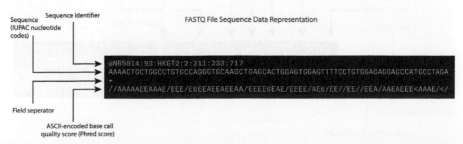

Fig. 2. Visualizes the sequence and base quality score data representation in a FASTQ file.

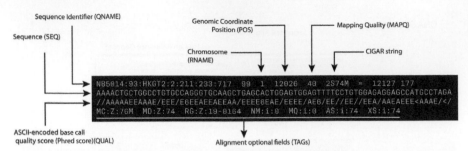

Fig. 3. Visualizes the sequence alignment data and metadata representation in a BAM file.

can be counted to identify and quantify the gene fusion.[8] Alternatively, the cDNA sequences can be aligned against the human genome reference, and fusion (chimeric) reads can be detected and quantified by either identifying spanning read pairs that map to the different fusion gene partners or by identifying junction reads (single read spanning the fusion breakpoint junction) or a combination of both methods (see **Fig. 1**).[9]

The results of variant identification are stored in one of the variant call formats, including VCF (**Fig. 4**), gVCF, GFF, and others. Such formats allow encoding quantitative information about the variant, such as variant allele fraction (VAF), depth of coverage at the variant position, strand bias, zygosity, and genotype quality. Given the more complex representation of copy number alterations and large structural variants, including gene fusions, there is ongoing work on using alternative file formats to represent such data appropriately.[10] For DNA sequence variants, the downstream bioinformatics analyses involve cross-referencing to multiple genomic databases to extract meaningful information about gene symbol, variant (HGVS) nomenclature, variant prevalence, functional impact, and assertion of clinical significance. Annotated DNA sequence variants, copy number alterations, structural variants, and other genetic alterations are rendered and visualized by a user interface.[4,6] Such a user interface allows trained molecular professionals to interpret the clinical significance of the genetic alterations and release a comprehensive molecular report.

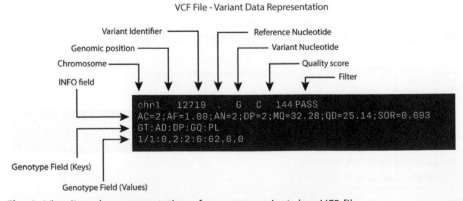

Fig. 4. Visualizes the representation of sequence variants in a VCF file.

Additional important applications of bioinformatics in molecular laboratory operations include quality control (QC) monitoring of sequencing data across runs, identification of background sequencing noise to reduce false-positive results, validation of upgrades to the bioinformatics pipeline, and the development and validation of novel algorithms for sequence data processing and variant interpretation.

DISCUSSION

Practical Considerations for Bioinformatics Pipeline Implementation and Validation in Cancer Next-Generation Sequencing Testing

Bioinformatics workflows in a clinical laboratory performing tumor testing are very complex. Raw sequence data to a clinical report is a multistep analytical process, much of which happens behind the scenes. To have high confidence in the performance of a bioinformatics pipeline and the tumor NGS results, a thorough validation as described in the recently published guidelines[1,11] and following the CAP NGS bioinformatics checklist should be performed. Subsequent updates to the bioinformatics pipeline should undergo appropriate revalidation and systematic version control. Bioinformatics pipeline and the related software interoperate closely with other devices, such as laboratory instrumentations, sequencing platforms, high-performance computing clusters (HPC), persistent storage resources, and other software such as laboratory information system (LIS), and electronic medical records (EMR). It is therefore important that the pipeline validation includes such interface functions, if applicable. In addition, the security of protected health information (PHI), including genetic data, and accreditation and regulatory compliance is necessary for the implementation of bioinformatics resources in a clinical laboratory.[4] The results of an NGS test are one or more genomic alterations identified by the bioinformatics pipeline. Detection, accurate representation, and generation of HGVS variant nomenclature can be challenging depending on the variant type, sequence context, and other factors. It is therefore critical to understand the evaluated region of the genome sequence by the NGS assay for accurate clinical reporting. Appropriate automation of bioinformatics resource development and deployment in clinical production contributes to optimized test turnaround time, better productivity of the bioinformatics team, and maintainable infrastructure.[12,13]

Life cycle of pipeline validation

An important requirement for the implementation of a bioinformatics pipeline is proper clinical validation in the context of the entire NGS assay. The recent guidelines from the Association for Molecular Pathology (AMP) recommend an end-to-end validation of the NGS assay that includes the bioinformatics pipeline.[1,11] The process of NGS bioinformatics pipeline validation involves a phase of optimization and familiarization (O&F) during which different software tools are evaluated, custom code developed, and optimized to build the bioinformatics pipelines. Once the bioinformatics pipeline is determined to be at the appropriate performance level during the O&F phase, all configuration, command line parameters, and assets, such as reference genome, panel BED files, and genomic databases, are locked down before the start of the validation phase. The performance characteristic of the bioinformatics pipeline is determined during the validation phase using a cohort of samples that appropriately represents the spectrum of genomic alterations that are expected to be detected in clinical testing. If the validation phase identifies issues with variant identification, the laboratory can make necessary modifications to the bioinformatics pipeline as part of the O&F phase and perform the validation again after locking down all configurations of the pipeline. If the change is limited to the bioinformatics pipeline, validation can be performed on the raw data from the same sequencing run. Full resequencing of the sample is not required. The clinical laboratory, with the assistance of bioinformatics professionals, must review, understand, and document each component of the pipeline, the data dependencies, input/output requirements, and constraints, and develop mechanisms to alert any unanticipated errors. After validation is complete, the entire process and the performance characteristics of the bioinformatics pipeline should be documented in compliance with the appropriate accreditation entity (for example CAP in the United States).[1]

Validation cohort

The performance characteristic of the bioinformatics pipeline should be determined based on the types of variants that the NGS assay intends to detect in clinical samples. For example, if the clinical NGS test is expected to detect SNV, Indels, and CNAs, the validation cohort should constitute samples that harbor these representative types of genomic alterations. Importantly, the variants in each category should predominantly be clinically significant rather than benign variants. From a bioinformatics pipeline standpoint, the categorization of the variant types is influenced by the algorithm(s) used for detecting them. If a subset of complex Indels requires the use of specialized algorithms outside of a general-purpose variant caller, then such a set of complex variants should be categorized separately when constructing the validation cohort. Internal tandem duplication (ITD) variants seen in FLT3 (**Fig. 5**) and BCOR genes are typical examples of such complex variants. The sequence characteristic of a region of the human genome can also impact the performance characteristics of the pipeline and therefore variants, regardless of the type, should be included in the validation cohort if such variants are expected to be detected in clinical testing. Low complexity regions of the genome that are GC rich (*TERT* promoter, *CEBPA*) tend to sequence poorly, resulting in reduced sensitivity for the detection of all variant types,

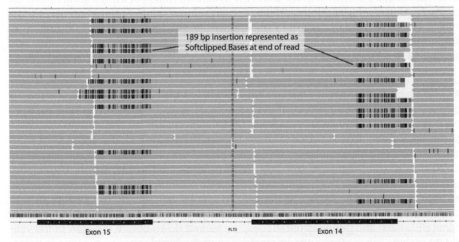

Fig. 5. Integrated Genome Viewer (IGV) snapshot demonstrates the sequence pileup in the region of exons 14 and 15 of the *FLT3* gene that harbors a 189 bp internal tandem duplication (ITD) variant. Multiple reads demonstrate soft clipped reads at one of the ends (multicolor bars) due to the largely duplicated sequence mismatching with the reference genome. Only specialized variant calling algorithms can correctly identify such large Indels using the soft clipped sequences and other relevant information from these reads.

including SNVs as well as increased possibility of false-positive variant calls (**Figs. 6**). The AMP validation guidelines recommend that an appropriate minimum number of variants, based on desired confidence and reliability, for each variant type must be part of the validation cohort to validate the bioinformatics pipeline. The readers are encouraged to refer to the AMP guidelines for further details of the mathematical approach to determine the minimum sample/variant cohort size.[1,11]

The sample matrix, such as fresh tissue, peripheral blood, formalin-fixed paraffin-embedded tissue (FFPE), and body fluids, should also be considered when determining the performance characteristics of the bioinformatics pipeline based on the sample types to be expected during clinical testing. Certain sample types may contain PCR inhibitors, such as bile and melanin pigment, that may result in a lower-than-expected depth of coverage and the bioinformatics pipeline should be validated to ensure that the performance characteristics of the pipeline are not compromised for such sample types. In other sample types, such as pancreatic cyst fluids, the number of neoplastic cells is inherently low resulting in lower input nucleic acid and potentially variant with VAF less than 10%. If such samples are expected to be tested using the NGS assay, the bioinformatics pipeline should be validated for such sample types.[11]

Many of the complex or challenging variants, including Indels, SVs (Structural Variants), and fusions, are rare and difficult to procure for a validation cohort in sufficient numbers. In such scenarios, in silico variants introduced into sequence data generated from real samples can be used to augment the validation of the bioinformatics pipeline. However, it is important to remember that in silico approach should only be used for supplementing rare and challenging variants rather than constitute most of the validation cohort.[1]

Limits of detection
When validating an NGS test, it is critical to establish a lower limit of detection based on the assay design, sequencing chemistry, bioinformatics pipeline configuration,

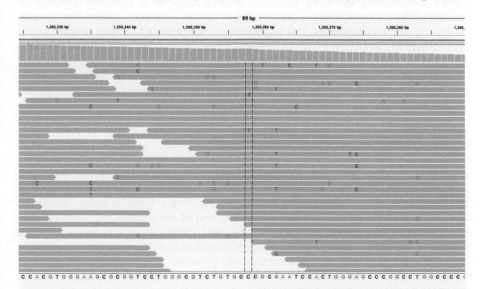

Fig. 6. IGV snapshot of the region of the *TERT* promoter sequence. Note the GC rich sequence that leads to multiple random mismatches and propensity for a high rate of false-positive variant calls.

variant, and sample types expected to be sequenced during clinical testing. The lower limits of detection (LOD) for an NGS test includes the lowest sequencing read depth at which a variant can be reliably identified and the lowest VAF that a variant can be consistently identified given a read depth threshold.[1] This is particularly important when validating the bioinformatics pipeline for tumor sequencing as it is not uncommon to expect variants present in tumor samples at VAF less than 10% often due to the low proportion of tumor cells in a sample or clonal heterogeneity within the tumor. In addition, the presence of inhibitory substances such as bile pigments, melanin, and necrotic tissue, can result in lower than expected or variable read depth across the sequenced regions. When establishing the lower LOD of detection for NGS assay, the validation cohort should include variants with VAF at or near the limits of detection.[1,11] This can be achieved by either sequencing samples that natively harbor desired variants at low VAF or using diluting the sample containing the variants of interest with genomic DNA from a nonneoplastic sample or reference material. Similarly, dilution studies to decrease the starting input DNA for NGS assay should be performed to establish the lower LOD for the read depth. In some cases, read depth LOD analysis can additionally be performed using in silico approach by random down-sampling of sequencing reads from a BAM file.

Somatic next-generation sequencing test results

Variant nomenclature. Variant nomenclature is an essential part of a clinical report and represents the fundamental element of a molecular test result. The Human Genome Variation Society (HGVS) variant nomenclature system is the de-facto representation of sequence variants in a clinical report, which is universally accepted as a standard by laboratory accreditation agencies and understood by molecular professionals, clinicians, and medical genetics professionals.[14] The synthesis of this nomenclature for variants identified by NGS testing requires a complex process of conversion of the coordinate system from the human reference genome to specific cDNA and protein transcripts. The alignment of the transcripts to the forward or the reverse genomic DNA strands and the HGVS 3′rule for variants in repeat sequence regions add additional complexity to the process. There are several annotation tools (open source and commercial) available that can generate HGVS nomenclature. However, they may render inconsistent HGVS nomenclature and therefore require the laboratory to optimize and validate for clinical use.[14,15]

Variant identification and manipulation. The ability to detect sequence variants determines the performance characteristics of a bioinformatics pipeline and the overall NGS assay. Several aspects of the pipeline can impact the performance characteristics, and therefore the components of the pipeline must be carefully reviewed and validated to ensure acceptable sensitivity of variant detection. During a validation of an NGS assay, it is challenging to estimate a pipeline's false-negative rate accurately. The identification of phased variants is one of the challenges. For example, EGFR in-frame variants in exon 19, which render tumors sensitive to tyrosine kinase inhibitors, are often identified as multiple variants that can be a variable combination of SNVs and Indels (**Fig. 7**). Such horizontally complex variants represent a haplotype, whereby the individual variants (primitives) are in-phase, that is, present on the same contiguous sequencing reads.[1] The correct identification of complex variants is vital for accurate clinical reporting and follow-up molecular testing on tumor relapse, including minimal residual disease (MRD) testing. Only some of the newer variant calling algorithms are haplotype-aware (eg, Mutect2,[16] VarDict,[17] Strelka2[18])

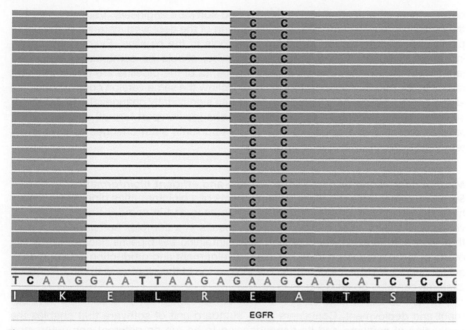

Fig. 7. IGV snapshot of the region of *EGFR* exon 19 from a lung adenocarcinoma sample demonstrates a horizontally complex variant. The primitive variant calls (1 deletion and 2 SNVs) are separated by a single nucleotide but are in phase, that is, all primitives are on the same reads. The most appropriate method is to report this finding as a single haplotype variant, instead of 3 separate variants in the clinical report.

and therefore, the clinical laboratories should carefully review their variant calling algorithms during the O&F and validation phases. VarGrouper is a software tool that was developed to primarily address the limitation of variant calling algorithms without haplotype-aware variant detection features.[19]

Another contributor to the pool of false-negative (missed) variants is the process of in silico masking targeted NGS panels. Clinical laboratories often mask a portion of an NGS panel to report a subset of genes on the panel. This approach is optimal for assay maintenance and is cost-effective. The process of masking involves the use of tools that intersect a variant call file with a BED (Browser Extensible Data) file that defines the regions of interest of the smaller reportable panel. The typical but undesirable behavior of some of these algorithms results in an empty but perfectly valid VCF file when the input BED file is missing instead of throwing an error. Consequently, for clinical testing, accidently missing a BED file due to inconsistent transfer from development to the production environment may silently produce false-negative results and significantly impact patient care. It is, therefore, prudent that the bioinformatics pipeline is designed to handle such intrinsic algorithm behavior and alert the end-user to unexpected results in clinical testing.

Version control
Version control is another important consideration when implementing the bioinformatics pipeline. Version control can be enforced using various software frameworks, such as git, mercurial, and source control, among others. These tools enable not only systematic management of the pipeline source code but also allow collaborative

development by a team of bioinformatics and software engineers. Version control of the pipeline should include semantic versioning of the deployed instance of the entire pipeline as well as the individual software tools in the pipeline. Every deployment, including an update to the production pipeline, should be semantically versioned (eg, v1.2.2 to v1.8.1). If one or more components of the pipeline are developed and managed by the clinical laboratory, it should follow the same version control principles as the entire pipeline. As pipeline upgrade often significantly changes the NGS test results (eg, ability to detect new variant types, change in report format) and the clinical report content, it is a good practice to communicate such changes to the clinical teams and clients, whenever appropriate.

Modern information technology for scalable and efficient bioinformatics

Software containers. The multiple components of a bioinformatics pipeline frequently have dependencies on different software runtimes and in some instances, different versions of the same software. This often results in a complex software ecosystem that results in unnecessary overhead for maintaining the pipeline, lack of portability of the pipeline, inconsistencies between development and production environments, and an increased chance of errors. The integration of the pipeline with other software systems can also be challenging.

Software container technology has revolutionized the practice of software development and deployment. Containers are a standard unit of software that enables the packaging of software and its dependencies to be run on different computers and operating systems with virtually no configuration changes. Unlike virtual machines (VM), containers are a lightweight Linux operating system process that can isolate the software running inside the container from all other running applications on the computer, allowing portability and avoiding software conflicts. As containers are typically small software units, they can be instantiated very quickly to execute a specific task. While web applications are the most common use case, with appropriate design considerations, containers can help streamline the development and deployment of the bioinformatics pipeline and enable portability across different IT platforms in health care systems and the cloud.[20] A recent study demonstrated the distinct advantage of using containers for the bioinformatics pipeline such that NGS data analyzed on various IT infrastructures and with different workflow managers produced the same results.[21] Containers support versioning and therefore help implement version control for the bioinformatics pipeline. Containers are available in different open-source projects such as Docker, Singularity, Podman, and LXC. Docker containers are the most popular and widely used general-purpose application containers. Singularity containers are designed specifically for bioinformatics applications on HPC systems.[22]

Containers can provide a framework for a distributive architecture of the bioinformatics pipeline, whereby each step of the pipeline is provisioned into a container or application service. This enables scalability and modularity in the bioinformatics pipeline. An individual component of the pipeline can be updated in isolation without impacting other components, resulting in more focused and efficient revalidation strategies. Similarly, different pipeline components can be horizontally scaled (increasing the number of containers) to remove performance bottlenecks in the pipeline.[20] A sophisticated software application that is deployed using several containers is typically managed in a production environment using container orchestration platforms such as Kubernetes, Mesos, Docker Swarm, or a cloud vendor-specific framework.

Automation. The lifecycle of pipeline development, testing, and deployment to production infrastructure is a complicated task. Any upgrades to the pipeline must be revalidated to ensure the expected behavior of the intended changes and no unintended impact on test results. Manual testing and validation of updates to the bioinformatics pipeline is time-consuming and, in some instances, inconsistent. Automation in managing bioinformatics resources and workflows helps with streamlining day-to-day bioinformatics operations. The advantages of automation include more thorough and consistent enforcement of validation policies, regular testing, and validation of pipeline upgrades, standardized version control, and codebase integration. Documentation of the results from each of the steps in the lifecycle of pipeline development is critical for compliance with clinical laboratory regulations. For example, the audit trail of codebase changes and pipeline upgrades, including the identity of the bioinformatic team member, should be documented to allow systematic troubleshooting in the event of software malfunction or unintended impact on NGS test results. Automation, coupled with appropriate logging, can help generate the necessary documentation and audit trail. Pipeline development and deployment automation can provide support for upgrades to clinical production systems with minimal impact on ongoing laboratory operations, including rollback in the instance of failed updates. Finally, an important use case of automation is the real-time monitoring of deployed bioinformatics pipelines in production. Edge-case scenarios related to the nature of sequencing data or unexpected changes in the deployment environment can significantly, often silently, impact NGS test results. In such scenarios, continuous monitoring and automated alert mechanisms are important to avert unanticipated downtimes and erroneous test results.[20] These advantages of automation come along with the burden of the time for the initial setup of the infrastructure and learning curve of the bioinformatics team with automation tools. Therefore, automation should be strategically planned by the laboratory, depending on the available bioinformatics resources, IT infrastructure, and bioinformatics personnel.

SUMMARY

In summary, the article highlighted various practical considerations and strategies for developing robust bioinformatics infrastructure in a clinical laboratory. Laboratory directors need to consider a multidisciplinary approach when developing bioinformatics resources. Key stakeholders should include clinical, laboratory, and hospital informatics teams, cloud and/or system architects, molecular pathologists, laboratory personnel, and the laboratory quality assurance team. It is essential to understand that building a robust bioinformatics infrastructure requires staff with expertise and training in bioinformatics and software engineering, strategic planning, and phased implementation including validation and version control before clinical testing is performed. Additionally, the use of container technology can be incorporated in the development and deployment of the bioinformatics pipeline either at the beginning or phased to a later stage, based on the size of the bioinformatics team, and the availability of relevant expertise and resources.

CLINICS CARE POINTS

- Bioinformatics pipeline performance impacts the overall accuracy of the NGS test result that has direct impact on clinical care of patients.
- Validation of the NGS bioinformatics pipeline as part of the end-to-end assay validation is critical.

- Validation cohort should consist of variants that are representative of sample types, different genomic regions, and variant complexity that is exected during routine clinical testing.

- The clincial report of an NGS test should indicate the limits of detection of the assay for important variant types as well as other limitations of the assay, including those due to the bioinformatics pipeline, that can result in reduced variant detection sensitivity.

DISCLOSURE

The author has nothing to disclose.

REFERENCES

1. Roy S, Coldren C, Karunamurthy A, et al. Standards and guidelines for validating next-generation sequencing bioinformatics pipelines: a joint recommendation of the Association for Molecular Pathology and the College of American Pathologists. J Mol Diagn 2018;20:4–27.
2. Wang X, Liotta L. Clinical bioinformatics: a new emerging science. J Clin Bioinforma 2011;1:1.
3. Mantere T, Kersten S, Hoischen A. Long-read sequencing emerging in medical genetics. Front Genet 2019;10:426.
4. Roy S, LaFramboise WA, Nikiforov YE, et al. Next-generation sequencing informatics: challenges and strategies for implementation in a clinical environment. Arch Pathol Lab Med 2016;140:958–75.
5. Hsi-Yang Fritz M, Leinonen R, Cochrane G, et al. Efficient storage of high throughput DNA sequencing data using reference-based compression. Genome Res 2011;21:734–40.
6. Kadri S. Advances in next-generation sequencing bioinformatics for clinical diagnostics: taking precision oncology to the next level. Adv Mol Pathol 2018;1: 149–66.
7. Abel HJ, Duncavage EJ. Detection of structural DNA variation from next generation sequencing data: a review of informatic approaches. Cancer Genet 2013; 206:432–40.
8. Kirchner M, Neumann O, Volckmar AL, et al. RNA-based detection of gene fusions in formalin-fixed and paraffin-embedded solid cancer samples. Cancers (Basel) 2019;11.
9. Sun L, McNulty SN, Evenson MJ, et al. Clinical implications of a targeted RNA-sequencing panel in the detection of gene fusions in solid tumors. J Mol Diagn 2021;23:1749–60.
10. Lubin IM, Aziz N, Babb LJ, et al. Principles and recommendations for standardizing the use of the next-generation sequencing variant file in clinical settings. J Mol Diagn 2017;19:417–26.
11. Jennings LJ, Arcila ME, Corless C, et al. Guidelines for validation of next-generation sequencing-based oncology panels: a joint Consensus recommendation of the Association for Molecular Pathology and College of American Pathologists. J Mol Diagn 2017;19:341–65.
12. Leipzig J. A review of bioinformatic pipeline frameworks. Brief Bioinform 2017;18: 530–6.
13. Fjukstad B, Bongo LA. A review of scalable bioinformatics pipelines. Data Sci Eng 2017;2:245–51.

14. Callenberg KM, Santana-Santos L, Chen L, et al. Clinical implementation and validation of automated human genome variation society (HGVS) nomenclature system for next-generation sequencing-based assays for cancer. J Mol Diagn 2018; 20:628–34.
15. Yen JL, Garcia S, Montana A, et al. A variant by any name: quantifying annotation discordance across tools and clinical databases. Genome Med 2017;9:7.
16. Van der Auwera GA, O'Connor BD. Genomics in the cloud: using Docker, GATK, and WDL in Terra. 1st edition. Sebastopol: O'Reilly Media; 2020.
17. Lai Z, Markovets A, Ahdesmaki M, et al. VarDict: a novel and versatile variant caller for next-generation sequencing in cancer research. Nucleic Acids Res 2016; 44:e108.
18. Kim S, Scheffler K, Halpern AL, et al. Strelka2: fast and accurate calling of germline and somatic variants. Nat Methods 2018;15:591–4.
19. Schmidt RJ, Macleay A, Le LP. VarGrouper: a bioinformatic tool for local haplotyping of deletion-insertion variants from next-generation sequencing data after variant calling. J Mol Diagn 2019;21:384–9.
20. Kadri S, Sboner A, Sigaras A, et al. Containers in bioinformatics: applications, practical considerations, and best practices in molecular pathology. J Mol Diagn 2022;24(5):442–54.
21. Kadri S, Roy S. Platform-agnostic deployment of bioinformatics pipelines for clinical NGS assays using containers, infrastructure orchestration, and workflow manager (Abstract #I031). J Mol Diagn 2019;21:1119–249.
22. Kurtzer GM, Sochat V, Bauer MW. Singularity: scientific containers for mobility of compute. PLoS One 2017;12:e0177459.

Best Practice for Clinical Somatic Variant Interpretation and Reporting

Jeffrey Schubert, PhD[a,1], Jinhua Wu, PhD[a,1], Marilyn M. Li, MD[a,b,c], Kajia Cao, PhD[a,*]

KEYWORDS

- Somatic variant classification • Reporting criteria • Variant oncogenicity
- Clinical impact

KEY POINTS

- A standardized system of classification for somatic variants is necessary to facilitate communication between laboratory professionals and clinicians as tumor sequencing becomes more common.
- A robust bioinformatics pipeline incorporating tools that can detect multiple variation events is needed to capture the diverse types of somatic alterations.
- Maintaining an internal variant database can streamline analysis efficiency by facilitating variant prioritization and classification.
- Thorough data analysis should combine interpretation of a variant's oncogenicity in addition to its predicted clinical impact in order to accurately classify it.

INTRODUCTION

During the past decade, there has been an increased push toward the development of precision cancer medicine, in hopes of tailoring treatments that effectively induce a therapeutic response based on the genomic profile of an individual's tumor.[1–3] Concurrently, there have been tremendous improvements in reducing cost and increasing the speed and capacity of next generation sequencing (NGS) technologies, as well as in the development of sophisticated bioinformatics tools. As NGS-based clinical tests have become more accessible and widely used, the amount of data generated has increased substantially.[4,5] Although tumor sequencing previously focused on variants in known hotspot regions, more recently these small targeted

[a] Division of Genomic Diagnostics, Department of Pathology & Laboratory Medicine, The Children's Hospital of Philadelphia, 3615 Civic Center boulevard, 706 ARC, Philadelphia, PA 19104, USA; [b] Perelman School of Medicine, University of Pennsylvania, Philadelphia, PA, USA; [c] Department of Pediatrics, Children's Hospital of Philadelphia, Philadelphia, PA, USA
[1] Contributed equally.
* Corresponding author.
E-mail address: CaoK@chop.edu

Clin Lab Med 42 (2022) 423–434
https://doi.org/10.1016/j.cll.2022.04.006
0272-2712/22/© 2022 Elsevier Inc. All rights reserved.

labmed.theclinics.com

hotspot panels are being replaced by much broader strategies, ranging from panels with hundreds of cancer-associated genes to much more open-ended methods such as whole genome sequencing, creating an explosion of cancer genomic data.[6,7] With such an increase in the breadth of tumor sequencing, it is now critical to have an efficient, reliable, and reproducible method of interpreting how a patient's variants may inform cancer care.

The 2017 Association for Molecular Pathology, American Society of Clinical Oncology, and College of American Pathologists (AMP/ASCO/CAP) standards and guidelines for the interpretation and reporting of sequence variants in cancer[8] are the first set of professional recommendations for laboratories to share a common system of somatic variant classification, similar to the American College of Medical Genetics and Genomics (ACMG)/AMP guidelines for constitutional variants.[9] A standardized and more universal approach is necessary to avoid inconsistencies in variant interpretation and reporting, as different clinical laboratories and institutions had established their own sets of standards with unique terminologies before the release of the 2017 guidelines.[10–12] Additionally, considering that specific genetic patterns or abnormalities are now included in official tumor classification and treatment guidelines,[13–15] it is increasingly important for laboratory professionals to share a common language with oncologists to accurately define the genetic context of a patient's tumor.

The 2017 AMP/ASCO/CAP guidelines proposed the following 4-tiered system of variant classification to serve as this common language: Tier I, variants of strong clinical significance; Tier II, variants of potential clinical significance; Tier III, variants of unknown clinical significance; and Tier IV, benign or likely benign variants. To assign the appropriate tier, the guidelines suggest using clinical and experimental evidence that would directly inform patient care or drive clinical decision-making. There are 4 proposed levels of evidence, A, B, C, and D, which have decreasing degrees of significance regarding 3 considerations on clinical impact: (1) therapeutic response or resistance, (2) diagnosis, and (3) prognosis. A visual representation and explanation of variant tiers and levels of evidence can be seen in **Fig. 1**.

At present, there are 329 PubMed citations of the 2017 guidelines, suggesting their increased implementation in laboratory settings.[16–18] However, it is important to recall the AMP/ASCO/CAP guidelines are the first set of professional standards for somatic variant interpretation, and their adoption into practice is still a work in progress. For example, interlaboratory surveys have demonstrated discordances in classification between participants asked to use the 2017 guidelines on sets of test variants, which were partly attributed to lack of practice or familiarity with the guidelines.[19,20] Individual clinical laboratories seeking to adopt the AMP/ASCO/CAP guidelines may benefit from comparing their previous classifications to new ones made with the 2017 guidelines; one group recently laid an elegant framework for using this strategy and demonstrated high concordance between classification methods while identifying factors that led to discordance.[21]

Ultimately, the 2017 guidelines should be used as a framework to meet both physician and laboratory needs and can be modified as necessary. For example, based on the high frequency of germline pathogenic variants identified in pediatric cancer patients, our laboratory refined classification of Tier I variants into Tier IA, somatic variants with A or B level evidence, and Tier IB, confirmed pathogenic/likely pathogenic germline variants. This review article will discuss the best practice for clinical somatic variant interpretation and reporting with a focus on (1) resources and tools for variant classification and interpretation, (2) basic bioinformatics pipelines for variant filtration, annotation, and prioritization, and (3) establishing an efficient variant classification and interpretation workflow.

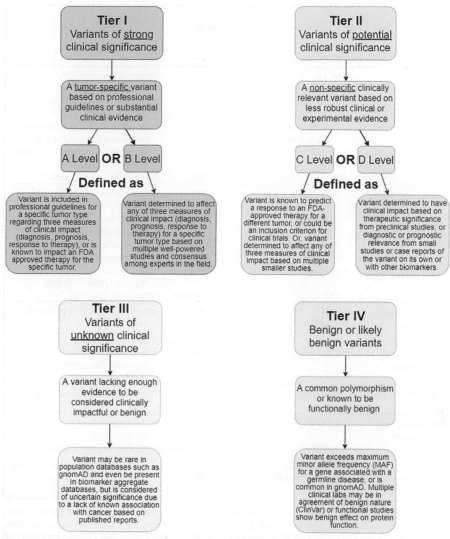

Fig. 1. Flow chart of tier and evidence-based classification for somatic variants based on 2017 AMP/ASCO/CAP guidelines. FDA, Food and Drug Administration.

RESOURCES AND TOOLS FOR SOMATIC VARIANT CLASSIFICATION AND INTERPRETATION

Familiarity and working knowledge of relevant tools and resources is necessary to properly analyze and classify somatic variation. **Table 1** contains a list of the most commonly used resources and tools, although it is by no means comprehensive. For more complete lists of resources that cover other areas such as *in silico* variant pathogenicity and splice site predictions, refer to prior guidelines.[8,9] When available, guidelines concerning diagnosis, prognosis, or treatment issued by professional organizations and workgroups should be used as primary sources of evidence for the assessment of a variant's clinical impact.[22,23]

Table 1
Tools and resources to aid in somatic variant interpretation

Function	Tool or Resource	Free Access	Link
Professional guidelines and related resources	NCCN	Yes	https://www.nccn.org/guidelines/category_1
	WHO classification online	No	https://tumourclassification.iarc.who.int/welcome
	FDA-approved therapies	Yes	https://www.cancer.gov/about-cancer/treatment/types/targeted-therapies/targeted-therapies-fact-sheet
	Clinical Trials	Yes	https://clinicaltrials.gov/
Cancer variant databases	COSMIC[28]	Yes	https://cancer.sanger.ac.uk/cosmic
	cBioPortal[29]	Yes	https://www.cbioportal.org/
	CIVIC[30]	Yes	https://civicdb.org/home
	TCGA	Yes	https://www.cancer.gov/tcga
	OncoKB[31]	Yes	https://www.oncokb.org/
	My Cancer Genome	Yes	https://www.mycancergenome.org/
	JAX CKB[32]	Limited	https://ckb.jax.org/
Cancer variant database aggregator	VICC Meta-Knowledgebase[25]	Yes	https://search.cancervariants.org/
Cancer variant interpreter	CGI[27]	Yes	https://www.cancergenomeinterpreter.org/home
Population database	gnomAD[33]	Yes	https://gnomad.broadinstitute.org/
General variant databases	ClinVar[34]	Yes	https://www.ncbi.nlm.nih.gov/clinvar/
	HGMD[35]	Limited	http://www.hgmd.cf.ac.uk/ac/index.php
Variant visualization and analysis	Alamut Visual	No	https://www.interactive-biosoftware.com/

Abbreviations: AD, genome aggregation database; CGI, cancer genome interpreter; gnom; CIVIC, clinical interpretation of variants in cancer; COSMIC, catalog of somatic mutations in cancer; FDA, Food and Drug Administration; HGMD, Human Gene Mutation Database; JAX CKB, Jackson Clinical Knowledgebase; NCCN, National Comprehensive Cancer Network; OncoKB, precision oncology knowledge base; TCGA, The Cancer Genome Atlas; VICC, the variant interpretation for cancer consortium; WHO, World Health Organization.

The included cancer variant databases (see **Table 1**) offer a wide range of information and summarize salient information from professional organizations, including gene and variant level associations with specific tumor types, response to Food and Drug Association (FDA)-approved therapies, clinical trial results, literature summaries, and more. Although many of these databases are curated, results should be critically interpreted because some of these databases also contain passenger or benign germline variants. Additionally, a variant may not be seen across all databases, which is why it is best practice to query at least 2, or use one that aggregates data from multiple sources, such as the Variant Interpretation for Cancer Consortium Meta-Knowledgebase.[24,25] With increasingly large datasets, it will also be useful to integrate information from these resources into bioinformatics tools and pipelines, allowing automatic identification of a list of clinically significant variants.[26,27]

BIOINFORMATICS TOOLS AND CLINICAL PIPELINES FOR SOMATIC VARIANT ANALYSIS

Because tumors often harbor diverse types of alterations in multiple different genes and/or genomic regions, NGS-based panels that target hundreds of genes to evaluate single nucleotide variants (SNVs)/small insertions or deletions (indels), copy number alterations (CNAs), and fusion genes have emerged to be a common choice for tumor testing. Further, the tumor sample can be sequenced together with normal tissue and the sequencing data can be merged to streamline somatic variant detection, evaluate tumor mutation burden and microsatellite instability, and identify potential germline pathogenic variants. Achieving these goals requires the knowledge of available bioinformatics tools and adequate application of these tools to build robust bioinformatics pipelines that are highly efficient, accurate, and reproducible for somatic variant detection.

Bioinformatics Tools for Variant Identification and Filtration

There are many choices of publicly available somatic variant callers for NGS data processing. For example, MuTect[28] provides highly sensitive SNV calls; Scalpel[29] aims at small deletions and indels; whereas, FreeBayes[30] and VarScan2[31] detect both SNVs and indels. Pindel,[32] however, offers the capability of detecting breakpoints of large-sized duplications enabling the identification of recurrent internal tandem duplications (ITDs). For somatic variant analysis, it is important to select the right tools to integrate into the bioinformatics pipelines based on the gene content of the panels and the variant types intended to be detected. This will require not only bioinformatics expertise but also knowledge about tumor biology and associated genes and mutations, emphasizing the importance of collaboration among bioinformaticians, oncologists, and molecular professionals.

Pros and Cons of Bioinformatics Approaches

Different from cancer research, where variants called by multiple callers are usually intersected to boost up the confidence of positive findings,[33] in clinical settings, the union of results from multiple callers is preferred to compensate the low concordance of different variant callers[34] and minimize the chance of missing potential positive findings. We studied 1847 tumor samples sequenced in our laboratory and found that 1.4% of samples harbor clinically significant variants that are uniquely called by only one caller, emphasizing that intersected approaches may miss variants critical for patient care.

This approach may lead to an overwhelming number of variants. Multiple levels of filtration can be built into the pipeline to remove unwanted variants. These include (1) variants with variant allele fraction (VAF) less than the detection limit of the test (ours is 3%), (2) sequencing artifacts, and (3) variants of no clinical significance such as rare polymorphisms. To effectively remove noise, laboratories should establish multiple laboratory-specific managed variant lists (MVLs), such as variants of clinical significance, artifacts, polymorphisms, and pseudogenes. These MVLs can be built into the bioinformatic pipeline to automatically retain clinically significant variants and eliminate unwanted noise. For example, our laboratory uses a machine learning-based method, named aiQC, to distinguish bona fide SNVs from artifacts/pseudogenes with 99.3% sensitivity and 100% specificity using MVLs collected from hundreds of tumors sequenced in our laboratory.[35]

SOMATIC VARIANT CLASSIFICATION AND INTERPRETATION

Cancers often harbor multiple somatic variants and multiple types of genomic alterations. Additionally, different tumors may carry the same mutations with similar or different clinical significance, making somatic variant classification and interpretation much more challenging than germline variant interpretation. Somatic variant analysis includes evaluating variant oncogenicity and clinical impact. Oncogenicity evaluation includes gene-tumor associations, variant-tumor associations, types of variants (SNVs, indels, frameshift, splicing, CNAs, or fusions) and functional effects (gain or loss of function). The clinical impact of variants comprises therapeutic implication, diagnostic influence, and prognostic significance, as well as the strength of the impact. Tumor sequencing may uncover germline variants associated with cancer predisposition. Presumed germline pathogenic variants, if confirmed germline via tumor/normal paired analysis or targeted germline confirmation, should be classified based on the ACMG/AMP guidelines for germline variant interpretation.[8]

The Oncogenicity of Somatic Variants

Genes that contain mutations causally implicated in cancer are referred to as cancer genes, and their dysfunction drives cancer development and progression.[36–38] The Cancer Gene Census (CGC) is an ongoing effort to catalog cancer genes. Genes in the CGC are divided into 2 tiers: tier 1, genes that possess a documented activity relevant to cancer, along with evidence of mutations in cancer that change the activity of the gene product in a way that promotes oncogenic transformation and tier 2, genes with strong indications of having a role in cancer but with less extensive available evidence. The current version of CGC (v94) contains 723 cancer genes with 576 classified as tier 1 and 147 tier 2. Of these, 90% contain somatic mutations in cancer, 20% display germline mutations that predispose an individual to cancer, and 10% show both somatic and germline mutations (https://cancer.sanger.ac.uk/cosmic/census?tier=2).[39,40] A cancer gene may be causally implicated in multiple different tumors and a given cancer can be associated with mutations in multiple genes.

The oncogenicity of a somatic variant depends on its effect on the protein. A variant can lead to gain of function (activation) of an oncogene, resulting in a protein with increased function or the acquisition of a different function. Alternatively, a variant can lead to loss of function of a tumor suppressor, resulting in the loss of the protein or one that suppresses normal protein function, which is also known as dominant negative.[41] Most gain-of-function variants are missense or in-frame indels in protein functional domains, resulting in autophosphorylation of the protein, which dysregulates downstream signaling pathways leading to uncontrolled cell growth and proliferation.[42] Another type of gain-of-function mutation, including some of TP53 mutations, changes the protein function and promotes a cell proliferative effect.[43] Intragenic alterations, including ITDs,[44,45] kinase domain duplications,[46–48] or skipping,[49] is often activating mutations. Other types of gain-of-function mutations include gene amplifications and fusion genes. Gene amplifications lead to increased gene expression and protein production.[50] Fusion genes are often oncogenic through the elimination of the autosuppressor of the protein kinase or promoter/enhancer hijacking.[51,52] Conversely, mutations in tumor suppressor genes are often loss-of-function mutations, including nonsense, frameshift indels, and splice-site mutations, giving rise to a truncated protein. CNAs that delete or disrupt tumor suppressor genes are also common loss-of-function changes that often present as a second hit, leading to loss of heterozygosity.

Clinical laboratories should set up a system for somatic variant oncogenicity evaluation. According to the AMP/ASCO/CAP somatic variant interpretation guidelines, our laboratory established a laboratory standard procedure for somatic variant oncogenicity evaluation, which includes assessing the quality of the variant, VAF, the location of the variant in the protein, the presence and the frequency of the variant in the general population databases and germline or somatic mutation databases, variant functional prediction, and literature search. To determine if a variant is true or false, we implemented the aiQC system in our bioinformatics pipeline. aiQC uses machine learning tools to create an algorithm based on multiple variant features from approximately 12,000 manually curated variants.[35] aiQC automatically labels each variant true or false. When a variant is labeled false, it will be marked as artifact, polymorphism, or pseudogene.

VAF, in combination with tumor content and CNAs, can help to determine if a variant is somatic or germline and the size of the tumor cell clone. The presence and frequency of a variant in general population databases can help determine whether it is a benign polymorphism. Further, the presence and frequency of a variant in germline or somatic variant databases provides evidence regarding whether the variant is likely germline or somatic, recurrent or rare, or is located in a mutation hotspot. The location of a variant in an important functional domain increases the odds of it being oncogenic. Functional studies provide experimental evidence of oncogenicity. However, the type of the study (such as in vivo vs in vitro) and the reproducibility of the assays used should be considered to determine the strength of the evidence.[8]

The classification of CNAs and fusions is quite different from SNVs/indels. If a CNA involves a single gene, then considering gene function only could be sufficient; however, CNAs are often observed in multiple chromosomes in a specific pattern; for example, a high-hyperdiploid genome with gains of multiple specific chromosomes in pediatric B-lymphoblastic leukemia is diagnostic for B-lymphoblastic leukemia/lymphoma (B-ALL) with hyperdiploidy and is associated with a favorable prognosis.[53] Fusion genes are often oncogenic drivers, therefore, the function of the chimeric oncoprotein is critical in the classification of fusions. For instance, although the 5'-partner genes may vary, the 3'-partners of oncogenic neurotrophic tyrosine receptor kinase (NTRK) fusions always retain the tropomyosin receptor kinase domains of TRK-A, TRK-B, and TRK-C.[54] As mentioned earlier, promoter hijacking that dramatically increases the expression of the gene is another common oncogenic mechanism of fusion genes. The *P2RY8::CRLF2* fusion, for example, leads to *CRLF2* overexpression through juxtaposition of *CRLF2* to the promoter of *P2RY8*.[55]

Clinical Impact of Somatic Variants

The clinical impact of somatic variants can be categorized into 3 areas, prediction of responses to targeted therapies, diagnosis of a specific type or subtype of tumor, and stratification of patient risk and disease outcomes.

Somatic variants in tumors may predict the response or resistance to specific therapies. These therapies may be biomarker-based. For example, *BRAF^V600E* predicts response to the US FDA-approved BRAF-inhibitor vemurafenib in melanoma.[56] NTRK fusion-positive patients may be treated with FDA-approved TRK inhibitors larotrectinib or entrectinib.[56] Response to therapies could also be risk-based. For example, *ETV6::RUNX1* fusion in B-ALL predicts an excellent response to standard risk chemotherapy for B-ALL. Somatic variants can also be biomarkers for diagnosing specific tumors or tumor subtypes. For example, *PML::RARA* fusion is pathognomonic for promyelocytic leukemia.[57] In many tumors, somatic variants are required as part of the diagnostic criteria. In juvenile myelomonocytic leukemia, in addition to hematological findings, the presence of somatic variants in *PTPN11*, *KRAS* or *NRAS*, or monosomy 7 is part of the requirement for diagnosis.[58] Somatic variants

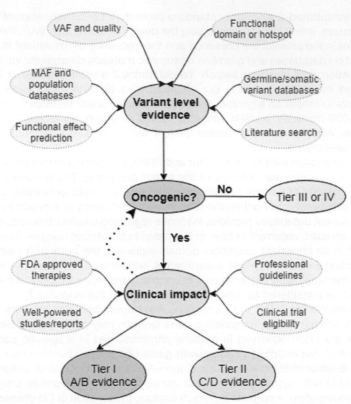

Fig. 2. When classifying a new variant, many lines of evidence (dotted-lined ovals) are collected to determine potential oncogenicity (see **Table 1** for resources). A variant's effect (gain or loss of function) should be considered in the context of the gene (oncogene vs tumor suppressor) and tumor type. Nononcogenic variants may be classified as Tier III or IV. Further information (see **Fig. 1**) is needed to determine the strength of the clinical impact (Tier I vs II) based on available evidence (A/B vs C/D). The dotted-line arrow represents that variant level evidence is not always necessary to demonstrate oncogenicity; for example, variants with a known response to FDA-approved therapies would automatically be considered Tier I. FDA, Food and Drug Administration; MAF, minor allele frequency; VAF, variant allele fraction.

may carry prognostic significance and can be used to stratify patient risk. The importance of stratifying a patient's risk is to determine the best treatment strategy for the patient avoiding overtreatment or undertreatment. For instance, *BCR::ABL1* fusions are associated with a poor prognosis in B-ALL, which is essential in determining therapeutic regimens.[59]

The strength of evidence for the clinical impact of a variant should also be evaluated. Biomarkers that predict responses to FDA-approved drugs or those listed in professional guidelines for diagnosis, prognosis, or treatment decision-making bear the highest strength (level A or B). In addition to World Health Organization or National Comprehensive Cancer Network guidelines, guidelines from specific professional groups, such as Children's Oncology Group and disease-specific workgroups, like International Working Group for the Prognosis of MDS, also publish biomarker-based disease-specific guidelines. Somatic variants, which lead to off-label use of FDA-approved therapies or qualify for clinical trials for investigative drugs or therapies are weaker evidence, level C or D, depending on the stage of clinical trials. The determination of the strength of diagnostic/prognostic significance can be subjective if not specifically listed in the professional guidelines and may require the integration of variant oncogenicity and clinical impact based on thorough database and literature search.

Integrated Genomic Variant Classification

Somatic variant classification should integrate the oncogenicity with the clinical impact of the variant. However, highly oncogenic variants, such as a *TP53* mutation, may not have the strongest clinical impact in some tumors, and alternatively a noncausal alteration, such as high tumor mutation burden, may have a strong clinical impact due to its therapeutic implications. In general, the known clinical impact of a variant outweighs its strength of oncogenicity but the oncogenicity of a variant weighs more when its clinical impact is unclear. These considerations could be built into variant analysis procedures to streamline processes and increase efficiency, a comprehensive somatic variant classification workflow is illustrated in **Fig. 2**.

FUNDING

This research is partially supported by Department of Pathology and Laboratory Medicine at the Children's Hospital of Philadelphia.

SUMMARY

Because the clinical impact of cancer genomics is being increasingly recognized, tumor sequencing will likely continue to expand in breadth and scope. Therefore, it is vital for laboratory professionals to adopt the AMP/ASCO/CAP guidelines and create a standardized system of classification and nomenclature for somatic variants. Combining robust bioinformatics pipelines with thorough data analysis is necessary to efficiently and reproducibly identify and assess the impact of clinically relevant variants. Following the recommendations listed here and within the AMP/ASCO/CAP guidelines will allow physicians and laboratories to share a common language when reporting the impact of somatic variants on diagnosis, prognosis, or treatment of a tumor.

REFERENCES

1. Forrest SJ, Geoerger B, Janeway KA. Precision medicine in pediatric oncology. Curr Opin Pediatr 2018;30(1):17–24.
2. Sicklick JK, Kato S, Okamura R, et al. Molecular profiling of cancer patients enables personalized combination therapy: the I-PREDICT study. Nat Med 2019; 25(5):744–50.
3. Tsimberidou AM, Fountzilas E, Nikanjam M, et al. Review of precision cancer medicine: Evolution of the treatment paradigm. Cancer Treat Rev 2020;86: 102019.
4. van Dijk EL, Auger H, Jaszczyszyn Y, et al. Ten years of next-generation sequencing technology. Trends Genet 2014;30(9):418–26.
5. Wong KC. Big data challenges in genome informatics. Biophys Rev 2019; 11(1):51–4.
6. ITP-CAoWG Consortium. Pan-cancer analysis of whole genomes. Nature 2020; 578(7793):82–93.

7. Sabour L, Sabour M, Ghorbian S. Clinical applications of next-generation sequencing in cancer diagnosis. Pathol Oncol Res 2017;23(2):225–34.

8. Li MM, Datto M, Duncavage EJ, et al. Standards and guidelines for the interpretation and reporting of sequence variants in cancer: a joint consensus recommendation of the association for molecular Pathology, American Society of clinical oncology, and College of American Pathologists. J Mol Diagn 2017; 19(1):4–23.

9. Richards S, Aziz N, Bale S, et al. Standards and guidelines for the interpretation of sequence variants: a joint consensus recommendation of the American College of medical genetics and genomics and the association for molecular Pathology. Genet Med 2015;17(5):405–24.

10. Cottrell CE, Al-Kateb H, Bredemeyer AJ, et al. Validation of a next-generation sequencing assay for clinical molecular oncology. J Mol Diagn 2014;16(1): 89–105.

11. Sukhai MA, Craddock KJ, Thomas M, et al. A classification system for clinical relevance of somatic variants identified in molecular profiling of cancer. Genet Med 2016;18(2):128–36.

12. Van Allen EM, Wagle N, Stojanov P, et al. Whole-exome sequencing and clinical interpretation of formalin-fixed, paraffin-embedded tumor samples to guide precision cancer medicine. Nat Med 2014;20(6):682–8.

13. Krzyszczyk P, Acevedo A, Davidoff EJ, et al. The growing role of precision and personalized medicine for cancer treatment. Technology (Singap World Sci) 2018;6(3–4):79–100.

14. Louis DN, Perry A, Reifenberger G, et al. The 2016 World Health organization classification of tumors of the Central Nervous system: a summary. Acta Neuropathol 2016;131(6):803–20.

15. Zhong Y, Xu F, Wu J, et al. Application of next generation sequencing in laboratory medicine. Ann Lab Med 2021;41(1):25–43.

16. Nie Q, Hsiao MC, Chandok H, et al. Molecular profiling of CNS tumors for the treatment and management of disease. J Clin Neurosci 2020;71:311–5.

17. Özdoğan M, Papadopoulou E, Tsoulos N, et al. Comprehensive tumor molecular profile analysis in clinical practice. BMC Med Genomics 2021;14(1):105.

18. Surrey LF, MacFarland SP, Chang F, et al. Clinical utility of custom-designed NGS panel testing in pediatric tumors. Genome Med 2019;11(1):32.

19. Gao P, Zhang R, Li Z, et al. Challenges of providing concordant interpretation of somatic variants in non-small cell Lung cancer: a Multicenter study. J Cancer 2019;10(8):1814–24.

20. Sirohi D, Schmidt RL, Aisner DL, et al. Multi-institutional evaluation of Interrater Agreement of variant classification based on the 2017 association for molecular Pathology, American Society of clinical oncology, and College of American Pathologists standards and guidelines for the interpretation and reporting of sequence variants in cancer. J Mol Diagn 2020;22(2):284–93.

21. Parikh BA, Love-Gregory L, Duncavage EJ, et al. Identification of challenges and a framework for implementation of the AMP/ASCO/CAP classification guidelines for reporting somatic variants. Pract Lab Med 2020;21:e00170.

22. Irwin MS, Naranjo A, Zhang FF, et al. Revised neuroblastoma risk classification system: a Report from the Children's oncology group. J Clin Oncol 2021. JCO2100278.

23. Lindeman NI, Cagle PT, Aisner DL, et al. Updated molecular testing guideline for the selection of Lung cancer patients for treatment with targeted tyrosine kinase inhibitors: Guideline from the College of American Pathologists, the International

association for the study of Lung cancer, and the association for molecular Pathology. Arch Pathol Lab Med 2018;142(3):321–46.

24. Banck H, Dugas M, MÜller-Tidow C, et al. Comparison of open-access databases for clinical variant interpretation in cancer: a Case study of MDS/AML. Cancer Genomics Proteomics 2021;18(2):157–66.

25. Wagner AH, Walsh B, Mayfield G, et al. A harmonized meta-knowledgebase of clinical interpretations of somatic genomic variants in cancer. Nat Genet 2020; 52(4):448–57.

26. He MM, Li Q, Yan M, et al. Variant Interpretation for Cancer (VIC): a computational tool for assessing clinical impacts of somatic variants. Genome Med 2019; 11(1):53.

27. Tamborero D, Rubio-Perez C, Deu-Pons J, et al. Cancer Genome Interpreter annotates the biological and clinical relevance of tumor alterations. Genome Med 2018;10(1):25.

28. Cibulskis K, Lawrence MS, Carter SL, et al. Sensitive detection of somatic point mutations in impure and heterogeneous cancer samples. Nat Biotechnol 2013; 31(3):213–9.

29. Fang H, Bergmann EA, Arora K, et al. Indel variant analysis of short-read sequencing data with Scalpel. Nat Protoc 2016;11(12):2529–48.

30. Garrison E, Marth G. Haplotype-based variant detection from short-read sequencing. arXiv preprint arXiv:12073907. 2012.

31. Koboldt DC, Zhang Q, Larson DE, et al. VarScan 2: somatic mutation and copy number alteration discovery in cancer by exome sequencing. Genome Res 2012;22(3):568–76.

32. Ye K, Schulz MH, Long Q, et al. Pindel: a pattern growth approach to detect break points of large deletions and medium sized insertions from paired-end short reads. Bioinformatics 2009;25(21):2865–71.

33. The I, of Whole TP-CA, Consortium G. Pan-cancer analysis of whole genomes. Nature 2020;578(7793):82.

34. Kroigard AB, Thomassen M, Laenkholm AV, et al. Evaluation of nine somatic variant callers for detection of somatic mutations in exome and targeted Deep sequencing data. PLoS One 2016;11(3):e0151664.

35. Wu C, Zhao X, Welsh M, et al. Using machine learning to identify true somatic variants from next-generation sequencing. Clin Chem 2020;66(1):239–46.

36. Futreal PA, Coin L, Marshall M, et al. A census of human cancer genes. Nat Rev Cancer 2004;4(3):177–83.

37. Sever R, Brugge JS. Signal transduction in cancer. Cold Spring Harb Perspect Med 2015;5(4).

38. Sondka Z, Bamford S, Cole CG, et al. The COSMIC Cancer Gene Census: describing genetic dysfunction across all human cancers. Nat Rev Cancer 2018;18(11):696–705.

39. Agnarsson BA, Jonasson JG, Bjornsdottir IB, et al. Inherited BRCA2 mutation associated with high grade breast cancer. Breast Cancer Res Treat 1998;47(2): 121–7.

40. Klein AP. Genetic susceptibility to pancreatic cancer. Mol Carcinog 2012;51(1): 14–24.

41. Goh AM, Coffill CR, Lane DP. The role of mutant p53 in human cancer. J Pathol 2011;223(2):116–26.

42. Du Z, Lovly CM. Mechanisms of receptor tyrosine kinase activation in cancer. Mol Cancer 2018;17(1):58.

43. van Oijen MG, Slootweg PJ. Gain-of-function mutations in the tumor suppressor gene p53. Clin Cancer Res 2000;6(6):2138–45.
44. Nakao M, Yokota S, Iwai T, et al. Internal tandem duplication of the flt3 gene found in acute myeloid leukemia. Leukemia 1996;10(12):1911–8.
45. Astolfi A, Fiore M, Melchionda F, et al. BCOR involvement in cancer. Epigenomics 2019;11(7):835–55.
46. Gallant JN, Sheehan JH, Shaver TM, et al. EGFR kinase domain duplication (EGFR-KDD) is a Novel oncogenic driver in Lung cancer that is clinically responsive to Afatinib. Cancer Discov 2015;5(11):1155–63.
47. Chen HY, Brady DC, Villanueva J. Double Trouble: kinase domain duplication as a new path to drug resistance. Pigment Cell Melanoma Res 2016;29(5):493–5.
48. Jones DT, Hutter B, Jager N, et al. Recurrent somatic alterations of FGFR1 and NTRK2 in pilocytic astrocytoma. Nat Genet 2013;45(8):927–32.
49. Heist RS, Shim HS, Gingipally S, et al. MET Exon 14 skipping in non-small cell Lung cancer. Oncologist 2016;21(4):481–6.
50. Dzieran J, Rodriguez Garcia A, Westermark UK, et al. MYCN-amplified neuroblastoma maintains an aggressive and undifferentiated phenotype by deregulation of estrogen and NGF signaling. Proc Natl Acad Sci U S A 2018;115(6): E1229–38.
51. Hecht JL, Aster JC. Molecular biology of Burkitt's lymphoma. J Clin Oncol 2000; 18(21):3707–21.
52. Jain P, Surrey LF, Straka J, et al. BRAF fusions in pediatric histiocytic neoplasms define distinct therapeutic responsiveness to RAF paradox breakers. Pediatr Blood Cancer 2021;68(6):e28933.
53. Sutcliffe MJ, Shuster JJ, Sather HN, et al. High concordance from independent studies by the Children's cancer group (CCG) and pediatric oncology group (POG) associating favorable prognosis with combined trisomies 4, 10, and 17 in children with NCI standard-risk B-precursor acute lymphoblastic leukemia: a Children's oncology group (COG) initiative. Leukemia 2005;19(5):734–40.
54. Cocco E, Scaltriti M, Drilon A. NTRK fusion-positive cancers and TRK inhibitor. therapy. Nat Rev Clin Oncol 2018;15(12):731–47.
55. Harvey RC, Mullighan CG, Chen IM, et al. Rearrangement of CRLF2 is associated with mutation of JAK kinases, alteration of IKZF1, Hispanic/Latino ethnicity, and a poor outcome in pediatric B-progenitor acute lymphoblastic leukemia. Blood 2010;115(26):5312–21.
56. Table of Pharmacogenomic biomarkers in drug labeling. 2021. Available at: https://www.fda.gov/drugs/science-and-research-drugs/table-pharmacogenomic-biomarkers-drug-labeling. Accessed September, 2021.
57. Zhang JW, Wang JY, Chen SJ, et al. Mechanisms of all-trans retinoic acid-induced differentiation of acute promyelocytic leukemia cells. J Biosci 2000; 25(3):275–84.
58. Locatelli F, Niemeyer CM. How I treat juvenile myelomonocytic leukemia. Blood 2015;125(7):1083–90.
59. Taylor J, Xiao W, Abdel-Wahab O. Diagnosis and classification of hematologic malignancies on the basis of genetics. Blood 2017;130(4):410–23.

Molecular Detection of Oncogenic Gene Rearrangements

Zehra Ordulu, MD[a,b], Valentina Nardi, MD[b,*]

KEYWORDS

- Fusion • Rearrangement • Cytogenetics • FISH • Sequencing • Molecular testing
- Fusion detection

KEY POINTS

- Detection of oncogenic rearrangements has a pivotal role for the diagnosis and treatment of multiple cancer types. Therefore, understanding the advantages and limitations of each molecular technology used for detection of gene rearrangements becomes fundamental for precision medicine.
- Gene rearrangements can be detected with DNA, RNA, and protein-based technologies that range from conventional cytogenetics to high-throughput sequencing and immunohistochemistry.
- The optimal method for gene fusion detection usually depends on the clinical scenario. A high-throughput comprehensive method such as massively parallel sequencing might be desirable if there is limited material for a tumor with an unknown oncogenic driver, whereas a rapid single gene assay such as RT-PCR may be sufficient for cases with high a priori clinical suspicion.

INTRODUCTION

The description of the first gene rearrangements goes back to the 1980s,[1,2] approximately a decade after the discovery of chromosome banding.[3] Since then, advances in molecular technologies for the detection of oncogenic gene rearrangements have revolutionized the field of precision medicine in a range of different clinical settings, from assisting diagnosis to targeted therapy options for many tumor types. The functional consequence of gene rearrangements is production of a chimeric protein or deregulation of the involved genes. These consequences result from structural DNA

There are no commercial or financial conflicts of interest for either of the authors.

[a] Department of Pathology, Immunology and Laboratory Medicine, University of Florida, Box 100275, Gainesville, FL 32610, USA; [b] Department of Pathology, Massachusetts General Hospital, Harvard Medical School, Boston, MA, USA

* Corresponding author. Department of Pathology, Massachusetts General Hospital, Warren 219, 55 Fruit street, Boston, MA 02114.

E-mail address: Vnardi@partners.org

changes, such as translocations, inversions, and even copy number alterations (eg, gene deletions) (**Fig. 1**), as opposed to single nucleotide variants commonly referred to as mutations. In fact, it has been recently recommended that gene fusions should be described with a double colon (::) separator (eg, *BCR::ABL1*)[4] akin to the International System for Human Cytogenetic Nomenclature chromosome break and reunion symbol highlighting the importance of structural alterations in their development. Therefore, the methods used in gene fusion detection are designed to capture these larger-scale changes, now to/at the nucleotide-level resolution via high-throughput sequencing technologies. Herein, the genomic tools identifying gene fusions are discussed from conventional low-resolution to high-throughput high-resolution methods (**Fig. 2**). Albeit immunohistochemical detection of gene fusions at the protein level is beyond the scope of this review, it is worth noting that there are successful examples used in routine clinical practice, particularly in the setting of non–small cell lung carcinoma.[5]

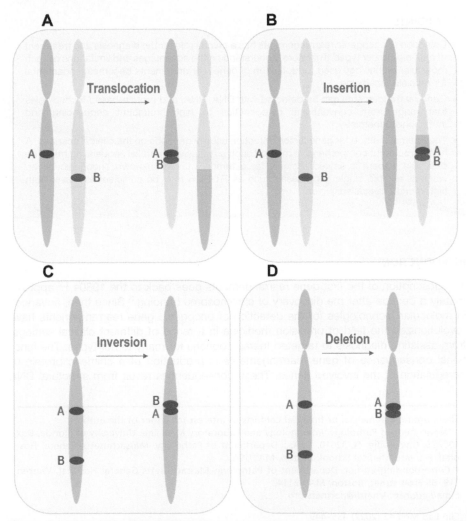

Fig. 1. Structural alterations leading to oncogenic rearrangements: (*A*) Translocation, (*B*) insertion, (*C*) inversion, and (*D*) deletion.

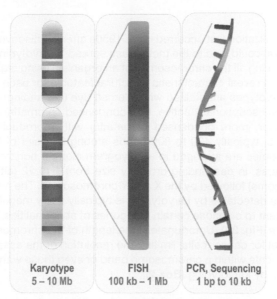

Karyotype
5 – 10 Mb

FISH
100 kb – 1 Mb

PCR, Sequencing
1 bp to 10 kb

Fig. 2. Resolution of commonly used technologies for oncogenic rearrangement detection.

PREANALYTICAL CONSIDERATIONS

The material (DNA or RNA; fresh or formalin-fixed paraffin-embedded [FFPE]) being used and the regions targeted in the genome (1 or 2 genes versus multiplex [small or comprehensive panels]) are important to consider while choosing the methodology for the detection of these oncogenic alterations. For example, patients with advanced stage disease may only have a limited cytology-based material, in which case, multiplex testing might be more advantageous given the exponential increase in predictive biomarkers (unless there is a high suspicion/prior history for a known genomic alteration). Although RNA-based methods might be more sensitive (there are multiple copies of RNA per cell) and easier to get high coverage given there is less genomic targeting (exon only), RNA is a labile molecule that is easily affected by environmental factors, type, and age of the specimen. In comparison, DNA is more stable; however, usually there is only 1 copy of the rearrangement per nucleus, and capturing rearrangements at their intronic breakpoints is more challenging in terms of their genomic coverage, sequencing-related issues, and postanalytical bioinformatics pipelines.[6] In fact, introns are much larger than exons where recurrent hotspot mutations occur: average size of a human intron is 6355 bp in protein-coding genes and the average size of an exon is 309 bp in protein-coding genes.[7] In addition, introns are inherently more difficult to sequence due to their repetitive and homologous sequence content.[8] Therefore, a cost-effective approach with high sensitivity for detecting both rearrangement breakpoints at introns and hotspot mutations at exons using the same DNA-based method may become cumbersome for clinical laboratory settings. Last, the functional significance of an incidental fusion detected by a DNA-based approach may not be as predictable as detection of an expressed fusion transcript by an RNA-based method. On the other hand, rearrangements resulting from exchange of promoter elements yielding transcriptional upregulation without a chimeric fusion cannot be detected by an RNA-based approach (**Box 1**).

KARYOTYPING

Chromosome visualization first occurred in the 1950s after the discovery that hypotonic treatment of cells could lead to the metaphase spread.[9] Karyotyping is the process of pairing and ordering all the chromosomes of an organism using standardized staining procedures that reveal characteristic structural features for each chromosome.

Today most karyotypes are stained with Giemsa dye (G-banding) resulting in light bands (GC rich, transcriptionally active, less condensed chromatin) and dark bands (AT-rich, gene poor, more condensed chromatin) with reproducible patterns for each chromosome, typically 400 to 800 bands among 23 pairs of human chromosomes. Chromosomes are arranged in a karyogram along a horizontal axis, shared by their centromeres, in descending order by size from 1 to 22 (although 21 is the smallest chromosome) followed by the X and Y chromosomes. The resolution of chromosomal changes detectable by karyotyping is typically a few megabases; however, this can be sufficient to diagnose certain categories of abnormalities, including recurrent translocations (**Fig. 3**A). Unfortunately, the length of the chromosome spreads is usually suboptimal for cancer cells, limiting the resolution of the assay. Intrachromosomal rearrangements within a chromosome band or even those within the same arm are usually cryptic by karyotyping (**Box 2**).

FLUORESCENCE IN SITU HYBRIDIZATION

First developed in the 1980s, fluorescence in situ hybridization (FISH) technique is still used as a routine clinical tool in which fluorescent probes are used to localize DNA targets both in fresh and fixed material, including FFPE. In the setting of oncogenic gene rearrangements, break-apart fusion probes are designed 5' and 3' of the recurrent breakpoint in the target gene and will be split apart if there is a rearrangement of that gene. Fusion probes target 2 different genomic regions that are spatially away from each other in their constitutional state but come together in the setting of a gene rearrangement (**Fig. 3**B–D). Therefore, high suspicion for at least one of the regions involved is necessary for the use of FISH probes (**Table 1**). FISH has the

---

Box 1
Sample material (DNA vs RNA)

DNA based:
- Advantages: More stable to environmental changes and easily obtained from a variety of sample types including FFPE material or cell-free tumor DNA
- Limitations: Difficult to capture; more limited sensitivity (1 rearranged allele per nucleus, unless amplified at DNA level) leading to false-negative results for low-tumor-cellularity specimens. Given that rearrangements usually occur at large intronic regions that are not always recurrent to the nucleotide level, large genomic regions need to be baited and sequenced increasing costs and requiring sophisticated/complex bioinformatic pipelines. Last, this approach does not give information about expression of the rearrangement and may identify incidental bystander rearrangements that are not oncogenic.

RNA-based:
- Advantages: More sensitive (many copies of fusion transcripts per nucleus), requires less genomic coverage (exon only), detects expressed transcripts
- Limitations: RNA quality is easily affected by specimen type, environmental factors, and fixation. Rearrangements resulting in transcriptional deregulation without a chimeric fusion cannot be detected.

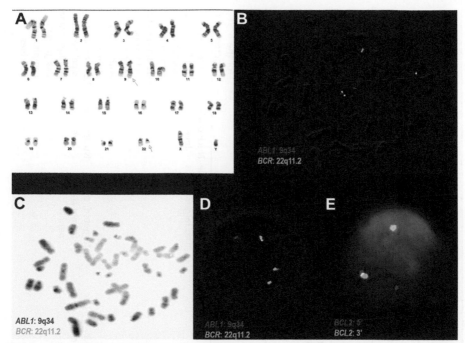

Fig. 3. Cytogenetic techniques used for rearrangement detection. (*A*) Karyogram showing t(9;22) (*arrows*). (*B*) Metaphase FISH of a *BCR::ABL1* fusion probe highlighting the derivative 9 and 22 chromosomes in fused (*yellow*) signal and uninvolved ones in individual red and green. (*C*) Inverted metaphase image of the previous FISH to better visualize chromosome architecture. (*D*) Interphase FISH using the same fusion probe for the t(9;22) *BCR::ABL1*. (*E*) A break-apart *BCL2* FISH highlighting the normal *BLC2* in fused (*yellow*) signal, whereas rearranged *BCL2* in individual red and green showing the split between 5′ and 3′ ends of the genes. ([*A–D*] *Courtesy of* Paola Dal Cin, Brigham and Women's Hospital, Boston, MA.)

spatiotemporal advantage when performed on a 5-μm section from an FFPE sample because a direct comparison with the histologic morphology is possible, but several artifacts are also introduced by applying probes to sections of nuclei, which result in reduced analytical specificity and sensitivity. FISH probe design can be challenging

---

Box 2
Karyotyping

Advantages:
• Agnostic whole-genome assay
• Useful technique for the laboratories with only cytogenetic setup without the molecular genetic infrastructure

Limitations:
• Requires fresh tissue
• Resolution limited to ~3 to 10 Mb, depending on the quality of the metaphases and banding. Intrachromosomal same-arm or band-level genetic rearrangements are usually undetectable (cryptic) by karyotype analysis
• Labor intensive and requires expertise, especially in the setting of complex alterations that can mask the recurrent fusion rearrangement

Table 1
Fusion detection

Method		Sample	Cost	Turnaround Time	Unknown Partner[b]		Genome Coverage	Level of Detection	Assay-Specific Issues
					Rearrangement Detection	Unknown Gene Detection			
Karyotype		Fresh (DNA)	$$	Cultured: days to weeks	Yes	No	Whole	Chromosome band (5–10 Mb)	Labor intensive, low resolution
FISH		Fresh, FFPE (DNA)	$	Cultured: days to weeks No culture: 1–3 d	Break-apart: Yes Fusion: No	Break-apart: No Fusion: No	Targeted regions (usually up to 2 genes; gives spatiotemporal information)	FISH probe size (100 kb –1 Mb)	Labor intensive, need to have high suspicion for the targeted gene
PCR[a] (nested, quantitative)		Fresh, FFPE (DNA/RNA)	$	1–3 d	No	No	Targeted regions (usually up to 2 genes)	Nucleotide level	Need to have high suspicion for the targeted gene
Massively parallel sequencing	Hybrid capture	Fresh, FFPE DNA/RNA (moderate input, 40–50 ng)	$$	7–21 d (usually longer than amplicon based)	Yes	Yes	Targeted, scalable to larger panels	Nucleotide level	Bioinformatics pipeline, data storage, difficult to detect fusions in intronic regions with repeat elements
	Classical amplicon	Fresh, FFPE RNA (low input, 10 ng)	$$	3–14 d (usually faster than hybrid capture)	Maybe (5'-3' imbalance)	No	Targeted, small- to mid-size panels	Nucleotide level	Bioinformatics pipeline, data storage, primer design more complicated, PCR bias

| Anchored multiplex PCR | Fresh, FFPE RNA (moderate input 100–200 ng) | $$ | 7–14 d (usually faster than hybrid capture) | Yes | Yes | Targeted, small- to mid-size panels | Nucleotide level | Bioinformatics pipeline, data storage, primer design more complicated, PCR bias |

Abbreviations: PCR, polymerase chain reaction; RACE, rapid amplification of cDNA ends.

[a] Excluding RACE as too labor intensive to use in clinical practice.

[b] All methods except for karyotyping need to have at least one of the partners being targeted to detect the rearrangement, so this part is referring to the unknown partner that may or may not be targeted depending on the technology.

especially for small intrachromosomal alterations that may be beyond the resolution of the assay and result in false-negative results, because it can occur with the subtle *ALK* rearrangements in lung cancer.[10] Alternatively, a complex alteration that does not result in a fusion may cause a false-positive result if, for example, genetic material inserts between the probes upstream the gene of interest.[11] Also, occasionally complex genetic events leading to a gene fusion may not result in the expected FISH pattern for that fusion (**Box 3**).[12]

Reverse Transcription Polymerase Chain Reaction

Reverse transcription polymerase chain reaction (RT-PCR) requires generation of complementary DNA (cDNA) from RNA, and to detect a fusion transcript, primer pairs need to be designed for both 5′ and 3′ partners. RT-PCR can be performed as a qualitative assay (**Fig. 4**) or a quantitative assay (real-time PCR) (**Fig. 5**). Nested PCR requires 2 sets of reactions with first primer pair annealing to sequences upstream to the target region, whereas the second pair uses the former set's product as a template. This approach reduces the nonspecific binding and increases specificity while enriching for the targeted region's sequence. Nested PCR does not objectively provide information about the quantity, whereas real-time PCR can be used for quantification, particularly for measurable residual disease (MRD) when the fusion gene is known to be involved for the tested cancer. Nested PCR can be highly sensitive (in the appropriate setting can detect MRD as low as 0.0001%).[13] RT-PCR approach depends on the RNA quality, which could be poor in FFPE specimens and is not highly scalable when there are multiple candidate regions. RT-PCR can also miss fusions with novel partners or unusual breakpoints, even when one of the targets is known (**Box 4**).

MASSIVELY PARALLEL SEQUENCING

Massively parallel sequencing (also referred to as next-generation sequencing) is commonly done via sequence-by-synthesis through the detection of fluorescence or flow of hydrogen ions as the bases incorporate during the sequencing process.[14] The generated data are later analyzed by bioinformatic pipelines. At present, for clinical oncology testing, targeted panels are more widely used than whole genome, exome, or transcriptome sequencing for several reasons including lower input requirement, enrichment of the clinically valuable regions, and quicker data analysis and interpretation. Therefore, one of the most critical steps is target enrichment during library preparation before sequencing. This step is essential for high coverage of the

---

Box 3
Fluorescence in situ hybridization

Advantages:
- Spatiotemporal information
- Break-apart probes are agnostic in regard to the rearrangement partner
- Rapid turnaround time
- Useful technique for the laboratories with only cytogenetic setup without the molecular genetic infrastructure

Limitations:
- False-positive or false-negative results due to location of the probes or other alterations not resulting in or masking the fusions
- Need to have high suspicion for at least one of the involved regions/genes

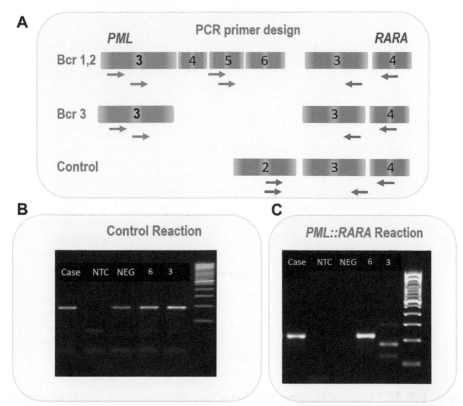

Fig. 4. *PML::RARA* nested PCR. (*A*) Three pairs of nested PCR primers are designed to capture bcr1, 2, and 3 isoforms. The 3′ *RARA* primers are constant in every reaction (exon 4 for the first amplification and exon 3 for the nested second round), whereas 5′ *PML* exon 3 primer sets can capture all isoforms and 5′ *PML* exon 5 primer sets only bcr 1 and 2. The third pair is used for control reaction and targets uninvolved *RARA* allele with the 5′ *RARA* exon 2 primer set. (*B*) Control reaction for the uninvolved *RARA* shows amplification in all except for the nontemplate control (NTC). (*C*) *PML::RARA* reaction shows that the "case" amplifies to a product that is sized as "6" (control sample with a breakpoint on intron 6), which is longer than the "3" (control sample with a breakpoint on intron 3). As expected, the negative control without the fusion and NTC are not amplified in this reaction.

desired regions while avoiding offtarget reads. Each target enrichment method (**Fig. 6**) has different performance characteristics as detailed in later discussion, with a note that the repeat regions or pseudogenes are difficult to sequence regardless of the target enrichment method being used currently in the clinical settings.

Classical Amplicon Capture

In classical amplicon capture, multiplexed PCR is performed using primers targeting each end of the region of interest. This method is RNA based and cannot use DNA as a template due to the complexity of primer design in the intronic breakpoint regions.[15] Albeit the detection of the fusion gene depends on primers capturing both partners, the presence of a fusion may be inferred by looking at the 5′ and 3′ expression imbalance even when one of the partners is unknown.

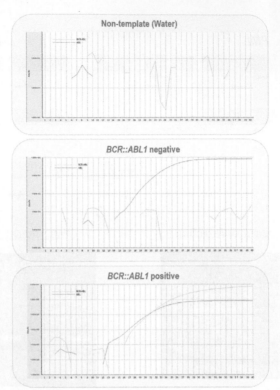

Fig. 5. *BCR::ABL1* quantitative assay. (*Top*) A reaction with no template creates nonspecific signals with no meaningful PCR product. (*Middle*) A case with no *BCR::ABL1* fusion, only has a positive reaction for the wild-type *ABL* (*red line*). (*Bottom*) A case with *BCR::ABL1* fusion has a reaction with both wild-type *ABL1*, and *BCR::ABL1*. (x-axis: cycle number, y-axis: delta Rn: the fluorescent reaction signal for the experiment minus the baseline signal generated by the instrument).

Hybrid Capture

Hybrid capture uses long oligonucleotide baits, which are longer than amplicon primers and hybridized to targeted regions. In this setting, targeting one of the fusion partners is enough to detect the rearrangement and the unknown partner.[15] Although

---

Box 4
Reverse transcription polymerase chain reaction

Advantages:
- Sensitive for MRD (when combined with real-time PCR)
- Rapid turnaround time
- Low cost per assay
- Low input requirement

Limitations:
- Can be affected by poor RNA quality
- Requires a priori knowledge of both fusion partners
- Not appropriate for multiple/unknown candidate fusions

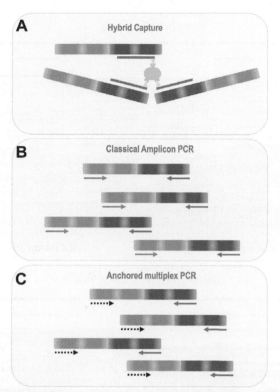

Fig. 6. Simplified schematic diagrams for massively parallel sequencing target enrichment methods. (*A*) Hybrid capture using labeled oligonucleotide baits (*blue rods*), where targeting only one of the involved genes is enough for fusion detection and PCR is not part of the library preparation. (*B*) Amplicon-based PCR: Both ends of the oncogenic rearrangement are targeted by PCR primers (*blue and orange arrows*) for amplification. (*C*) Anchored multiplex PCR: Gene-specific primers (*blue arrows*) target one of the involved partners, whereas the other end is amplified by universal primers (*black dotted arrow*) and therefore could be unknown.

both RNA and DNA specimens may be enriched by hybrid capture, hybrid capture of DNA is more widely used, as can detect mutations, structural rearrangements (**Fig. 7**), and copy number alterations all together. However, the sensitivity of fusion detection at large intronic DNA breakpoints is lower when compared with RNA-based approaches.[16,17] Another limitation is the longer workflow when compared with amplicon-based methods.

Anchored Multiplex Polymerase Chain Reaction

Anchored multiplex PCR is akin to classical amplicon sequencing with the use of multiplex PCR; however, it has an initial universal adapter ligation step helping with the amplification without prior knowledge of the gene fusion partner. Although gene-specific primers are anchored to an exon-intron boundary or within the exon of a target gene, universal reverse primers can bind to both known and unknown ends of the targeted regions (**Box 5**).[18]

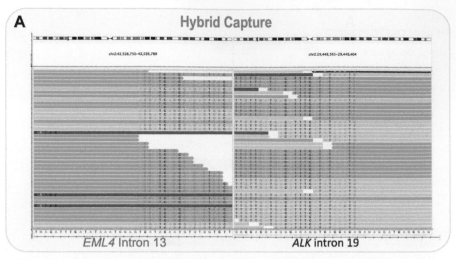

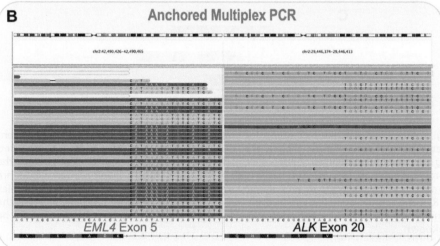

Fig. 7. Two different *EML4::ALK* fusions detected following (*A*) hybrid capture and (*B*) anchored multiplex PCR. Note that both techniques target *ALK,* and hypothetically an unknown fusion partner can also be detected. Hybrid capture breakpoints are from introns (DNA based), whereas the anchored multiplex PCR reads are from exons (RNA based). (The mismatched nucleotides highlighted as individual letters in both figures represent soft clipped bases in the sequence belonging to the partner gene).

OTHER EMERGING TECHNOLOGIES
Multiplex Digital Color Coding

This technique involves direct quantification of nucleic acids without reverse transcription or amplification,[19] which makes this application suitable for clinical samples with suboptimal RNA quality that may not survive PCR amplification. This technique can target multiple genes, and by 3′-5′ expression imbalance, fusions of the targeted genes with unknown partners can also be inferred, and therefore might be a good multiplex test alternative to FISH particularly in the setting of limited specimens.[20]

> **Box 5**
> **Massively parallel sequencing**
>
> - Amplicon-based sequencing
>   - RNA template (lowest input)
>   - Highly sensitive with focused gene panels with hotspot mutation detection
>   - Typically faster turnaround than hybrid capture, but smaller panels
>   - PCR-related artifacts
>   - Cannot detect promoter swap events (ie, immunoglobulin gene rearrangements) or unknown fusion partner of a targeted gene (needs a priori knowledge of both gene fusion partners)
>   - Could infer fusion based on 5'-3' expression imbalance in the setting of an unknown partner of a targeted gene.
> - Hybrid capture:
>   - DNA and RNA template (higher RNA input than classical amplicon based)
>   - Typically longer turnaround time than amplicon based
>   - Limited sensitivity with more comprehensive profiling (up to whole genome)
>   - Can detect promoter swap events (ie, immunoglobulin gene rearrangements) and unknown fusion partner of a targeted gene
>   - Does not require complex primer design and easier to expand the targeted regions
>   - Coverage is more uniform and is not biased by PCR artifacts
> - Anchored multiplex PCR-based sequencing:
>   - RNA template (higher input than classical amplicon or hybrid capture)
>   - Typically faster turnaround than hybrid capture, but smaller panels
>   - PCR artifacts
>   - Cannot detect promoter swap events (ie, immunoglobulin gene rearrangements); however, can detect unknown fusion partner of a targeted gene.

Long-Read Sequencing

Previously described sequencing technologies analyze sequences in short reads (<1000 nt). Long-read sequencing is an emerging field that may overcome some of the issues of these former sequencing methods such as repetitive and homologous regions that are difficult to sequence, and therefore can more easily target the large intronic regions in DNA where rearrangement breakpoints occur. Although they can be a good alternative technology for fresh or frozen samples, one caveat with these platforms is that generating long-read sequences is not plausible with FFPE specimens yielding average fragment sizes of 300 to 400 bp.

Long-read sequencing can be done via sequence-by-synthesis using nanochambers containing a single polymerase using phospho-linked nucleotides that release a signal with each addition.[21] Another approach is using protein nanopores measuring changes in the electronic conductance as each nucleotide of the molecule passes through.[22]

There are also a few technologies that can provide long-range information while still using short-range sequencing. For example, long genomic DNA fragments can be partitioned using microfluidics and short sequences developed from them can be barcoded to retain the long-range information. These barcoded libraries can then be computationally reconstructed for detection of structural alterations.[23] Another method is to generate large-insert, "jumping" libraries by shearing the genomic DNA into 2- to 4-kb-sized fragments. These fragments can then be circularized and digested again to sequence the shorter reads on the "paired ends" of these larger fragments.[24]

Optical Mapping

In this technology, a genome map is generated by massively parallel fluorescent detection of endonuclease motif sites from a single DNA molecule. The sample genome maps are then assembled de novo and compared with a reference genome, which can help visualization of structural variants resulting in oncogenic fusions.[25]

CLINICS CARE POINTS

- Highly sensitive and rapid turnaround time tests such as RT-PCR may be preferred for patients with known driver fusions for disease monitoring, whereas more extensive panels covering a wide variety of regions might be more useful for the first-time diagnosis of samples with limited material.

- Currently the ideal approach for most clinical settings may be the combination of rapid single gene/small panel tests with a comprehensive massively parallel sequencing. This way, the most essential known biomarkers can be tested rapidly while screening for other alterations not covered in the former is still underway. However, this approach is limited by the adequacy of the specimen and the financial resources of the clinical laboratory.

REFERENCES

1. Leder P. Translocations among antibody genes in human cancer. IARC Sci Publ 1985;60:341–57.
2. Shtivelman E, Lifshitz B, Gale RP, et al. Fused transcript of abl and bcr genes in chronic myelogenous leukaemia. Nature 1985;315(6020):550–4.
3. Caspersson T, Zech L, Johansson C. Differential binding of alkylating fluorochromes in human chromosomes. Exp Cell Res 1970;60(3):315–9.
4. Bruford EA, Antonescu CR, Carroll AJ, et al. HUGO Gene Nomenclature Committee (HGNC) recommendations for the designation of gene fusions. Leukemia 2021. https://doi.org/10.1038/s41375-021-01436-6.
5. Mino-Kenudson M, Chirieac LR, Law K, et al. A novel, highly sensitive antibody allows for the routine detection of ALK-rearranged lung adenocarcinomas by standard immunohistochemistry. Clin Cancer Res 2010;16(5):1561–71.
6. Garcia EP, Minkovsky A, Jia Y, et al. Validation of OncoPanel: a targeted next-generation sequencing assay for the detection of Somatic variants in cancer. Arch Pathol Lab Med 2017;141(6):751–8.
7. Piovesan A, Caracausi M, Antonaros F, et al. GeneBase 1.1: a tool to summarize data from NCBI gene datasets and its application to an update of human gene statistics. Database (Oxford) 2016. https://doi.org/10.1093/database/baw153.
8. Treangen TJ, Salzberg SL. Repetitive DNA and next-generation sequencing: computational challenges and solutions. Nat Rev Genet 2011;13(1):36–46.
9. Hsu TC. Mammalian chromosomes in vitro: I. The karyotype of man. J Hered 1952;43(4):167–72.
10. Camidge DR, Kono SA, Flacco A, et al. Optimizing the detection of lung cancer patients harboring anaplastic lymphoma kinase (ALK) gene rearrangements potentially suitable for ALK inhibitor treatment. Clin Cancer Res 2010;16(22):5581–90.
11. Uguen A, Marcorelles P, De Braekeleer M. Searching for ROS1 rearrangements in lung cancer by fluorescent in situ hybridization: the importance of probe design. J Thorac Oncol 2015;10(8):e83–5.
12. Ordulu Z, Avril S, Nardi V, et al. Low-grade endometrial stromal sarcoma with sex cord-like differentiation and phf1-jazf1 fusion with deletions: a diagnostic pitfall of JAZF1 FISH. Int J Gynecol Pathol 2021. https://doi.org/10.1097/PGP.0000000000000795.

13. Cassinat B, Zassadowski F, Balitrand N, et al. Quantitation of minimal residual disease in acute promyelocytic leukemia patients with t(15;17) translocation using real-time RT-PCR. Leukemia 2000;14(2):324–8.
14. Quail MA, Smith M, Coupland P, et al. A tale of three next generation sequencing platforms: comparison of Ion Torrent, Pacific Biosciences and Illumina MiSeq sequencers. BMC Genomics 2012;13:341.
15. Heyer EE, Blackburn J. Sequencing strategies for fusion gene detection. Bioessays 2020;42(7):e2000016.
16. Davies KD, Le AT, Sheren J, et al. Comparison of molecular testing modalities for detection of ROS1 rearrangements in a Cohort of positive patient samples. J Thorac Oncol 2018;13(10):1474–82.
17. Solomon JP, Benayed R, Hechtman JF, et al. Identifying patients with NTRK fusion cancer. Ann Oncol 2019;30(Suppl 8):viii16–22.
18. Zheng Z, Liebers M, Zhelyazkova B, et al. Anchored multiplex PCR for targeted next-generation sequencing. Nat Med 2014;20(12):1479–84.
19. Geiss GK, Bumgarner RE, Birditt B, et al. Direct multiplexed measurement of gene expression with color-coded probe pairs. Nat Biotechnol 2008;26(3): 317–25.
20. Ali G, Bruno R, Savino M, et al. Analysis of fusion genes by NanoString System: a role in lung cytology? Arch Pathol Lab Med 2018;142(4):480–9.
21. Korlach J, Bjornson KP, Chaudhuri BP, et al. Real-time DNA sequencing from single polymerase molecules. Meth Enzymol 2010;472:431–55.
22. Chen P, Gu J, Brandin E, et al. Probing single DNA molecule transport using fabricated nanopores. Nano Lett 2004;4(11):2293–8.
23. Spies N, Weng Z, Bishara A, et al. Genome-wide reconstruction of complex structural variants using read clouds. Nat Methods 2017;14(9):915–20.
24. Hanscom C, Talkowski M. Design of large-insert jumping libraries for structural variant detection using Illumina sequencing. Curr Protoc Hum Genet 2014;80:7 22 1–9.
25. Chan EKF, Cameron DL, Petersen DC, et al. Optical mapping reveals a higher level of genomic architecture of chained fusions in cancer. Genome Res 2018; 28(5):726–38.

Copy Number Analysis in Cancer Diagnostic Testing

Tara Spence, MSc, PhD[a],*, Adrian M. Dubuc, PhD, FACMG[b]

KEYWORDS

- Copy number analysis • Clinical oncology • Cytogenomics • Genome diagnostics

KEY POINTS

- Somatic CNAs yield a wealth of clinically relevant and actionable information, with an enormous potential to refine personalized cancer medicine for solid tumors and hematologic malignancies.
- As the diversity of approaches for CNA detection rapidly evolves, selection of the most appropriate technology may be a challenge, confounded by competing advantages and limitations in any given clinical context.
- This review describes the unique technical and interpretative considerations that are encountered in the detection and analysis of somatic CNAs.

INTRODUCTION

Comprehensive genomic characterization of cancers has rapidly transitioned from research innovations to diagnostic applications. Increasingly, in accordance with continual revisions to the World Health Organization (WHO), many solid tumors and hematologic malignancies alike require the detection or exclusion of pathognomonic single-nucleotide variants (SNV), structural variants (SVs) and copy number variants (CNVs) to achieve diagnosis and/or appropriate clinical management.

Somatic CNVs, referred to as copy number alterations (CNAs) in this review, have long been recognized as an important component of neoplastic transformation, resulting in the activation of proto-oncogenes, or disruption of tumor suppressor genes. CNAs can be observed in ~50% of cancers, substantiating a greater degree of alteration than any other type of somatic variation[1–3] and CNAs that are of potential clinical actionability are identified frequently in tumor specimens lacking single-nucleotide driver variants.[4] CNAs range dramatically in size–from highly targeted focal alterations,

^a Cytogenomics Laboratory, Vancouver General Hospital, Jim Pattison South, 899 12th Avenue West, Vancouver, British Columbia, V5Z 1M9, Canada; ^b Brigham and Women's Hospital, BWH Center for Advanced Molecular Diagnostics (CAMD), 75 Francis Street, BWH Shapiro Bldg 5th Floor, Boston MA 02115, USA
* Corresponding author.
E-mail address: tara.spence@vch.ca

Clin Lab Med 42 (2022) 451–468
https://doi.org/10.1016/j.cll.2022.05.003   labmed.theclinics.com
0272-2712/22/Crown Copyright © 2022 Published by Elsevier Inc. All rights reserved.

less than ~5 megabases (Mb) in size, to whole-genome doubling events–and amplitude–from homozygous deletions resulting in biallelic inactivation to amplifications.

Essential to our understanding of the detection of CNAs in cancer is the knowledge that the mechanism, size, and functional consequence of these alterations are highly variable,[2] thus necessitating diverse approaches to the detection of these alterations depending on the tumor context (summarized in **Table 1**). There is a tendency for similar CNAs to be found in a spectrum of distinct cancer types, suggesting that the neoplastic process that gives rise to many CNVs is often tumor-agnostic.[1] Many cancer cells also demonstrate polyploidy (ie, a gain or loss of a complete haploid or diploid set of chromosomes), whereby the relative imbalance of large chromosomal gains or losses is attenuated by gains of a near-complete chromosome complement.[5] It has also been demonstrated that the level of allelic imbalance or overall CNA burden, which can be defined as the degree to which a tumor cell genome is altered, is directly associated with prognosis, recurrence, and disease outcome in some cancer types[6] and that there is a direct correlation between CNAs and differential gene expression across cancer types.[7]

Clinically, the detection of a specific CNA alteration (eg, *ERBB2* gene amplification in breast cancer), or collective pattern of alterations (eg, 1p/19q whole-arm codeletion in oligodendroglioma) may determine disease management. A number of key classes of somatic alterations exist, many of which have observable changes in focal, whole-chromosome, or whole-genome copy number (**Table 2**), and significant efforts have been devoted to delineating the correlation between specific CNAs and biological or clinical characteristics of distinct cancer types.[8–10] However, the feasibility of the detection of the diversity of known and novel alterations in the routine standard-of-care clinical setting remains a practical challenge due to financial, infrastructure, technical and interpretative limitations. Presently, the assessment of CNAs in hematologic malignancies and solid tumors is accomplished using conventional G-banded karyotype analysis, fluorescent *in situ* hybridization (FISH), chromosomal microarray, or next-generation sequencing (NGS), or a combination of these methodologies. Selection of the appropriate assay is guided by the specific clinical scenario, tumor type, availability of tissue source material, cost, available infrastructure, and available technical and interpretative expertise.

This review will focus on the utility of classic, emerging, and future technologies for the detection of CNAs, including challenges and limitations faced in the routine clinical application of these methodologies.

Classical Cytogenetics and the Detection of Copy Number Alterations

Karyotype analysis

A foundational component of cytogenetics is chromosome analysis of G-banded karyotypes. This method was established as the cornerstone of hematologic oncology in the 1960s with the discovery of the Philadelphia chromosome[11]; the pathogenic derivative of the recurrent t(9;22) (q34.1;q11.2) translocation resulting in the oncogenic *BCR::ABL1* gene fusion, a driving event of chronic myeloid leukemia (CML). Karyotype analysis enables genome-wide, single-cell assessment in its chromosomal form, albeit at a low resolution (maximally achieved at ~5–10 Mb on optimal metaphases spreads). Metaphases are evaluated for copy number gains or losses, polysomy (gains or losses of partial or whole chromosomes), polyploidy, and balanced or unbalanced chromosomal rearrangements, which may aid in the diagnostic classification of the specific neoplasms or demonstrate evidence of a clonal process.

The longstanding use of karyotyping in oncology settings has created a wealth of information regarding CNAs and their associations with individual cancer types.

Table 1
Summary of current, emerging, and future techniques for the evaluation of copy number alterations in cancer

Technique	Applications	Limitations
Karyotype	• Detects large chromosomal losses and gains across the entire genome, at a maximal resolution of ~5–10 Mb • Detects polyploidy, polysomy, marker and ring chromosomes, balanced translocations and inversions • Detection of clonal populations and clonal evolution • Low infrastructure requirements and relatively low cost	• Requires chromosome preparation from fresh tissue that is amenable to cell culture, harvest and banding conditions • Cannot detect copy number alterations < ~5–10 Mb, loss of heterozygosity, or cryptic translocations • Low throughput • Requires high-technical skill
Fluorescence *in situ* hybridization	• Accurate detection of targeted copy number losses, gains, and amplifications > ~150 kb • Targeted detection of recurrent translocations, including cryptic translocations not visible on karyotype analysis • Targeted identification of predetermined clonal populations and clonal evolution, including the detection of subclonal populations • Spatial tumor tissue architecture is preserved in FFPE specimens • Relatively low infrastructure requirements	• Cannot detect alterations in loci that are not predetermined and directly targeted • Cannot detect loss of heterozygosity, balanced translocations, copy number alterations < ~150 kb • Low throughput, nonscalable, generally requiring a single assay per targeted locus • Low to moderate cost per assay
Chromosomal microarray	• High-resolution detection of known and novel copy number losses and gains > ~50–100 kb across the entire genome, depending on array design • Detects polysomy • Can detect copy-neutral loss of heterozygosity, depending on array design • Relatively rapid throughput and nontargeted	• Cannot detect balanced translocations, copy number alterations < ~50–100 kb • Moderate cost • Performed on bulk DNA with limited ability to detect low-level clonal alterations

(*continued on next page*)

Table 1
(continued)

Technique	Applications	Limitations
Targeted next-generation sequencing	• Detects SNVs, small insertions/deletions, and targeted exon or gene-level copy number gains and losses • May detect focal loss of heterozygosity, depending on panel design and coverage of the region of interest • Rapid throughput, amenable to multiplexing • Low sample DNA input requirements • Low limit of detection for clonal alterations	• Limited ability to detect moderate to large copy number alterations • Accuracy of target detection may be influenced by PCR amplification bias due to GC content or repetitive regions • Moderate to high cost
Whole-exome and whole-genome sequencing	• Detects SNVs, small insertions/deletions, focal copy number gains and losses, and partial or whole-chromosome gains or losses • May detect structural rearrangements and loss of heterozygosity with appropriate design and bioinformatic algorithms • Amenable to multiplexing • PCR-free library preparations are available, reducing concerns related to amplification bias • Low limit of detection for clonal alterations	• Throughput and multiplexing ability are reduced compared with targeted NGS • Accuracy of target detection may be influenced by PCR amplification bias, depending on library preparation design • May be challenging to confirm variant calls • High cost and infrastructure requirements, including equipment and bioinformatic support • Analysis may be labor intensive and require interpretation expertise
Long-read sequencing	• Detects SNVs, small insertions/deletions, focal copy number gains and losses, and partial or whole-chromosome gains or losses • May detect loss of heterozygosity • Amenable to multiplexing • Detects complex structural rearrangements	• Typically, low base quality calling and typically lower accuracy for the identification of variants, compared with NGS • Lower throughput • High cost and infrastructure requirements, including equipment and bioinformatic support • Labor intensive analysis and requirement for interpretation time and expertise

(continued on next page)

Table 1 (continued)		
Technique	**Applications**	**Limitations**
Optical genome mapping	• Detects copy number losses, gains and amplifications >~500b across the entire genome • Detects polysomy, balanced translocations, and inversions • Can decipher complex structural variants, including chromothripsis, tandem duplications and cryptic insertions, at a high resolution • Rapid throughput, nontargeted, relatively low cost	• Cannot detect SNVs, polyploidy, or balanced rearrangements involving centromeric or p-arm acrocentric breakpoints • Current design cannot detect loss of heterozygosity • Requires high-quality, large fragment DNA from fresh or frozen specimens using a separate extraction protocol, and cannot be applied to FFPE source material • Labor intensive interpretation of the magnitude of variants detected • Moderate cost • Potentially limited detection of clonal alterations • Challenging to confirm variant calls

Abbreviations: CGH, comparative genomic hybridization; FFPE, formalin-fixed paraffin embedded; NGS, next-generation sequencing; SNP, single-nucleotide polymorphism; SNV, single-nucleotide variant.

Specific CNAs have been linked to specific histopathological diagnoses, such as the presence of supernumerary large ring and marker chromosomes in liposarcoma,[12] or unbalanced translocations resulting in loss of the chromosome 3 short arm in clear cell renal cell carcinoma.[13] Identification of CNAs on karyotype analysis may also aid in disease prognostication, such as the identification of terminal deletions of chromosome 5q or 7q as markers of good or intermediate prognosis, respectively, in myelodysplastic syndrome.[14] Moreover, this perspective of the genome has provided invaluable information regarding a variety of genomic mechanisms that drive or contribute to malignant transformation, such as chromothripsis events in the rapidly evolving cancer genome identified by karyotype analysis,[15] or double minute formation as a mechanism for oncogene amplification.[16]

Oncology karyotype analysis is performed on direct or short-term cultured cells, generally harvested in the presence of a chromosome resolution additive to prevent chromosome compaction and a mitotic inhibitor to arrest cells in metaphase by obstructing spindle formation. Subsequent treatment with a hypotonic solution causes cells to swell, enhancing chromosome spreading, followed by fixation and slide preparation. Banding and staining are then performed using an appropriate protocol, commonly G-banding using trypsin and Giemsa stain, and visualized using light microscopy or automated image analysis. This procedure results in the reproducible formation of a series of consistent landmark "bands" along the length of chromosomes, allowing for the delineation of alterations as differences in the expected observable banding pattern.

Table 2
Classes of somatic alterations identified in acquired cancer and method of detection in routine clinical analysis

Alteration Type	Example Variant	Primary Method of Routine Clinical Detection
Single nucleotide variant	EGFR L858 R in nonsmall cell lung cancer[59]	Targeted next-generation sequencing
Small insertions and/or deletions	FLT3 internal tandem duplication (ITD) in acute myeloid leukemia[60]	Targeted PCR with sizing by capillary electrophoresis
Copy number alterations		
Exon-level	Single exon deletions or duplications in BRCA1[61]	Targeted next-generation sequencing
Gene-level	ERBB2 gene amplification in breast cancer[62]	FISH
Aneuploidy		
Partial chromosome	Deletion of the region encompassing TP53 at 17p13 in acute myeloid leukemia[63]	Karyotype or FISH
Whole chromosome	Trisomy 8 in myelodysplastic syndrome[14]	Karyotype
Copy-neutral loss of heterozygosity	B-lymphoblastic leukemia/ lymphoma (B-ALL) with hypodiploidy[64]	SNP array
Structural variations (inversions, translocations)	Translocation between chromosome 4 and 14 resulting in t(4;14) (p16;q32) FGFR3::IGH fusions in plasma cell neoplasms[65]	FISH
Chromothripsis	Massive genomic rearrangements in cutaneous melanoma[66]	SNP array

Abbreviations: FISH, fluorescence in situ hybridization; MLPA, multiplex ligation-dependent probe amplification; PCR, polymerase chain reaction; SNP, single-nucleotide polymorphism.

From a diagnostics perspective, karyotyping precludes the need for a priori knowledge of expected CNAs. However, achieving an appropriate band resolution and chromosome spread is essential to effective chromosome analysis, necessitating the use of actively diving cells. As such, nonviable, frozen, or paraffin-embedded tissue is unsuitable for evaluation using this approach. Specimen types that may be acceptable for cancer cytogenetic analysis, guided by the clinical indication and specimen availability, may include bone marrow, blood, lymph node, solid tumor, fine needle aspirates, and plural effusions.[17–19] Chromosome preparation results are fundamentally unpredictable, influenced by a range of technical and biological factors that may yield variability in the accuracy and resolution of metaphase spreads. Therefore, routine karyotype analysis performed in clinical cytogenetic laboratories is typically restricted to neoplastic disorders that are most amenable to cytogenetic evaluation. Traditional karyotype analysis is best suited for the assessment of neoplasms of myeloid origin in particular, which rapidly divide in culture. Bone marrow-derived cells of lymphoid origin often fail to divide in culture, even in the presence of appropriate lymphoid cell stimulation. Suboptimal culture yielded by many other hematologic and lymphoid malignancies, as well as by solid tumors, results in low-resolution metaphases, which may preclude the detection of chromosomal abnormalities, and thus decrease the clinical utility. Moreover, the metaphases achieved may not necessarily represent the neoplastic component of the specimen, and thus normal karyotyping results may be carefully considered in the context of the other clinical and laboratory findings.

It is generally accepted that chromosome analysis should be performed for certain hematologic and lymphoid malignancies at diagnosis or initial assessment, with routine follow-up to evaluate for the persistence of a neoplastic clone, detection of clonal evolution, as well as postbone marrow transplant in a sex mis-matched donor to assess for engraftment success and recurrence.[17,19,20] Clinical laboratories typically analyze and karyotype a minimum number of metaphases per specimen at the time of initial evaluation, which will vary depending on the indication. This can be tedious and time-consuming contingent on the resolution achieved and clonal complexity. Each clinical laboratory is expected to comply with the minimal recommendations governed by their regional or national authority, and to establish standardized practices in-house for sample processing, analysis, turnaround time, and quality control based on the indication for referral.[17,20]

Fluorescence in situ hybridization

FISH analysis is a major component of cytogenetic testing. Introduced in the 1980s[21] and used routinely in clinical settings for the targeted evaluation of known chromosomal abnormalities present in a given indication, including recurrent structural rearrangements, focal copy number losses, gains or amplifications, as well as partial or whole-chromosome polysomy. FISH often represents a primary modality of cytogenetic testing for malignancies with specific/known cytogenetic features, such as highly recurrent/pathognomonic translocations or CNAs with known diagnostic or prognostic information. It is also useful in conjunction with chromosome studies, and specifically may clarify the presence or absence of cytogenetically cryptic alterations (ie, those not visible at the limit of resolution of karyotype analysis) and/or in the context of tumor types that fail to yield sufficient resolution and quality for chromosome analysis, as discussed above.

FISH analysis involves the application of DNA probes labeled with different colored fluorophores to visualize specific, targeted regions of the genome. Specimens are pretreated with a proteolytic enzyme to allow for probe penetration, followed by the denaturation of the double-stranded genomic DNA and hybridization of the complementary single-stranded DNA probes. A series of washes are performed to remove unbound probe and reduce nonspecific or artifactual binding. Probe signals are detected using fluorescence microscopy, whereby a targeted region of interest is assessed in relation to a control locus-specific probe. For instance, the detection of amplification of the *MDM2* locus, diagnostic for dedifferentiated liposarcoma or atypical lipomatous tumor/well-differentiated liposarcoma,[22] may be achieved using a fluorescently labeled locus-specific probe complementary to the *MDM2* gene at chromosome 12q15. Within a single interphase nucleus, the number of signals can be equated in relation to the control probe with an expected diploid signal, such as a chromosome 12 centromeric probe labeled with a differently colored fluorophore. This evaluation distinguishes *MDM2* amplified malignant liposarcomas from benign lipomas, the diagnosis of which is otherwise confounded by morphologic heterogeneity and histologic overlap between benign adipose tumors and malignant lesions.[23] Another such example is the detection of amplification of the locus containing the *MYCN* gene on chromosome 2p24 that is frequently observed in neuroblastoma as powerful prognostic markers, associated with high risk, aggressive disease and poor prognosis.[24] Furthermore, the specific pattern of *MYCN* CNAs by FISH provides further insight into clinical outcomes, with gain of the locus being associated with favorable outcome with respect to amplified tumors, but poorer prognosis in comparison to tumors with a diploid *MYCN* complement,[25] while heterogeneous amplification (ie, coexistence of amplified and nonamplified nuclei within a tumor region) is indicative of a somewhat favorable outcome in comparison to homogeneous amplification of the locus.[26]

Similarly, whole-chromosome polysomy can be inferred using a probe targeted to the centromeric region of a chromosome, whereby the identification of 3 signals in interphase nuclei may be deduced as trisomy for a particular chromosome. FISH using centromere-specific probes for the detection of trisomy 4, 10, and 17 can be used in this way to infer the presence of polysomy for these chromosomes as a prognostic marker in childhood acute lymphoblastic leukemia.[27] Copy number loss can also be detected using an enumeration probe, as in the evaluation for haploinsufficiency of the locus on chromosome 17p13, which contains the *TP53* gene, in tandem with a chromosome 17 centromere-specific control probe. In plasma cell myeloma (PCM), loss of this locus is a marker of disease progression,[28] justifying the WHO recommendation for its inclusion in the minimal testing panel for cytogenetic analysis in PCM.[22] Similarly, FISH using an enumeration probeset can be used for the detection of hemizygous and homozygous loss of the region containing the *CDKN2A* gene on chromosome 9p21; a frequent finding in low-grade gliomas.[29] Homozygous loss of the *CDKN2A* locus, in particular, is an independent marker of very poor prognosis in high-grade gliomas in the presence of *IDH1/IDH2* mutations.[30]

FISH can be performed on direct or cultured cells and tissue, including fixed interphase nuclei preservations of blood or bone marrow, complementary to the preparations used for routine karyotype analysis, but can also be performed on formalin-fixed paraffin-embedded (FFPE) tissue biopsies, surgical specimens, aspirates or effusions. Importantly, FISH can be performed on sample types not adequate or suitable for G-banded chromosome analysis. FFPE tissue has the key benefit of preserving tumor architecture and facilitates the evaluation of spatial CNAs by FISH in a heterogenous tissue specimen of mixed neoplastic, necrotic and normal cells. However, fluorescent signal patterns from paraffin-embedded tissue may be confounded by sectioning artifacts and diffuse, artifactual or weak signals depending on the tissue type and preservation quality.

A diversity of FISH probes targeting an array of known recurrently altered loci are available from a variety of supplies. All probes used in an accredited clinical laboratory must be validated in-house and cut-off values established before clinical use, in accordance with the American College of Medical Genetics (ACMG) and the College of American Pathologists (CAP) recommendations, or similar guidelines based on local governing standards. Disease-specific FISH panels that detect recurrent, clinically significant abnormalities are typically offered based on the histopathological suspicion of a given diagnosis. Additionally, multicolour or multiplex FISH (M-FISH) or spectral karyotyping (SKY) may be useful for the delineation of marker chromosomes of unknown origin, or cryptic and variant chromosome rearrangements. However, these preparations tend to be costly, and the clinical yield of characterizing various nonrecurrent abnormalities may be debated when compared with individually targeting well-characterized, clinically informative chromosome anomalies using FISH for single loci.

FISH enables both a rapid analysis and increased sensitivity over G-banded chromosome assessment and may enable quick risk stratification and/or confirmation of diagnosis, whereby applicable. As such, a timely diagnosis may be achieved at the initial presentation, facilitating decision making for appropriate treatment stratification. Specifically, FISH can then be used in disease monitoring by routinely evaluating for the presence of the known diagnostic CNA or rearrangement detected in the diagnostic specimen, and for the assessment of maintenance or reemergence of a neoplastic clone, by quantitating minimal residual disease longitudinally over the course of the disease, or to evaluate for recurrence postbone marrow transplant.

Despite the accuracy, accessibility, and ability for the clonal assessment offered by FISH, this approach to CNA detection is not readily scalable as it requires the evaluation of a single targeted region in each assay. Another key limitation of FISH analysis is the targeted nature of predefined loci, and a fundamental limitation to the use of FISH analysis is, therefore, the inability to detect abnormalities not directly targeted by the FISH probes used. The assay requires a predetermined clinical suspicion of particular disease subtypes, such as the confirmation of the BCR::ABL1 translocation in the context of a suspected diagnosis of CML. FISH probes are designed to target specific loci of sufficient size to enable probe binding and therefore small copy number gains or losses, less than approximately 150 kilobases (kb), are below the limit of resolution for this method of detection. Furthermore, assessment and interpretation of FISH signal patterns may often prove challenging. Given the unstable chromosome complement of neoplastic cells, signal patterns often seem atypical and heterogenous within a specimen, making the interpretation of such patterns complex, and requiring expertise and in-depth knowledge of structural rearrangements in neoplasia. A subtle deviance from the typically observed signal pattern or intensity may also be indirectly suggestive of structural alterations in the genome in a given neoplastic specimen, such as an uncharacteristically dim signal or signals that reproducibly seem in proximity. False-negative signal patterns may also occur in the presence of underlying polymorphic variations or somatic alterations in the targeted region that prevent fidelity in probe hybridization.

Expanding Technologies for Copy Number Variant Assessment

Chromosomal microarray

While chromosome analysis and FISH remain the primary approaches used by clinical cancer cytogenetics laboratories for diagnosis, prognosis, and monitoring of malignancies, appropriate integration of chromosomal microarray analysis (CMA) into the testing paradigm can add clinically significant information in a way that is complementary to traditional methods. CMA has many advantages over conventional techniques for copy number evaluation, such as scalable, high-resolution, genome-wide coverage that allows for the detection of both known and novel CNAs and loss of heterozygosity (LOH), depending on the platform used, and may be performed on DNA extracted from fresh, cultured, frozen or FFPE specimens. The 2 most common array-based technologies include; array comparative genomic hybridization (CGH) and single-nucleotide polymorphism (SNP) array. Although platform designs vary, in general array CGH offers a rapid, cost-effective, high-resolution platform for the evaluation of copy number changes,[31,32] but often is not designed to detect regions of copy-neutral loss of heterozygosity (CN-LOH).

It is also possible to detect many (but not all) ploidy states, which represent critically important features of certain disease types. For example, recent studies have demonstrated the utility of CMA in the detection of ploidy and the capability of distinguishing between hyperdiploid and endoreduplicated hypodiploid states in the context of

B-cell acute lymphoblastic leukemia, with substantial implications in prognosis and disease management.[33,34] CMA can likewise be used for the detection of concurrent loss of the short arm of chromosome 1 and the long arm of chromosome 19, termed 1p/19q codeletion, a unique pathognomonic biomarker for oligodendrogliomas[35,36] that is associated with significantly improved prognosis and better predictive response to therapy.[37] Detection of 1p/19q hemizygosity can be achieved using FISH panels or may be apparent in a single assay on CMA as copy number loss and LOH for the relevant regions.

While the use of CMA in clinical diagnostic analysis of cancers has expanded greatly over the past few years, the cost, limits of detection, inability to detect structural rearrangements, and increased complexity of interpretation have hindered its use as an upfront test. Also, due to the inherent use of bulk DNA as the input material, which can effectively dilute the abnormal tumor signal in heterogeneous specimens with low tumor cellularity, this technology may be unable to detect low-level clonal abnormalities below the limit of detection for a particular platform (often 10%–15%), that may be apparent in subclones using conventional G-banded karyotype analysis or FISH.

Targeted next-generation sequencing

Advances in informatics and decreasing sequencing costs have facilitated a rapid expansion of next-generation sequencing (NGS) in the context of clinical care. Increasingly, these modalities of testing are enabling the detection of CNAs. NGS is scalable, high-throughput, and covers a diverse range of targets in a single assay. Copy number assessment by NGS is an indirect estimate, whereby targeted regions of interest are amplified using a hybrid capture or amplicon-based strategy, then sequenced, aligned to the reference genome, and counted. Each targeted region has distinctive amplification efficiency based on GC content, length, and other extrinsic sources of variability. The sequence reads are, therefore, corrected and normalized informatically using one or a combination of available copy number algorithms to provide an estimate of gene dosage at the targeted region.[38] Targeted NGS platforms typically have low DNA input requirements, a key advantage for malignancies whereby only a biopsy specimen may be available for genetic analysis. Molecular barcoding also enables multiplexing and high throughput. However, CNA analysis from targeted NGS data is technically challenging, confounded by both the procedure selected for the capture and enrichment of the region of interest and by tumor purity and ploidy. Presently, there is a lack of standards in the clinical diagnostic community in regard to how CNAs are detected and reported, leading to considerable variability in the potential output of results.

The utility of simultaneous detection of various alteration types in a given specimen using a targeted NGS platform is exemplified by malignancies with recurrent CNAs in genes with established actionable SNVs. Simultaneous identification of *MET* amplification and *MET* exon 14 skipping variants can be achieved using large panel NGS for the detection of these recurrent, actionable alterations in nonsmall cell lung cancers, with either variant type equally resulting in potential eligibility for MET inhibitor therapy.[39] Other such examples include *KIT* alterations in lung cancer[40] and melanoma,[41] or *BRAF* alterations in melanoma.[4,42]

There are technical challenges associated with the fidelity of copy number calling on targeted NGS data, impacted by tumor cellularity, alteration size, sequencing coverage, and informatic pipeline applied. Technical challenges are also faced due to the inherent GC bias between genes and across exons of the same gene, as well as the presence of homologous regions and pseudogenes leading to bias in amplification and sequencing fidelity, capture, coverage, and mappability between target regions. The resolution of CNA size is also lost on targeted panels, whereby the size limit of detection is restricted by the size and chromosomal location of the targeted regions. Although informatic calling algorithms for the detection of gains and amplifications by NGS have improved drastically in recent years, accurate detection of CNAs associated with haploinsufficiency, including focal deletions (single exon, multi-exon, or whole-gene deletions) in tumor suppressor genes, such as *BRCA1* and *BRCA2*, remains a particular challenge. Many NGS platforms have difficulty in calling deletions, particularly in the context of lower tumor cellularity. However, concurrent detection of single nucleotide and CNAs in *BRCA1* and *BRCA2* would enable streamlined testing for the purpose of PARP inhibitor therapy eligibility,[43,44] necessitating the need for improvements in this area.

With these considerations, detection of small intragenic gains or losses on targeted sequencing panels has more become feasible with sufficient depth of sequencing coverage and improved bioinformatic CNA calling algorithms. The utility of this approach is unquestionable, enabling simultaneous detection of various alteration types using a single, rapid, cost-effective technology. Appropriate validation of the NGS panel for CNA detection is essential, ensuring that data meet strict quality metrics for base quality score and sufficient read depth to ensure adequate coverage across regions of interest.

Emerging Approaches and Future Directions in Copy Number Alteration Detection

Whole-exome, whole-genome, and long-read sequencing

Falling sequencing costs, increasing sequencing accuracy, and improving computational power is creating opportunity for the use of low pass whole-exome sequencing (WES) and whole-genome sequencing (WGS) for the assessment of focal copy number gains or losses and whole-chromosome alterations in cancer. The greatest potential for the application of WGS approaches lies within the simultaneous capture of genome-wide SNVs, SVs, and CNAs within a single assay. Unlike targeted NGS, CNA breakpoints may be accurately delineated; particularly relevant to the evaluation of loci with multiple contiguous genes of interest. LOH may also be assessed from genome-wide sequencing data, as demonstrated by the evaluation of LOH in regions containing the *BRCA1* or *BRCA2* genes.[45]

As with WGS, long-read sequencing (LRS) similarly provides an opportunity for the detection of a range of variant types on a genome-wide scale (reviewed in[46]). LRS can uniquely elucidate allelic phasing of variants with simultaneous detection of complex structural alterations. However, in addition to a substantially higher cost, LRS has long been troubled with a significantly lower base quality rate compared with short-read sequencing, which has prohibited LRS from being relied on for routine clinical variant detection, particularly when alterations are observed at low variant allele frequencies. However, available technologies for LRS have made leaps and bounds in improved accuracy with the application of unique molecular identifiers (UMI) in recent years[47]), and are rapidly becoming feasible alternatives to both classical cytogenetics and WGS approaches.

In comparison to targeted approaches, genome-wide sequencing of genetic alterations generally results in a comparably longer turnaround time and lower multiplexing ability, at a significantly higher cost. WES, WGS, and LRS also require significantly greater computational power, storage capacity, bioinformatics capability, and interpretation time and expertise. Many key considerations associated with bioinformatics and accurate variant calling reviewed above for targeted NGS remain a challenge. However, broader coverage of the genome supports confidence in variant detection and allows for a more accurate assessment of alteration size and boundaries. It is important to acknowledge that technical issues related to artifactual PCR amplification bias and technical duplicates can confound copy number calling from sequencing data, particularly in the context of hybrid-capture platforms, whether targeted or whole exome. Recent introduction of PCR-free library preparation methods may combat this hurdle in the future.[48] The intricacies of copy number variant calling on sequencing data in oncology are discussed in detail elsewhere.[49,50] The field continues to evolve as sequencing technology and bioinformatics calling algorithms improve, yet accurate identification of CNAs by sequencing remains a challenge at present.

However, genome-wide sequencing offers a wealth of information, with the potential to replace multiple siloed assays into a single comprehensive pipeline for the detection of SNVs, insertions and deletions, SVs, CNAs, and chromosomal aneuploidies. When compared individually, the per-sample cost of these sequencing platforms is prohibitively higher relative to the alternative approaches discussed in previous sections. Yet, when other factors are taken into account, including the cost of infrastructure, training and technical expertise, routine proficiency testing for each test and maintenance of accreditation, as well as the expertise required to interpret and report each individual assay, the overall cost as a replacement for multiple individual assays becomes relatively more reasonable. Not only does a single-assay approach afford the opportunity to more readily and rapidly detect the totality of genomic alterations that define disease, WGS and LRS may also yield novel discoveries and associations which may refine our understanding of cancer diagnoses and treatment.

Optical genome mapping

Our current testing approach of karyotype analysis, FISH, and CMA leave significant gaps in our ability to detect CNAs greater than ~500 bp in size (**Fig. 1**). This limitation may be resolved using WGS or LRS, yet these technologies have limitations and are not readily available in most clinical cancer genetics laboratories. An alternative approach–Optical Genome Mapping (OGM) – has become of rapidly increasing interest.

OGM has an enormous potential to revolutionize the paradigm of classical cytogenetics testing approaches, by resolving the limit of resolution between targeted NGS and FISH or array-based testing. OGM can reliably detect CNAs and SVs down to an

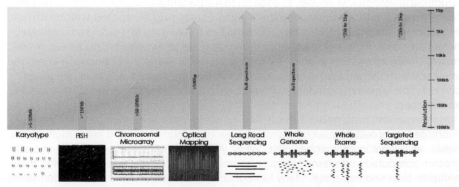

Fig. 1. Resolution of classic, emerging, and future technologies in the detection of copy number alteration in cancer.

incredibly low resolution, enabling focused delineation of genomic breakpoints, while providing additional resolution of SV orientation; a distinct advantage over both NGS and CMA. The technology itself is not sequencing-based; rather it is an imaging technology with a mechanistically simple approach of enzymatically labeling high molecular weight, ultra-long DNA molecules in a unique, reproducible pattern, followed by electrophoresis on a nanochannel chip and imaging.[51] A *de novo* assembly is generated informatically from the ultrahigh-resolution imaged DNA molecules and aligned to a reference genome for the detection of deletions and tandem, inverted or intrachromosomal gains.[52] This approach allows for rapid detection of a range of complex SVs and CNAs simultaneously, in a single, cost-effective assay, including the identification of balanced and unbalanced translocations and inversions, and CNAs ranging from approximately 500 bp to whole-chromosome polysomy, according to the manufacturer.

At present OGM is not capable of detecting LOH, limiting its applicability with respect to some array-based platforms. In addition, the reliance on a reference genome creates hurdles in terms of defining normal population variation, as well as oncogenic variation that accumulates as a passenger effect of the disease process. Furthermore, due to the necessity for ultra-long DNA molecules, OGM requires a unique DNA extraction procedure, distinct from other available technologies, necessitating a fresh or frozen source material. This is a potentially significant hurdle for solid tumor testing using OGM, which has fundamentally relied on FFPE source material, as well as for variant confirmation testing and for workflows requiring tandem or reflex testing using other methodologies.

Recent publications have demonstrated the feasibility and potential utility of OGM in profiling hematologic malignancies[53–55] and solid tumors.[56] It will be interesting and exciting to observe how clinical laboratories adopt OGM as a potential replacement for current, classical testing approaches, particularly in the context of hematologic malignancies.

DISCUSSION

With the breadth of new technologies enabling CNA detection, a critical challenge lies in the translation of our knowledge of specific CNAs into informative, clinically useful findings. Due to the diversity and sheer number of CNAs identified in tumor specimens, combined with variable breakpoints and difficulty in detection by any one particular method, accurate and consistent testing and interpretation of CNAs remains a significant hurdle. The ACMG has released technical standards for the analysis of chromosomal alterations in cancer,[57] in addition to specific guidance on the use of chromosome analysis, FISH and CMA in the context of hematologic neoplasms[17] and solid tumors.[18] This guidance is supported by more recently published comprehensive recommendations from the ACMG and Cancer Genomics Consortium (CGC) related to interpretation and reporting of acquired CNAs and loss of heterozygosity.[58] This platform-agnostic guidance is becoming widely adopted throughout clinical laboratories in North America, offering a framework to enable consistency in interpretation and reporting across individual centers.

Targeted approaches, such as conventional karyotype, FISH analysis and CMA remain mainstays in clinical laboratories. Yet, with the ever-decreasing cost, rapidly improving accuracy in detection, and increased access, evaluation of CNAs by emerging technologies such as WGS, LRS and OGM has been permitted in ways not previously possible on a routine basis. These novel approaches to the clinical analysis of copy number variations open the door to new possibilities for personalized medicine, which will undoubtedly impact routine clinical testing for CNAs, and ultimately, transform management for many hematologic malignancies and solid tumors.

CLINICS CARE POINTS

- Classical cytogenetic approaches of karyotype and FISH remain standard practice for the detection of CNAs in oncology.
- Emerging and future technologies, including whole genome sequencing, long-read sequencing and optical genome mapping will undoubtedly enhance diagnostic, prognostic and targeted therapeutic yield, replace existing approaches, and transform the landscape of CNA detection in oncology.
- The diversity and sheer number of CNAs identified in tumor specimens, combined with variable breakpoints and difficulty in detection by any single method, necessitates systematic, accurate and uniform interpretation criteria and laboratory reporting practices.

DISCLOSURE

The authors have nothing to disclose.

REFERENCES

1. Beroukhim R, Mermel CH, Porter D, et al. The landscape of somatic copy-number alteration across human cancers. Nature 2010;463(7283):899–905.
2. Zack TI, Schumacher SE, Carter SL, et al. Pan-cancer patterns of somatic copy number alteration. Nat Genet 2013;45(10):1134–40.
3. Ciriello G, Miller ML, Aksoy BA, et al. Emerging landscape of oncogenic signatures across human cancers. Nat Genet 2013;45(10):1127–33.
4. Vives-Usano M, García Pelaez B, Román Lladó R, et al. Analysis of copy number variations in solid tumors using a next generation sequencing custom panel. J Mol Pathol 2021;2(2):123–34.
5. Santaguida S, Amon A. Short- and long-term effects of chromosome mis-segregation and aneuploidy. Nat Rev Mol Cell Biol 2015;16(8):473–85.
6. Hieronymus H, Murali R, Tin A, et al. Tumor copy number alteration burden is a pan-cancer prognostic factor associated with recurrence and death. Elife 2018; 7:e37294.
7. Shao X, Lv N, Liao J, et al. Copy number variation is highly correlated with differential gene expression: a pan-cancer study. BMC Med Genet 2019;20(1):175.
8. Liang L, Fang JY, Xu J. Gastric cancer and gene copy number variation: emerging cancer drivers for targeted therapy. Oncogene 2016;35(12):1475–82.
9. Wang H, Liang L, Fang JY, et al. Somatic gene copy number alterations in colorectal cancer: new quest for cancer drivers and biomarkers. Oncogene 2016; 35(16):2011–9.
10. Nibourel O, Guihard S, Roumier C, et al. Copy-number analysis identified new prognostic marker in acute myeloid leukemia. Leukemia 2017;31(3):555–64.
11. Nowell P, Hungerford D. A minute chromosome in human chronic granulocytic leukemia. Science 1960;(132):1497.
12. Sueekantaiah C, Karakousis CP, Leong SPL, et al. Cytogenetic findings in liposarcoma correlate with histopathologic subtypes. Cancer 1992;69(10):2484–95.

13. Hsieh JJ, Le VH, Oyama T, et al. Chromosome 3p loss–orchestrated VHL, HIF, and epigenetic deregulation in clear cell renal cell carcinoma. J Clin Oncol 2018;36(36):3533–9.

14. Schanz J, Tüchler H, Solé F, et al. New comprehensive cytogenetic scoring system for primary myelodysplastic syndromes (MDS) and oligoblastic acute myeloid leukemia after MDS derived from an international database merge. J Clin Oncol 2012;30(8):820–9.

15. Leibowitz M, Zhang C, Pellman D. Chromothripsis: a new mechanism for rapid karyotype evolution. Annu Rev Genet 2015;49:183–211.

16. Verhaak RGW, Bafna V, Mischel PS. Extrachromosomal oncogene amplification in tumour pathogenesis and evolution. Nat Rev Cancer 2019;19(5):283–8.

17. Mikhail FM, Heerema NA, Rao KW, et al. Section E6.1-6.4 of the ACMG technical standards and guidelines: chromosome studies of neoplastic blood and bone marrow-acquired chromosomal abnormalities. Genet Med 2016;18(6):635–42.

18. Cooley LD, Morton CC, Sanger WG, et al. Section E6.5-6.8 of the ACMG technical standards and guidelines: chromosome studies of lymph node and solid tumor-acquired chromosomal abnormalities. Genet Med 2016;18(6):643–8.

19. Introduction. In: Wan TS, editor. Methods in. Cancer cytogenetics: methods and protocols, 220. Springer Protocols; 2016. https://doi.org/10.1385/1-59259-363-1:001.

20. Canadian College of Medical Geneticists (CCMG) Cytogenetics Committee. CCMG Practice Guidelines for Cytogenetic Analysis: Recommendations for the indications, analysis and reporting of cancer specimens. Published online 2010.

21. Chang S, Mark H. Emerging molecular cytogenetic technologies. Cytobios 1997; 90(360):7–22.

22. Swerdlow S, Campo E, Harris N, et al, editors. WHO classification of tumours of haematopoietic and lymphoid tissues. Revised 4t. International Agency for Research on Cancer; 2017.

23. Thway K, Wang J, Swansbury J, et al. Fluorescence in situ hybridization for MDM2 amplification as a routine ancillary diagnostic tool for suspected well-differentiated and dedifferentiated liposarcomas: experience at a tertiary center. Sarcoma 2015;812089.

24. Lee JW, Son MH, Cho HW, et al. Clinical significance of MYCN amplification in patients with high-risk neuroblastoma. Pediatr Blood Cancer 2018;65(10): e27257.

25. Campbell K, Gastier-Foster JM, Mann M, et al. Association of MYCN copy number with clinical features, tumor biology, and outcomes in neuroblastoma: a report from the Children's Oncology Group. Cancer 2017;123(21):4224–35.

26. Berbegall AP, Bogen D, Pötschger U, et al. Heterogeneous MYCN amplification in neuroblastoma: a SIOP europe neuroblastoma study. Br J Cancer 2018;118(11): 1502–12.

27. Enshaei A, Vora A, Harrison CJ, et al. Defining low-risk high hyperdiploidy in patients with paediatric acute lymphoblastic leukaemia: a retrospective analysis of data from the UKALL97/99 and UKALL2003 clinical trials. Lancet Haematol 2021; 8(11):e828–39.

28. Chin M, Sive JI, Allen C, et al. Prevalence and timing of TP53 mutations in del(17p) myeloma and effect on survival. Blood Cancer J 2017;7(9):e610.

29. Reis GF, Pekmezci M, Hansen HM, et al. CDKN2A loss is associated with shortened overall survival in lower-grade (World Health Organization Grades II-III) astrocytomas. J Neuropathol Exp Neurol 2015;74(5):442–52.

30. Appay R, Dehais C, Maurage CA, et al. CDKN2A homozygous deletion is a strong adverse prognosis factor in diffuse malignant IDH-mutant gliomas. Neuro Oncol 2019;21(12):1519–28.

31. Cantsilieris S, Baird PN, White SJ. Molecular methods for genotyping complex copy number polymorphisms. Genomics 2013;101(2):86–93.

32. Redon R, Carter NP. Comparative Genomic Hybridization: microarray design and data interpretation. Methods Mol Biol 2009;529:37–49.

33. Peterson JF, Van Dyke DL, Hoppman NL, et al. The utilization of chromosomal microarray technologies for hematologic neoplasms: an ACLPS critical review. Am J Clin Pathol 2018;150(5):375–84.

34. Mitrakos A, Kattamis A, Katsibardi K, et al. High resolution chromosomal microarray analysis (CMA) enhances the genetic profile of pediatric B-cell acute lymphoblastic leukemia patients. Leuk Res 2019;83:106177.

35. Louis DN, Perry A, Reifenberger G, et al. The 2016 World health organization classification of tumors of the central nervous system: a summary. Acta Neuropathol 2016;131(6):803–20.

36. Chamberlain MC, Born D. Prognostic significance of relative 1p/19q codeletion in oligodendroglial tumors. J Neurooncol 2015;125(2):249–51.

37. Van Den Bent MJ, Brandes AA, Taphoorn MJB, et al. Adjuvant procarbazine, lomustine, and vincristine chemotherapy in newly diagnosed anaplastic oligodendroglioma: long-term follow-up of EORTC brain tumor group study 26951. J Clin Oncol 2013;31(3):344–50.

38. Ho SS, Urban AE, Mills RE. Structural variation in the sequencing era. Nat Rev Genet 2020;21(3):171–89.

39. Wolf J, Seto T, Han J-Y, et al. Capmatinib in MET exon 14–mutated or MET -amplified non–small-cell lung cancer. N Engl J Med 2020;383(10):944–57.

40. Salomonsson A, Jönsson M, Isaksson S, et al. Histological specificity of alterations and expression of KIT and KITLG in non-small cell lung carcinoma. Genes Chromosom Cancer 2013;52(11):1088–96.

41. Carvajal RD, Antonescu CR, Wolchok JD, et al. KIT as a therapeutic target in metastatic melanoma. JAMA 2011;305(22):2327–34.

42. Kakadia S, Yarlagadda N, Awad R, et al. Mechanisms of resistance to BRAF and MEK inhibitors and clinical update of us food and drug administration-approved targeted therapy in advanced melanoma. Onco Targets Ther 2018;11:7095–107.

43. Friedlander M, Moore KN, Colombo N, et al. Patient-centred outcomes and effect of disease progression on health status in patients with newly diagnosed advanced ovarian cancer and a BRCA mutation receiving maintenance olaparib or placebo (SOLO1): a randomised, phase 3 trial. Lancet Oncol 2021;22(5): 632–42.

44. Tutt ANJ, Garber JE, Kaufman B, et al. Adjuvant olaparib for patients with BRCA1- or BRCA2-mutated breast cancer. N Engl J Med 2021;384(25):2394–405.

45. Sokol ES, Pavlick D, Khiabanian H, et al. Pan-cancer analysis of BRCA1 and BRCA2 genomic alterations and their association with genomic instability as measured by genome-wide loss of heterozygosity. JCO Precis Oncol 2020;(4): 442–65.

46. Sakamoto Y, Sereewattanawoot S, Suzuki A. A new era of long-read sequencing for cancer genomics. J Hum Genet 2020;65(1):3–10.

47. Karst SM, Ziels RM, Kirkegaard RH, et al. High-accuracy long-read amplicon sequences using unique molecular identifiers with Nanopore or PacBio sequencing. Nat Methods 2021;18(2):165–9.

48. Gross AM, Ajay SS, Rajan V, et al. Copy-number variants in clinical genome sequencing: deployment and interpretation for rare and undiagnosed disease. Genet Med 2019;21(5):1121–30.

49. Zare F, Dow M, Monteleone N, et al. An evaluation of copy number variation detection tools for cancer using whole exome sequencing data. BMC Bioinformatics 2017;18(1):1–13.

50. Zaccaria S, Raphael BJ. Accurate quantification of copy-number aberrations and whole-genome duplications in multi-sample tumor sequencing data. Nat Commun 2020;11(1). https://doi.org/10.1038/s41467-020-17967-y.

51. Sahajpal NS, Barseghyan H, Kolhe R, et al. Optical genome mapping as a next-generation cytogenomic tool for detection of structural and copy number variations for prenatal genomic analyses. Genes (Basel) 2021;12(3):1–11.

52. Yuan Y, Chung CYL, Chan TF. Advances in optical mapping for genomic research. Comput Struct Biotechnol J 2020;18:2051–62.

53. Lühmann JL, Stelter M, Wolter M, et al. The clinical utility of optical genome mapping for the assessment of genomic aberrations in acute lymphoblastic leukemia. Cancers (Basel) 2021;13(17):4388.

54. Neveling K, Mantere T, Vermeulen S, et al. Next-generation cytogenetics: comprehensive assessment of 52 hematological malignancy genomes by optical genome mapping. Am J Hum Genet 2021;108(8):1423–35.

55. Lestringant V, Duployez N, Penther D, et al. Optical genome mapping, a promising alternative to gold standard cytogenetic approaches in a series of acute lymphoblastic leukemias. Genes Chromosomes Cancer 2021;60(10):657–67.

56. Goldrich DY, Labarge B, Chartrand S, et al. Identification of somatic structural variants in solid tumors by optical genome mapping. J Pers Med 2021;11(2):1–21.

57. Shao L, Akkari Y, Cooley LD, et al. Chromosomal microarray analysis, including constitutional and neoplastic disease applications, 2021 revision: a technical standard of the American College of Medical Genetics and Genomics (ACMG). Genet Med 2021;(April). https://doi.org/10.1038/s41436-021-01214-w.

58. Mikhail FM, Biegel JA, Cooley LD, et al. Technical laboratory standards for interpretation and reporting of acquired copy-number abnormalities and copy-neutral loss of heterozygosity in neoplastic disorders: a joint consensus recommendation from the American College of Medical Genetics and Genom. Genet Med 2019;21(9):1903–15.

59. Tsai MF, Chang TH, Wu SG, et al. EGFR-L858R mutant enhances lung adenocarcinoma cell invasive ability and promotes malignant pleural effusion formation through activation of the CXCL12-CXCR4 pathway. Sci Rep 2015;5:1–14.

60. Fröhling S, Schlenk RF, Breitruck J, et al. Prognostic significance of activating FLT3 mutations in younger adults (16 to 60 years) with acute myeloid leukemia and normal cytogenetics: a study of the AML study group Ulm. Blood 2002;100(13):4372–80.

61. Rizzolo P, Silvestri V, Falchetti M, et al. Inherited and acquired alterations in development of breast cancer. Appl Clin Genet 2011;4:145–58.

62. Kallioniemi OP, Kallioniemi A, Kurisu W, et al. ERBB2 amplification in breast cancer analyzed by fluorescence in situ hybridization. Proc Natl Acad Sci U S A 1992;89(12):5321–5.

63. Seifert H, Mohr B, Thiede C, et al. The prognostic impact of 17p (p53) deletion in 2272 adults with acute myeloid leukemia. Leukemia 2009;23(4):656–63.

64. Fang M, Becker PS, Linenberger M, et al. Adult low-hypodiploid acute B-lymphoblastic leukemia with IKZF3 deletion and TP53 mutation: comparison with pediatric patients. Am J Clin Pathol 2015;144(2):263–70.

65. Rasche L, Kortüm KM, Raab MS, et al. The impact of tumor heterogeneity on diagnostics and novel therapeutic strategies in multiple myeloma. Int J Mol Sci 2019;20(5):1248.

66. Cortés-Ciriano I, Lee JJK, Xi R, et al. Comprehensive analysis of chromothripsis in 2,658 human cancers using whole-genome sequencing. Nat Genet 2020;52(3): 331–41.

Molecular Biomarkers of Response to Cancer Immunotherapy

Lauren L. Ritterhouse, MD, PhD*, Tasos Gogakos, MD, PhD

KEYWORDS

- Immunotherapy • Biomarkers • Immune checkpoint inhibitors
- Tumor mutational burden • Microsatellite instability • PD-L1

KEY POINTS

- The lack of uniform responses to immunotherapy has necessitated the development of biomarkers predictive of response to immune checkpoint inhibitors.
- Three Food and Drug Administration (FDA)-approved biomarkers have shown important, yet heterogenous, utility in clinical practice.
- The development of predictive biomarkers has created a shift in clinical practice, with drug approvals based on biomarker status alone and not tumor type or site.
- Currently, there is no ideal biomarker that can accurately predict the response of every patient to ICIs.
- Development of novel and combination of multiple biomarkers may benefit more patients in the future.

INTRODUCTION

Harnessing the immune system to advance cancer therapy has offered a new weapon in the quiver of clinical oncology. The lack of uniform, robust, or durable responses in many patients has necessitated the development of approaches for accurate prediction of subgroups that are most likely to benefit from immunotherapy. This has led to the development and regulatory approval of predictive biomarkers, as well as associated companion diagnostics. Despite these strides, there still exists great heterogeneity in the choice of biomarkers, the laboratory assays that generate them, and their overall clinical utility. This article surveys broadly the predictive biomarkers of response to cancer immunotherapy, focusing on the biomarkers with current FDA approval, and raising awareness of issues that may affect their broad applicability.

Center for Integrated Diagnostics, Department of Pathology, Massachusetts General Hospital, Harvard Medical School, Jackson Building, 10th Floor, Suite 1015, 55 Fruit Street, Boston, MA 02114, USA
* Corresponding author.
E-mail address: lritterhouse@mgh.harvard.edu

Clin Lab Med 42 (2022) 469–484
https://doi.org/10.1016/j.cll.2022.05.004
0272-2712/22/© 2022 Elsevier Inc. All rights reserved.

Immune Checkpoint Inhibitors

Immune checkpoints inhibitors (ICIs) have evolved to maintain homeostasis and protect against autoimmunity. They are established by the interaction of surface proteins on immune cells (T cells) with antigen-presenting or antigen-expressing cells. Productive binding between these members of these 2 classes of proteins results in immunosuppressive signaling that attenuates the activation of T cells, keeping them in an "off" state.

The discovery of such immunosuppressive mechanisms provided a possible path to the activation of the immune system against tumor cells that, owing to their underlying mutational processes, express neoantigens.[1–3] In order for such therapies to be effective, the immune system has to be able to recognize the tumor as antigenically different from self. In principle, the more antigenic the tumor, the more potent the effect of such therapies. The demonstration that inhibitory antibodies against such molecules can elicit an antitumor response ushered in a new era in clinical oncology.[4]

Immunotherapy has essentially resulted in a paradigm shift in cancer treatment. Instead of targeting tumor vulnerabilities by direct cytotoxic or targeted therapies, ICIs use the host's immune system for the elimination of cancer cells. Since the approval of the first ICI targeting CLTA-4 inhibition for the treatment of melanoma,[5] several other agents have become available, either as single or combination therapies, in at least 15 different tumor types.[5–8] Available ICIs in clinical practice include monoclonal antibodies against the programmed cell death protein (PD-1), its ligand (PD-L1), and the cytotoxic T-lymphocyte antigen 4 (CTLA-4).[9]

Additional immune checkpoints are also being investigated in clinical trials. Lymphocyte activating gene 3 (LAG-3) negatively regulates the lymphocytic response by inhibiting several ligands, acting synergistically with PD-1,[10,11] making it a promising target for overcoming resistance to PD-1-based immunotherapy[12,13] As of this writing, 69 clinical trials on LAG-3 are currently active or recruiting (http://www.clinicaltrials.gov/). T-cell immunoglobulin and mucin domain 3 (TIM-3) is expressed on multiple immune cell types as well as leukemic stem cells, and marks terminally exhausted CD8-positive T cells.[14–16] Expression of TIM-3 in tumor-infiltrating immune cells may correlate with worse prognosis or more advanced metastasis in multiple cancers.[17] Concurrent blockade of TIM-3 and PD-1 has shown promising results in preclinical trials in solid and hematologic malignancies.[18–20]

Even though ICIs have taken center stage in immunotherapy, and are the main focus of this article, it should be noted that there exist multiple other modalities of exploiting the immune system against cancer. These include T-cell transfer therapy of tumor-infiltrating lymphocytes (TILs), chimeric antigen receptor T-cell (CAR-T) cell therapies, tumor-specific monoclonal antibodies, cancer vaccines, and immune modulators, such as cytokine therapy.[3,21] In the context of this blooming field, it is essential that the development of accurate biomarkers keep up with the pace of treatment advances, to ensure maximal benefit for patients.

FOOD AND DRUG ADMINISTRATION-APPROVED BIOMARKERS

Despite impressive rates of durable clinical response in multiple patients with advanced cancer, not all patients benefit from ICI treatment. The range of response rates varies widely with approximately 20% response rates across all indications.[22] In addition, patients can experience serious adverse events.[23] The variability of response rates among patients suggests the presence of biomarkers that could more accurately predict clinical responses in specific patient subgroups. Taken together the lack of uniform response and the associated toxicity of ICI therapy necessitate the deployment of predictive biomarkers. The next section will focus on the 3 predictive biomarkers that are currently approved by the US Food and Drug Administration (FDA): PD-L1 expression, mismatch repair deficiency/microsatellite instability (dMMR/MSI), and tumor mutational burden (TMB).

PD-1/PD-L1

Expression of the members of the PD-1/PD-L1 axis emerged as the earliest predictive biomarkers for response to ICIs. PD-L1 expression as determined by immunohisto-chemistry was the first FDA-approved predictive biomarker in 2015 for NSCLC. Since then, this biomarker has been approved for additional tumor types (eg, melanoma, gastroesophageal junction, cervical, urothelial, head and neck squamous cell, esoph-ageal, and triple-negative breast cancer).

Early studies showed the efficacy of ICIs in PD-L1 expressing tumors of various types. For example, a study of 207 patients with various tumors demonstrated that PD-L1 positive tumors (60% of all tested tumors) had a 36% overall response rate (ORR) compared with 0% for PD-L1 negative tumors.[24] Various other studies have shown a correlation between PD-L1 expression in the tumor and/or immune cells and response to PD-1/PD-L1 inhibitors.[25] However, up to 20% of PD-L1 negative tu-mors also show response to therapy,[26–28] suggesting a poor negative predictive value for PD-L1 expression. In addition, some tumors, such as metastatic colon cancer showed no response irrespective of PD-L1 status.[25] Despite this heterogeneity in re-sponses, the correlation between PD-L1 expression and response to ICI administra-tion, either as a first or later line treatment has rendered PD-L1 expression a valuable predictive biomarker for clinical practice.[27,29,30]

There are currently 4 FDA-approved companion diagnostic assays for assessing PD-L1 tumor status, with additional ones being developed (**Table 1**;[31]). The presence of different assays, scoring systems, cut-offs, and drug-assay pairs has created a multi-layered reporting framework that results in great heterogeneity and precludes seamless harmonization across assays, trials, and treatments. Studies have demon-strated poor diagnostic concordance between certain antibodies. For example, com-parison between E1L3N and SP142 antibodies for PD-L1 scoring in NSCLC showed only 25% concordance.[32] A multi-institutional assessment of PD-L1 assays in NSCLC showed that the SP142 assay was associated with statistically significantly lower PD-L1 staining levels than 22C3, 28 to 8, and E1L3N for staining both tumor and immune cells.[33] The latter 3, however, showed almost perfect agreement for tumor-cell stain-ing and strong agreement for immune-cell staining.[33] The same study also demon-strated that on an individual basis, pathologists were able to score tumor cell expression reproducibly regardless of the antibody used, but performed poorly in scoring immune cells.[33] Multiple other studies have raised awareness for inconsis-tencies and pitfalls in the inter-assay correlation among PD-L1 assays.[34–38] It is also worth noting that in certain instances laboratory-developed tests, such as the E1L3N immunohistochemical assay may show great concordance with consensus scoring.

Despite the documented technical heterogeneity, PD-L1 IHC remains a widely used predictive biomarker for guiding ICI therapy. More data, however, will be required to ensure the scenarios in which drug-assay combinations can be interchangeable.

Mismatch Repair System and Microsatellite Instability

The DNA mismatch repair system (MMR) offers protection against mutations that occur during the lifecycle of DNA, including replication and recombination. In this pathway, MutS homologs recognize noncanonical basepairs and on the recruitment

Table 1
Approved PD-L1 immunohistochemistry assays

Drug	Ab Clone	Species	Tumor (Subset)	Scoring System	Cutoff
Pembrolizumab	22C3 PharmDx	Mouse monoclonal	First- or second-line in NSCLC	TPS	1% (lowered from 50% based on KEYNOTE-042; https://www.fda.gov/drugs/fda-expands-pembrolizumab-indication-first-line-treatment-nsclc-tps-1)
			First-line in urothelial, second-line in ESCC, first-line TNBC	CPS	10%
			First-line in SCCHN, second-line in CC	CPS	1%
Nivolumab ± Ipilimumab	28-8 PharmDx	Rabbit monoclonal	First-line in NSCLC	TPS	1%
Atezolizumab	SP142 Ventana	Rabbit monoclonal	First-line in NSCLC	TPS	50%
				IC	10%
			First-line in TNBC	IC	1%
			First-line in cisplatin-ineligible UC	IC	5%
Cemiplimab	22C3 PharmDx	Mouse monoclonal	First-line in NSCLC	TPS	50%
Durvalumab	SP263 Ventana	Rabbit monoclonal	Urothelial carcinoma	TPS	25%
				ICP and IC	1% and 25%
				ICP and IC	1% and 100%

Abbreviations: CC, cervical cancer; CPS, combined positive score (percentage of all PD-L1 staining cells tumor cells divided by the total number of viable tumor cells; ESCC, esophageal squamous cell carcinoma; IC, proportion of tumor area occupied by PD-L1 expressing tumor-infiltrating immune cells; ICP, immune cells present (percentage of tumor area occupied by immune cells); NSCLC, nonsmall cell lung cancer; SCCHN, squamous cell carcinoma of the head and neck; TNBC, triple-negative breast cancer; TPS, tumor proportion score (percentage of viable tumor cells showing partial or complete membrane staining relative to all viable tumor cells); UC, urothelial cancer.

of MutL homologs initiate appropriate replacement of the offending nucleotide in the newly synthesized strand via the nucleotide excision repair process.[39]

In humans, the 4 core MMR proteins function as 2 heterodimers, one consisting of the MutS homologs, MSH2 and MSH6; the other comprising 2 MutL homologs, MLH1 and PMS2. Inactivation of the MMR machinery results in up to a 1000-fold increase in mutation accumulation and is associated with an increased risk of tumorigenesis.[40] MMR deficiency (dMMR) can result from either germline inactivation, resulting in Lynch syndrome, or acquired (somatic) alterations, including the inactivation of *MLH1* via promoter methylation and loss-of-function mutations in any of the MMR genes.[41,42] dMMR was initially reported in the setting of colorectal cancer (CRC), whereby approximately 15% of all tumors have either germline or somatic inactivation of the pathway.[43]There is now evidence that dMMR is widespread and occurs in a variety of cancers with a variable frequency both across and within tumor types, and an overall prevalence of 4% across all adult solid tumors.[44–46]

Molecularly, dMMR results in an increased frequency of mismatches as well as small insertion or deletions (indels), particularly in homopolymer stretches. Short tandem repeats composed of repetitive motifs up to approximately 6 nucleotides, termed microsatellites, are particularly sensitive to dMMR. Microsatellites represent approximately 3% of the human genome and are enriched in noncoding sequences.[47–49] Replicative errors due to the misalignment of the newly synthesized strand lead to changes in the lengths of microsatellites. Such alterations are subject to repair by the MMR system. In the context of dMMR, though, there is a cumulative change in the length distribution of microsatellites over time, resulting in high MSI (MSI-H).[41,48,50] Consequently, MSI is the molecular manifestation of dMMR.

In an initial small cohort of patients with progressive metastatic colorectal cancer treated with ICIs, dMMR/MSI-H tumors showed an overall response rate (ORR) of 40% compared with MMR proficient ones.[51] This study was followed by a larger collection of uncontrolled, single-arm, phase 2 trials totaling 149 patients across 14 cancer types, that demonstrated ORR in 53% of patients.[52] These findings prompted the approval of ICI treatment of patients with dMMR tumors that had progressed and for which there were no better alternative treatment[53] (https://www.fda.gov/drugs/ resources-information-approved-drugs/fda-grants-accelerated-approval-pembrolizumab-first-tissuesite-agnostic-indication). This marked the first time a cancer drug was approved based exclusively on a biomarker and not on the tumor site or histology. It should be noted that the study engendering the FDA approval included only 2 tumor types with sample sizes greater than 10 patients, while 7 of the 14 tumor types were represented by only one patient, raising concern for the broader applicability of dMMR/MSI as a biomarker. Further studies focusing on colorectal cancer confirmed that patients with dMMR/MSI-H tumors showed a response to ICI treatment.[54] These findings culminated in the 2020 FDA approval of ICIs as first-line treatment of unresectable or metastatic dMMR/MSI-H colorectal cancer (https://www.fda.gov/drugs/ drug-approvals-and-databases/fda-approves-pembrolizumab-first-line-treatment-msi-hdmmr-colorectal-cancer).

Screening for dMMR occurs by IHC, site-specific polymerase chain reaction (PCR), next-generation sequencing (NGS), or a combination thereof. IHC testing relies on the loss of nuclear staining for any of the 4 core MMR proteins. It is an indirect assessment of underlying MSI, is dependent on adequate tissue quantity and processing quality, and can yield false-negative results in the setting of inactivating mutations that do not affect the epitopes recognized by antibodies. PCR-based testing measures the length of microsatellites in PCR-amplified genomic regions that contain them. A difference in the length distributions of microsatellites between tumor and normal tissue signifies

MSI. The National Cancer Institute has established a panel of 5 microsatellite markers and set criteria for evaluating MSI, while additional panels with comparable performance characteristics have also been developed.[51] A tumor is classified as MSI-H if at least 30% of tested sites are unstable, as MSI low if at least one, but less than 30% of sites, is unstable, and as MSI stable if no site is unstable.[55] The studies that led to the FDA approval of ICIs for dMMR/MSI-H tumors determined MMR and MSI status by IHC and PCR testing, respectively. These assays have been shown to be complementary and concurrent testing can overcome the limitations of each assay.[56]

An alternative approach for the assessment of MSI is NGS-based methods. These can use either direct sequencing of microsatellite regions or bioinformatic inference of MSI by identifying statistical enrichment in total mutations or specifically indels in homopolymeric regions.[57–61] NGS is capable of providing a global picture of microsatellite instability across the genome and therefore can be more sensitive for noncolorectal carcinomas with MSI than PCR-based assays.[62] NGS methods can offer confirmation of dMMR by direct sequencing of the MMR genes. They also inherently enable assaying multiple other genetic events that could contribute to the diagnostic and prognostic classification of the tested tumor. Finally, they can be directly or sequentially coupled with germline testing to inform genetic counseling for possible inherited causes of MSI. By setting cut-offs for the number of either total mutations or indels in repeat regions per total sequenced space, such methods achieve high sensitivity and specificity.[58,59,61,63,64]

The NCCN recommends that all patients with colon and endometrial cancer be screened for dMMR/MSI. Most laboratories perform screening by using IHC for MMR genes or PCR for MSI or both, with additional testing involving *MLH1* promoter methylation and/or sequencing often added in a sequential testing algorithm.

Tumor Mutational Burden

The conceptual underpinning of the responsiveness of dMMR tumors to ICI therapy is the formation of neoantigens resulting from mutations in the open reading frame of protein-coding genes. By extension, a direct measurement of the number of mutations in coding sequences should be independently representative of the neoantigen load of a tumor. Tumor mutational burden (TMB) describes this aggregate collection of possible immunogenic mutations.

TMB is defined as the number of mutations per megabase of sequenced genomic territory. TMB varies widely both across and within tumors, with melanoma, lung, and bladder cancer showing on average the highest TMB.[65,66] The range of TMB across different tumor types is representative of both the underlying molecular mechanisms of tumorigenesis, as well as the effects of environmental exposures on different tumor types, such as melanoma, lung, and head and neck cancer.[65,66] Despite the conceptual relationship between TMB and dMMR/MSI, the 2 biomarkers do not show full overlap. Most dMMR/MSI-H tumors also have high TMB, but tumors can have high TMB without being dMMR/MSI-H.[61]

The first clinical indication that TMB correlates with response to ICIs was in the setting of melanoma treated with CTLA-4 blockade,[67] followed by multiple other studies in various tumor types.[68–70] Studies in relatively large patient cohorts have shown that TMB is an independent predictor of response to ICIs.[71] The positive correlation between TMB status and mean response rate has been demonstrated in a meta-analysis of 27 different cancer types.[72]

The correlation of TMB with ICI response culminated in the FDA approval of a commercial companion diagnostic for determining eligibility for ICI treatment in patients with unresectable or metastatic solid tumors with high TMB that have progressed following prior treatment and who have no satisfactory alternative therapies (https://www.fda.gov/drugs/drug-approvals-and-databases/fda-approves-pembrolizumab-adults-and-children-tmb-h-solid-tumors). The approval was based on a multicenter noncontrolled trial of 10 cohorts of patients, 13% of whom (n = 102) had TMB-H tumors (as defined by at least 10 mut/Mb) and showed 29% ORR.[73] Concerns regarding the scope of the approval were raised shortly afterward.[74] First, TMB-H status was not predictive of improved overall survival (OS) but only of ORR. Second, only 10 tumor types, excluding very common cancers, such as CRC, NSCLC, breast, and prostate were studied. Third, the possible confounding presence of a specific underlying biological process accounting for high TMB was not evaluated. When a separate large cohort of patients was stratified for dMMR and pathogenic mutations in POLE or POLD1 genes, there was no difference in overall survival among patients with dMMR and TMB-H as compared with low TMB.[74] However, in hypermutated tumors associated with environmental carcinogen exposure there was a clinical benefit from ICI treatment regardless of the tumor genetic subtype.[74]

The benchmark studies that led to TMB approval as a predictive biomarker via its correlation with clinical response were conducted using whole-exome sequencing (WES).[67–70] This practice is still cost-ineffective for the vast majority of clinical laboratories, which typically rely on targeted gene panels for economic and logistical reasons. Panel testing has shown good concordance with, and can be a suitable alternative to, WES, when it exhibits reasonable genomic coverage (>1 Mb) and uses germline variant filtering.[71,75–77] In particular, panels with approximately more than 300 genes tend to show similar performance characteristics compared with WES, while panels with fewer than 150 genes suffer from low predictive accuracy.[78] Data from a commercially available companion diagnostic for TMB based on a 395-gene panel also indicate a correlation between TMB-H status and response to ICIs in a sizable cohort of approximately 4000 patients with NSCLC.[79] Therefore, even though data are still accruing, it seems that tumor panel sequencing can serve as a clinically meaningful surrogate for TMB estimation.[79,80] It is worth highlighting that there is still great variability in the methods used to estimate TMB and the clinically meaningful cut-offs for predicting treatment response. There is, therefore, still a great need for harmonization on how to determine TMB, as well as the cut-offs set for treatment eligibility across tumors[81,82]; Hellmann:2018gm.[69,83,84]

An additional advantage of TMB over other biomarkers is that, assuming a stochastic distribution of mutations along the genome, cell-free DNA (cfDNA) testing could inform the TMB status of a patient. This can overcome issues with solid tumor sampling and intratumoral heterogeneity. Retrospective analysis of randomized clinical trials showed that blood-based estimation of TMB using cfDNA sequencing is predictive of clinical benefit from ICI treatment independent of PD-L1 expression.[82]

It is worth mentioning that if the rationale of ICI effectiveness in TMB-high tumors is through the presence of immunogenic tumor neoantigens, then one would expect that correlation to play out in the tumor microenvironment (TME). Indeed, evidence suggests that the neoantigen load (the number of mutations targeted by T cells) may be directly related to ICI response, with clonal neoantigen burden being associated with longer overall survival in patients with lung adenocarcinoma.[85] The clonal aspect of neoantigens seems to be an additive predictor of response, as there is a correlation between combined TMB and low intratumoral heterogeneity (<1%) and overall survival.[85] This suggests that the combination of the 2 may confer higher predictive accuracy than each biomarker alone.

EMERGING BIOMARKERS

Since currently, no single biomarker can predict the population that will respond to ICIs with very high accuracy, there is a need for the development of additional biomarkers in parallel with the improvement of currently approved ones. The following section summarizes briefly the landscape of emerging predictive biomarkers.

Tumor-Infiltrating Lymphocytes and Tumor Microenvironment

Tumor-infiltrating lymphocytes (TILs) were identified as a possible prognostic biomarker first in breast cancer. In 2011, it was shown that the increased presence of CD8+ lymphocytes was associated with improved outcomes,[86] while in colorectal cancer, the presence of TILs in the tumor center and margin was indicative of recurrence.[87] As the presence of TILs suggests an inflamed TME, TILs have also been evaluated as a predictive biomarker of response to ICIs. The density of CD8+ TILs in pretreatment biopsies has been associated with increased responses to PD-1/PD-L1 or CTLA-4 blockade in breast cancer and melanoma.[88–91] However, to date, there is no established cut-off for separating responders and nonresponders.

Expanding on the characterization of the TME, the development of multiplexed immunohistochemistry or immunofluorescence panels has allowed the concurrent characterization of multiple immune markers on both the tumor and the TME.[91–93] Such methods have—to a certain extent—enabled the correlation between immune–tumor cell interactions and response to ICIs.[94,95] Improvements in assay standardization and result interpretation will likely increase the value of TILs and TME characterization as predictive biomarkers.

Gene Expression Profiling

The complexity of tumor–immune cell interactions can also be elucidated by the overall gene expression profile of the tumor and its immune environment. Composite signatures are being developed to assess the possible effectiveness of ICIs.

Gene expression profiles (GEP) that reflect transcriptional states and are compiled from the integrated expression levels of a panel of genes, such as the IFN-γ inflamed signature, have shown a correlation with response to ICIs. Retrospective assessment of GEP scores from multiple clinical trials suggests that higher scores may correlate with better rates of clinical responses,[96,97] independently of other biomarkers, such as TMB and PD-L1 expression. Such findings suggest the likely presence of additional immune-cell characteristics that may not be accurately reflected by the currently approved biomarkers.

Tumor Neoantigens

The theoretic backdrop behind the development of TMB, MSI-H, and dMMR is the concept of neoantigen formation in the tumor that can breach immune tolerance and elicit a neoantigen and tumor-specific immune response. The FDA-approved biomarkers essentially serve essentially as proxies for the neoantigen load of a tumor. Coupling tumor DNA sequencing with bioinformatic prediction tools enables the direct assessment of tumor neoantigens whose immunogenicity can be evaluated directly and independently in an *ex vivo* setting. Indeed, experimental evidence suggests that only a small fraction of tumor neoantigens are immunoreactive and that neoantigens seem to be unique to each patient.[98–103] These findings raise the possibility of nominating highly personalized biomarkers in the future. However, as of now, the lack of robust computational and experimental methods, the complexity of the underlying tumor biology, and the purported uniqueness of neoantigens render tumor neoantigens unripe for direct clinical biomarker utilization.

Microbiome

The interplay between the gut microbiome and the immune system has attracted attention as a possible modulator of ICI efficacy. It has been shown that the perturbation of the microbiome by antibiotic treatment is inversely correlated with response to ICIs.[104] Instead, a highly diverse microbiome may correlate with improved treatment outcomes.[105] Intriguingly, several studies have identified the enrichment of specific species in the microbiome of ICI responders.[104–106] This suggests the possible presence of specific beneficial bacterial species that can modulate the host immune response in a way that enhances the effects of ICIs. Despite these promising observations, the lack of standardized studies limits the current utility of the microbiome as a predictive biomarker.

Germline and Human Leukocyte Antigen Variants

Through their function in mediating the interaction between tumor and immune cells, human leukocyte antigen (HLA)-I genes play a key role in the host immune response. The diversity and repertoire of these highly polymorphic genes may, therefore, impact response to ICIs. Indeed, preliminary studies have indicated a correlation between high HLA-I diversity and increased survival in ICI-treated patients.[107] Extensive or complete heterozygosity of the HLA-I alleles has been postulated to impact such responses positively via increased expansion of the T-cell receptor repertoire.[107] Conversely, the high incidence of loss of heterozygosity in HLA-I loci in tumors is thought to represent a mechanism of immune escape and thus, resistance to ICIs.[108] In the future, sequencing and accurate characterization of the HLA-I immunopeptidome may result in improved predictions of response to ICI treatment. Apart from HLA-I genes, polymorphisms and variation in other immunity-related genes, such as HLA-II, NF-κB, and members of the JAK-STAT pathway have been identified in association with response to ICIs.[109]

Combination Biomarkers and Machine Learning

There may be no single biomarker or test that is highly predictive for identifying patients that will respond to immunotherapy. Among the existing FDA-approved biomarkers, there is some overlap in patients that are identified by each biomarker, yet also distinct populations that each of them identify.[61,110] Therefore, using existing and novel biomarkers in concert with each other may improve our ability to accurately predict outcomes. One retrospective analysis demonstrated the power of a machine learning model in achieving high sensitivity and specificity in predicting clinical response to immunotherapy across different cancer types in which an ensemble learning random forest classifier with 16 different input features was used that included both genomic, clinical, and demographic data points in the model.[111]

SUMMARY

Overall, there is still great variability in the use, application, and interpretation of the currently approved biomarkers for ICI treatment. At this stage, there is still no ideal biomarker that can accurately predict the response of every patient to ICIs. The limited predictive accuracy is due to multiple factors, including the intrinsic variability of tumor biology, the heterogeneity of the TME, as well as the technical aspects in both preanalytical assay standardization and postanalytical clinicopathological interpretation.

Despite the still unmet needs for standardization, the development of dMMR/MSI and TMB as biomarkers for immunotherapy has marked a striking shift in the practice of pathology. It has signaled the transition from standalone (single) to synergistic (aggregate) biomarkers and has led to the first approved cancer treatments based solely on biomarker status and not tumor site or histology. As the number of patients receiving immunotherapy continues to rise, the improvement of the currently approved biomarkers and the adoption of complementary or superior emerging biomarkers will be of paramount importance in ensuring the appropriate choice of treatment that will maximize benefits and minimize toxicities in these patients.

CLINICS CARE POINTS

- PD-1/PD-L1, microsatellite instability/mismatch repair deficincy, and tumor mutational burden are the only FDA-approved biomarkers for response to immunotherapy.
- The application of biomarkers for response to immunotherapy should be carried out with caution, due to variation across assays and tumor types.

REFERENCES

1. Ishida Y, Agata Y, Shibahara K, et al. Induced expression of PD-1, a novel member of the immunoglobulin gene superfamily, upon programmed cell death. EMBO J 1992;11:3887–95.
2. Krummel MF, Allison JP. CD28 and CTLA-4 have opposing effects on the response of T cells to stimulation. J Exp Med 1995;182:459–65.
3. Sharma P, Allison JP. The future of immune checkpoint therapy. Science 2015; 348:56–61.
4. Leach DR, Krummel MF, Allison JP. Enhancement of antitumor immunity by CTLA-4 blockade. Science 1996;271:1734–6.
5. Cameron F, Whiteside G, Perry C. Ipilimumab: first global approval. Drugs 2011; 71:1093–104.
6. Davis AA, Patel VG. The role of PD-L1 expression as a predictive biomarker: an analysis of all US Food and Drug Administration (FDA) approvals of immune checkpoint inhibitors. J Immunother Cancer 2019;7(1):278.
7. Postow MA, Chesney J, Pavlick AC, et al. Nivolumab and ipilimumab versus ipilimumab in untreated melanoma. N Engl J Med 2015;372:2006–17.
8. Vaddepally RK, Kharel P, Pandey R, et al. Review of indications of FDA-approved immune checkpoint inhibitors per NCCN guidelines with the level of evidence. Cancers 2020;12(738 12):738.
9. Ribas A, Wolchok JD. Cancer immunotherapy using checkpoint blockade. Science 2018;359:1350–5.
10. Woo S-R, Turnis ME, Goldberg MV, et al. Immune inhibitory molecules LAG-3 and PD-1 synergistically regulate T-cell function to promote tumoral immune escape. Cancer Res 2012;72:917–27.
11. Xu F, Liu J, Liu Di, et al. LSECtin expressed on melanoma cells promotes tumor progression by inhibiting antitumor T-cell responses. Cancer Res 2014;74: 3418–28.
12. Ascierto PA, Bono P, Bhatia S, et al. LBA18 - efficacy of BMS-986016, a monoclonal antibody that targets lymphocyte activation gene-3 (LAG-3), in combination with nivolumab in pts with melanoma who progressed during prior

anti–PD-1/PD-L1 therapy (mel prior IO) in all-comer and biomarker-enriched populations. Ann Oncol 2017;28:v611–2.

13. Long L, Zhang X, Chen F, et al. The promising immune checkpoint LAG-3: from tumor microenvironment to cancer immunotherapy. Genes Cancer 2018;9: 176–89.

14. Acharya N, Sabatos-Peyton C, Anderson AC. Tim-3 finds its place in the cancer immunotherapy landscape. J Immunother Cancer 2020;8:e000911.

15. Fourcade J, Sun Z, Benallaoua M, et al. Upregulation of Tim-3 and PD-1 expression is associated with tumor antigen-specific CD8+ T cell dysfunction in melanoma patients. J Exp Med 2010;207:2175–86.

16. Rezaei M, Tan J, Zeng C, et al. TIM-3 in leukemia; immune response and beyond. Front Oncol 2021;11:753677.

17. Gao X, Zhu Y, Li G, et al. TIM-3 expression characterizes regulatory T cells in tumor tissues and is associated with lung cancer progression. PLoS One 2012;7:e30676.

18. Ngiow SF, Scheidt, von B, Akiba H, et al. Anti-TIM3 antibody promotes T cell IFN-γ-mediated antitumor immunity and suppresses established tumors. Cancer Res 2011;71:3540–51.

19. Sakuishi K, Apetoh L, Sullivan JM, et al. Targeting Tim-3 and PD-1 pathways to reverse T cell exhaustion and restore anti-tumor immunity. J Exp Med 2010;207: 2187–94.

20. Zhou Q, Munger ME, Veenstra RG, et al. Coexpression of Tim-3 and PD-1 identifies a CD8+ T-cell exhaustion phenotype in mice with disseminated acute myelogenous leukemia. Blood 2011;117:4501–10.

21. Pan C, Liu H, Robins E, et al. Next-generation immuno-oncology agents: current momentum shifts in cancer immunotherapy. J Hematol Oncol 2020;. https://doi.org/10.1186/s13045-020-00862-w.

22. Carretero-González A, Lora D, Ghanem I, et al. Analysis of response rate with ANTI PD1/PD-L1 monoclonal antibodies in advanced solid tumors: a meta-analysis of randomized clinical trials. Oncotarget 2018;9:8706–15.

23. Kourie HR, Klastersky J. Immune checkpoint inhibitors side effects and management. Immunotherapy 2016;8:799–807.

24. Brahmer JR, Tykodi SS, Chow LQM, et al. Safety and activity of anti-PD-L1 antibody in patients with advanced cancer. N Engl J Med 2012;366:2455–65.

25. Khunger M, Jain P, Rakshit S, et al. Safety and efficacy of PD-1/PD-L1 inhibitors in treatment-naive and chemotherapy-refractory patients with non-small-cell lung cancer: a systematic review and meta-analysis. Clin Lung Cancer 2018; 19:e335–48.

26. Mahoney KM, Atkins MB. Prognostic and predictive markers for the new immunotherapies. Oncology (Williston Park) 2014;28(Suppl 3):39–48.

27. Robert C, Long GV, Brady B, et al. Nivolumab in previously untreated melanoma without BRAF mutation. N Engl J Med 2015;372:320–30.

28. Weber JS, D'Angelo SP, Minor D, et al. Nivolumab versus chemotherapy in patients with advanced melanoma who progressed after anti-CTLA-4 treatment (CheckMate 037): a randomised, controlled, open-label, phase 3 trial. Lancet Oncol 2015;16:375–84.

29. Brahmer J, Reckamp KL, Baas P, et al. Nivolumab versus docetaxel in advanced squamous-cell non-small-cell lung cancer. N Engl J Med 2015;373: 123–35.

30. Garon EB, Rizvi NA, Hui R, et al. Pembrolizumab for the treatment of non-small-cell lung cancer. N Engl J Med 2015;372:2018–28.

31. Walk EE, Yohe SL, Beckman A, et al, College of American pathologists personalized health care committee. The cancer immunotherapy biomarker testing landscape. Arch Pathol Lab Med 2020;144:706–24.
32. McLaughlin J, Han G, Schalper KA, et al. Quantitative assessment of the heterogeneity of PD-L1 expression in non-small-cell lung cancer. JAMA Oncol 2016;2: 46–54.
33. Rimm DL, Han G, Taube JM, et al. A prospective, multi-institutional, pathologist-based assessment of 4 immunohistochemistry assays for PD-L1 expression in non-small cell lung cancer. JAMA Oncol 2017;3:1051–8.
34. Haragan A, Field JK, Davies MPA, et al. Heterogeneity of PD-L1 expression in non-small cell lung cancer: implications for specimen sampling in predicting treatment response. Lung Cancer 2019;134:79–84.
35. Ilie M, Long-Mira E, Bence C, et al. Comparative study of the PD-L1 status between surgically resected specimens and matched biopsies of NSCLC patients reveal major discordances: a potential issue for anti-PD-L1 therapeutic strategies. Ann Oncol 2016;27:147–53.
36. Liu Y, Dong Z, Jiang T, et al. Heterogeneity of PD-L1 expression among the different histological components and metastatic lymph nodes in patients with resected lung adenosquamous carcinoma. Clin Lung Cancer 2018;19:e421–30.
37. Munari E, Rossi G, Zamboni G, et al. PD-L1 assays 22C3 and SP263 are not interchangeable in non-small cell lung cancer when considering clinically relevant cutoffs: an interclone evaluation by differently trained pathologists. Am J Surg Pathol 2018;42:1384–9.
38. Munari E, Zamboni G, Lunardi G, et al. PD-L1 expression comparison between primary and relapsed non-small cell lung carcinoma using whole sections and clone SP263. Oncotarget 2018;9:30465–71.
39. Iyer RR, Pluciennik A, Burdett V, et al. DNA mismatch repair: functions and mechanisms. Chem Rev 2006;106:302–23.
40. Modrich P, Lahue R. Mismatch repair in replication fidelity, genetic recombination, and cancer biology. Annu Rev Biochem 1996;65:101–33.
41. Buza N, Ziai J, Hui P. Mismatch repair deficiency testing in clinical practice. Expert Rev Mol Diagn 2016;16:591–604.
42. Peltomäki P, Vasen H. Mutations associated with HNPCC predisposition — update of ICG-HNPCC/INSiGHT mutation database. Dis Markers 2004;20:269–76.
43. Lynch HT, Snyder CL, Shaw TG, et al. Milestones of Lynch syndrome: 1895-2015. Nat Rev Cancer 2015;15:181–94.
44. Bonneville R, Krook MA, Kautto EA, et al. Landscape of microsatellite instability across 39 cancer types. JCO Precis Oncol 2017;2017. PO.17.00073.
45. Cortés-Ciriano I, Lee JJ-K, Xi R, et al. Comprehensive analysis of chromothripsis in 2,658 human cancers using whole-genome sequencing. Nat Genet 2020;52: 331–41.
46. Van de Water NS, Jeevaratnam P, Browett PJ, et al. Direct mutational analysis in a family with hereditary non-polyposis colorectal cancer. Aust N Z J Med 1994; 24:682–6.
47. Ellegren H. Microsatellites: simple sequences with complex evolution. Nat Rev Genet 2004;5:435–45.
48. Imai K, Yamamoto H. Carcinogenesis and microsatellite instability: the interrelationship between genetics and epigenetics. Carcinogenesis 2008;29:673–80.
49. Li Y-C, Korol AB, Fahima T, et al. Microsatellites within genes: structure, function, and evolution. Mol Biol Evol 2004;21:991–1007.

50. Lynch HT, Jascur T, Lanspa S, et al. Making sense of missense in Lynch syndrome: the clinical perspective. Cancer Prev Res (Phila) 2010;3:1371–4.
51. Boland CR, Thibodeau SN, Hamilton SR, et al. A National Cancer Institute Workshop on Microsatellite Instability for cancer detection and familial predisposition: development of international criteria for the determination of microsatellite instability in colorectal cancer. Cancer Res 1998;5248–57.
52. Le DT, Durham JN, Smith KN, et al. Mismatch repair deficiency predicts response of solid tumors to PD-1 blockade. Science 2017;357:409–13.
53. Prasad V, Kaestner V, Mailankody S. Cancer drugs approved based on biomarkers and not tumor type-FDA approval of pembrolizumab for mismatch repair-deficient solid cancers. JAMA Oncol 2018;4:157–8.
54. André T, Shiu K-K, Kim TW, et al. Pembrolizumab in microsatellite-instability-high advanced colorectal cancer. N Engl J Med 2020;383:2207–18.
55. Hegde M, Ferber M, Mao R, et al, Working Group of the American College of Medical Genetics and Genomics (ACMG) Laboratory Quality Assurance Committee. ACMG technical standards and guidelines for genetic testing for inherited colorectal cancer (Lynch syndrome, familial adenomatous polyposis, and MYH-associated polyposis). Genet Med 2014;16:101–16.
56. Funkhouser WK, Lubin IM, Monzon FA, et al. Relevance, pathogenesis, and testing algorithm for mismatch repair–defective colorectal carcinomas. J Mol Diagn 2012;14:91–103.
57. Gan C, Love C, Beshay V, et al. Applicability of next generation sequencing technology in microsatellite instability testing. Genes 2015;6:46–59.
58. Kautto EA, Bonneville R, Miya J, et al. Performance evaluation for rapid detection of pan-cancer microsatellite instability with MANTIS. Oncotarget 2017;8: 7452–63.
59. Nowak JA, Yurgelun MB, Bruce JL, et al. Detection of mismatch repair deficiency and microsatellite instability in colorectal adenocarcinoma by targeted next-generation sequencing. J Mol Diagn 2017;19:84–91.
60. Salipante SJ, Scroggins SM, Hampel HL, et al. Microsatellite instability detection by next generation sequencing. Clin Chem 2014;60:1192–9.
61. Vanderwalde A, Spetzler D, Xiao N, et al. Microsatellite instability status determined by next-generation sequencing and compared with PD-L1 and tumor mutational burden in 11,348 patients. Cancer Med 2018;7:746–56.
62. Hause RJ, Pritchard CC, Shendure J, et al. Classification and characterization of microsatellite instability across 18 cancer types. Nat Med 2016;22:1342–50.
63. Middha S, Zhang L, Nafa K, et al. Reliable pan-cancer microsatellite instability assessment by using targeted next-generation sequencing data. JCO Precis Oncol 2017.
64. Stadler ZK, Battaglin F, Middha S, et al. Reliable detection of mismatch repair deficiency in colorectal cancers using mutational load in next-generation sequencing panels. J Clin Oncol 2016;34:2141–7.
65. Alexandrov LB, Nik-Zainal S, Wedge DC, et al. Signatures of mutational processes in human cancer. Nature 2013;500:415–21.
66. Boot A, Covington KR, Islam SMA, et al. The repertoire of mutational signatures in human cancer. Nature 2020;1–28.
67. Snyder A, Makarov V, Merghoub T, et al. Genetic basis for clinical response to CTLA-4 blockade in melanoma. N Engl J Med 2014;371:2189–99.
68. Hellmann MD, Ciuleanu T-E, Pluzanski A, et al. Nivolumab plus ipilimumab in lung cancer with a high tumor mutational burden. N Engl J Med 2018;378: 2093–104.

69. Hellmann MD, Nathanson T, Rizvi H, et al. Genomic features of response to combination immunotherapy in patients with advanced non- small-cell lung cancer. Cancer Cell 2018;33:843–52.e844.

70. Rizvi NA, Hellmann MD, Snyder A, et al. Cancer immunology. Mutational landscape determines sensitivity to PD-1 blockade in non-small cell lung cancer. Science 2015;348:124–8.

71. Goodman AM, Kato S, Bazhenova L, et al. Tumor mutational burden as an independent predictor of response to immunotherapy in diverse cancers. Mol Cancer Ther 2017;16:2598–608.

72. Yarchoan M, Hopkins A, Jaffee EM. Tumor mutational burden and response rate to PD-1 inhibition. N Engl J Med 2017;377:2500–1.

73. Marabelle A, Fakih M, Lopez J, et al. Association of tumour mutational burden with outcomes in patients with advanced solid tumours treated with pembrolizumab: prospective biomarker analysis of the multicohort, open-label, phase 2 KEYNOTE-158 study. Lancet Oncol 2020;21:1353–65.

74. Rousseau B, Foote MB, Maron SB, et al. The spectrum of benefit from checkpoint blockade in hypermutated tumors. N Engl J Med 2021;384:1168–70.

75. Chalmers ZR, Connelly CF, Fabrizio D, et al. Analysis of 100,000 human cancer genomes reveals the landscape of tumor mutational burden. Genome Med 2017;19:94.

76. Mouw KW, Goldberg MS, Konstantinopoulos PA, et al. DNA damage and repair biomarkers of immunotherapy response. Cancer Discov 2017;7:675–93.

77. Rizvi H, Sanchez-Vega F, La K, et al. Molecular determinants of response to anti-programmed cell death (PD)-1 and anti-programmed death-ligand 1 (PD-L1) blockade in patients with non-small-cell lung cancer profiled with targeted next-generation sequencing. J Clin Oncol 2018;36:633–41.

78. Campesato LF, Barroso-Sousa R, Jimenez L, et al. Comprehensive cancer-gene panels can be used to estimate mutational load and predict clinical benefit to PD-1 blockade in clinical practice. Oncotarget 2015;6:34221–7.

79. Singal G, Miller PG, Agarwala V, et al. Association of patient characteristics and tumor genomics with clinical outcomes among patients with non-small cell lung cancer using a clinicogenomic database. JAMA 2019;321:1391–9.

80. Fang W, Ma Y, Yin JC, et al. Comprehensive genomic profiling identifies novel genetic predictors of response to anti-PD-(L)1 therapies in non-small cell lung cancer. Clin Cancer Res 2019;25:5015–26.

81. Balar AV, Galsky MD, Rosenberg JE, et al. Atezolizumab as first-line treatment in cisplatin-ineligible patients with locally advanced and metastatic urothelial carcinoma: a single-arm, multicentre, phase 2 trial. Lancet 2017;389:67–76.

82. Gandara DR, Paul SM, Kowanetz M, et al. Blood-based tumor mutational burden as a predictor of clinical benefit in non-small-cell lung cancer patients treated with atezolizumab. Nat Med 2018;24:1441–8.

83. Johnson DB, Frampton GM, Rioth MJ, et al. Targeted next generation sequencing identifies markers of response to PD-1 blockade. Cancer Immunol Res 2016;4:959–67.

84. Samstein RM, Lee C-H, Shoushtari AN, et al. Tumor mutational load predicts survival after immunotherapy across multiple cancer types. Nat Genet 2019;51: 202–6.

85. McGranahan N, Furness AJS, Rosenthal R, et al. Clonal neoantigens elicit T cell immunoreactivity and sensitivity to immune checkpoint blockade. Science 2016; 351:1463–9.

86. Mahmoud SMA, Paish EC, Powe DG, et al. Tumor-infiltrating CD8+ lymphocytes predict clinical outcome in breast cancer. J Clin Oncol 2011;29:1949–55.

87. Mlecnik B, Tosolini M, Kirilovsky A, et al. Histopathologic-based prognostic factors of colorectal cancers are associated with the state of the local immune reaction. J Clin Oncol 2011;29:610–8.

88. Chen P-L, Roh W, Reuben A, et al. Analysis of immune signatures in longitudinal tumor samples yields insight into biomarkers of response and mechanisms of resistance to immune checkpoint blockade. Cancer Discov 2016;6:827–37.

89. Schmid P, Salgado R, Park YH, et al. Pembrolizumab plus chemotherapy as neoadjuvant treatment of high-risk, early-stage triple-negative breast cancer: results from the phase 1b open- label, multicohort KEYNOTE-173 study. Ann Oncol 2020;31:569–81.

90. Tumeh PC, Harview CL, Yearley JH, et al. PD-1 blockade induces responses by inhibiting adaptive immune resistance. Nature 2014;515:568–71.

91. Wickenhauser C, Bethmann D, Feng Z, et al. Multispectral fluorescence imaging allows for distinctive topographic assessment and subclassification of tumor-infiltrating and surrounding immune cells. Methods Mol Biol 2019;1913:13–31.

92. Hofman P, Badoual C, Henderson F, et al. Multiplexed immunohistochemistry for molecular and immune profiling in lung cancer-just about ready for prime-time? Cancers 2019;12(738 11):283.

93. Parra ER, Francisco-Cruz A, Wistuba II. State-of-the-Art of profiling immune contexture in the era of multiplexed staining and digital analysis to study paraffin tumor tissues. Cancers 2019;12(738 11):247.

94. Giraldo NA, Nguyen P, Engle EL, et al. Multidimensional, quantitative assessment of PD-1/PD-L1 expression in patients with Merkel cell carcinoma and association with response to pembrolizumab. J Immunother Cancer 2018;6(1):99.

95. Johnson DB, Bordeaux J, Kim JY, et al. Quantitative spatial profiling of PD-1/PD-L1 interaction and HLA-DR/Ido-1 predicts improved outcomes of anti-PD-1 therapies in metastatic melanoma. Clin Cancer Res 2018;24:5250–60.

96. Cristescu R, Mogg R, Ayers M, et al. Pan-tumor genomic biomarkers for PD-1 checkpoint blockade-based immunotherapy. Science 2018;362:eaar3593.

97. Ott PA, Bang Y-J, Piha-Paul SA, et al. T-Cell-Inflamed gene-expression profile, programmed death ligand 1 expression, and tumor mutational burden predict efficacy in patients treated with pembrolizumab across 20 cancers: KEYNOTE-028. J Clin Oncol 2019;37:318–27.

98. Fritsch EF, Rajasagi M, Ott PA, et al. HLA-binding properties of tumor neoepitopes in humans. Cancer Immunol Res 2014;2:522–9.

99. Parkhurst MR, Robbins PF, Tran E, et al. Unique neoantigens arise from somatic mutations in patients with gastrointestinal cancers. Cancer Discov 2019;9:1022–35.

100. Schumacher TN, Schreiber RD. Neoantigens in cancer immunotherapy. Science 2015;348:69–74.

101. Tran E, Robbins PF, Rosenberg SA. "Final common pathway" of human cancer immunotherapy: targeting random somatic mutations. Nat Immunol 2017;18:255–62.

102. Van Bergen CAM, Rutten CE, Van Der Meijden ED, et al. High-throughput characterization of 10 new minor histocompatibility antigens by whole genome association scanning. Cancer Res 2010;70:9073–83.

103. van Buuren MM, Calis JJ, Schumacher TN. High sensitivity of cancer exome-based CD8 T cell neo-antigen identification. Oncoimmunology 2014;3:e28836.

104. Routy B, Le Chatelier E, Derosa L, et al. Gut microbiome influences efficacy of PD-1-based immunotherapy against epithelial tumors. Science 2018;359:91–7.
105. Matson V, Fessler J, Bao R, et al. The commensal microbiome is associated with anti-PD-1 efficacy in metastatic melanoma patients. Science 2018;359:104–8.
106. Gopalakrishnan V, Spencer CN, Nezi L, et al. Gut microbiome modulates response to anti-PD-1 immunotherapy in melanoma patients. Science 2018; 359:97–103.
107. Chowell D, Morris LGT, Grigg CM, et al. Patient HLA class I genotype influences cancer response to checkpoint blockade immunotherapy. Science 2018;359: 582–7.
108. Rosenthal R, Hiley CT, Rowan AJ, et al. Allele-specific HLA loss and immune escape in lung cancer evolution. Cell 2017;171:1259–71.e11.
109. Havel JJ, Chowell D, Chan TA. The evolving landscape of biomarkers for checkpoint inhibitor immunotherapy. Nat Rev Cancer 2019;19:133–50.
110. Luchini C, Bibeau F, Ligtenberg MJL, et al. ESMO recommendations on microsatellite instability testing for immunotherapy in cancer, and its relationship with PD-1/PD-L1 expression and tumour mutational burden: a systematic review-based approach. Ann Oncol 2019;30:1232–43.
111. Chowell D, Yoo S-K, Valero C, et al. Improved prediction of immune checkpoint blockade efficacy across multiple cancer types. Nat Biotechnol 2022;40: 499–506.

When Tissue Is the Issue
Expanding Cell-Free DNA "Liquid Biopsies" to Supernatants and Nonplasma Biofluids

Vera Paulson, MD, PhD[a,b,*], Eric Q. Konnick, MD, MS[a,b],
Christina H. Lockwood, PhD[a,b]

KEYWORDS

- Liquid biopsy • Cell-free DNA (cfDNA) • Biofluid • Cerebrospinal fluid (CSF)
- Circulating tumor DNA (ctDNA) • Urinary tumor DNA (utDNA) • Supernatant
- Preanalytical variables

KEY POINTS

- While there are no uniform standards for cfDNA testing in oncology, recommendations and guidelines concerning the processing of plasma-derived ctDNA can inform molecular diagnostics performed on cfDNA derived from supernatants and nonplasma biofluids.
- Preanalytical variables affecting cfDNA include biological considerations of the tumors and their communicating fluid compartment(s), as well as their collection, transport, storage, and extraction.
- Assays for cfDNA evaluation cover a range of targets, from allele-specific to broad whole exome or genome sequencing; assay selection primarily depends on the testing indication and required limit of detection.
- cfDNA acquisition results in fewer surgical complications, and assays using cfDNA demonstrate improved quality metrics, reduced turnaround time and expense, and higher sensitivity (potentially at the cost of specificity).

INTRODUCTION

Nearly 75 years ago, Mandel and Metais described the presence of fragments of cell-free DNA (cfDNA) in human peripheral blood.[1] While to date the mechanism of this phenomenon remains incompletely understood, cfDNA is thought to be the result of passive release of DNA during apoptosis, necrosis, NETosis, or physical cell damage and/or active secretion due to an underlying (patho)physiologic process, including pregnancy, organ transplant, autoimmune disease, trauma, infection, or neoplasia.[2]

[a] Department of Laboratory Medicine and Pathology, University of Washington, 1959 Northeast Pacific Street, Seattle, WA 98195, USA; [b] Brotman-Baty Institute for Precision Medicine, University of Washington, Seattle, WA
* Corresponding author.
E-mail address: vpauls@uw.edu

Clin Lab Med 42 (2022) 485–496
https://doi.org/10.1016/j.cll.2022.05.005
0272-2712/22/© 2022 Elsevier Inc. All rights reserved.

labmed.theclinics.com

The potential of cfDNA in evaluating neoplasia is substantial, with implications in cancer screening, diagnosis, prognosis, monitoring of disease progression, and the prediction of therapeutic response.

Cell-Free DNA in Peripheral Blood

The relative increase in serum cfDNA in patients with cancer compared with normal controls was first demonstrated in 1977.[3] Stroun and colleagues[4] would later report that at least some of this cfDNA was attributable to the cancer cells themselves, which was further supported by the identification of identical KRAS mutations in plasma-derived cfDNA of patients with pancreatic cancer and their corresponding tumor tissue.[5] This potential of tumor-derived cfDNA in peripheral blood, also known as circulating tumor DNA (ctDNA), to act as a surrogate for tissue led many to theorize that a "liquid biopsy" evaluating ctDNA might become the gold standard for tumor testing, at least in certain contexts. Advances in technology in the last decade have allowed the approval of multiple ctDNA liquid biopsy assays by the US Food and Drug Administration (FDA) and the European Medicines Agency (EMA).

Cell-Free DNA in Biofluids and Supernatants

cfDNA, however, is not limited to plasma, having been reported in bodily fluids (biofluids), including but not limited to cerebrospinal fluid (CSF), aqueous humor, tears, saliva, sputum, effusions, ascites, stool, urine, and organ-cyst fluid, as well as within interventional byproducts of lavage and fine-needle aspiration (FNA) (**Fig. 1**).[6–9] Rather than an exhaustive survey of the historic contributions and institutional experiences for each of these analytes, this review will instead focus on the preanalytical, analytical, and postanalytical considerations of cfDNA in oncology testing, as well as the limitations and benefits of cfDNA as a biomarker outside of the plasma compartment.

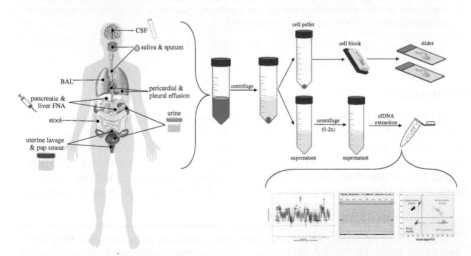

Fig. 1. A "liquid biopsy" can be performed on any biofluid (including CSF, saliva, sputum, effusions, ascites, stool, or urine) or supernatant obtained as a byproduct of an interventional procedure (including BAL, FNA, uterine lavage, or pap smear). These fluids are processed to obtain a cell pellet, which can be used for histologic diagnosis; following an additional 0 to 2 centrifugation steps, cfDNA can be extracted from the leftover supernatant for molecular studies including NGS and ddPCR.

PREANALYTICAL CONSIDERATIONS IN CELL-FREE DNA EVALUATION

Preanalytical variables in cfDNA testing include all steps preceding specimen analysis. These variables range from the biological considerations of the tumors themselves and the compartment from which cfDNA is derived to factors affecting specimen integrity including collection, transport, storage, and extraction. Although recommendations and guidelines concerning cfDNA processing and evaluation have predominantly focused on ctDNA, they can inform such matters regarding cfDNA in other fluids.[10,11]

Cell-Free DNA Characteristics

ctDNA was originally sized at ~185 to 200 base pairs (bp) by gel electrophoresis, but sequencing-based methods further refined the size to 166 bp, the combined length of nucleosome- and H1-histone-associated DNA.[12,13] Notably, ctDNA molecules are shorter than their nontumor cfDNA counterparts (~145 bp, range: 90–150 bp), possibly due to tissue-dependent nucleosome differences and/or nuclease action, a finding that has been exploited in several publications to predict tumor and/or tissue of origin.[2,8,13–16]

cfDNA from nonplasma fluids have also been reported to demonstrate patterns of 166bp-multiples, though some studies indicate wider variation, possibly secondary to nucleosome positioning, cellular disruption, and/or necrosis, which may generate longer fragments (1–10kb).[9,11,13,17,18] Tumor-derived cfDNA fragments in urine (utDNA) also diverge from plasma-derived cfDNA due to increased concentration of nucleases resulting in shorter cfDNA fragments.[6,19,20] Additionally, the glomerular filtration barrier restricts the passage of cfDNA fragments greater than 70 kDa (~100bp), essentially prohibiting nucleosome-associated cfDNA from entering urine.[20]

While the half-life of cfDNA in urine has been reported to be up to 5 hours, cfDNA in peripheral blood has a half-life of minutes to 1 to 2 hours, depending on patient factors and its association with cell membranes, extracellular vesicles, or proteins, which may increase stability.[2,6,13] These fragments are cleared from circulation via nuclease action and renal excretion into urine or through uptake by the liver and spleen, followed by degradation by macrophages.[2,13]

Physiologic Factors Affecting Cell-Free DNA

Factors impacting ctDNA concentration include tumor location/type, tumor burden/ stage, proliferative index, and the presence/absence of necrosis.[2,11,13,17] The patient's clinical condition, exposure to chemotherapy and radiation, and the time of sampling can also influence ctDNA levels.[2,11,17] These variables are likely to affect the quantity of tumor-derived cfDNA in other biofluids, along with the degree of communication between the tumor and extracted biofluid.

Of equal importance is the fraction of nontumor DNA in a specimen, either cfDNA or genomic DNA (gDNA) released from nonneoplastic cells. CSF is typically paucicellular, resulting in an enrichment of tumor-derived cfDNA, though quantities are frequently limited, particularly in low-grade tumors and tumors that are not in direct contact with CSF.[8] In contrast, effusions can contain both inflammatory and mesothelial cells that may vastly outnumber the tumor cells, resulting in a significant dilution of tumor-derived cfDNA.[17] Urine poses an additional challenge– although bladder tumors release nucleic acid directly into the urine, select cfDNA also passes through the glomerular filtration barrier and could be the source of utDNA or dilute tumor-derived cfDNA from another source.[20]

Saliva and gastrointestinal fluids pose additional challenges. Food may contain analytical inhibitors and/or carcinogens such as alcohol or tobacco products.[19] Other considerations include the effects of physical manipulation (brushing), exposure to digestive enzymes, or the presence of microorganisms in select biological compartments.[19] Despite these additional variables, biofluids in contact with tumor-containing tissue, organs, or organ systems may be the best source of tumor-derived cfDNA.

Nonbiological supernatants are another potential source of tumor-derived cfDNA.[7,9] While minimally invasive procedures such as FNAs produce limited material, which is frequently insufficient for molecular testing, substantial amounts of nucleic acid, both cfDNA and gDNA from centrifugation-disrupted cells, can be extracted from supernatant after centrifugation and cell-pelleting.[9] Moreover, molecular studies using supernatant-derived cfDNA demonstrate superior sequencing metrics and sensitivity compared with some cytology specimens alone.[7,9]

Collection, Transport, and Storage of Cell-Free DNA

The analytical sensitivity of cfDNA evaluation depends on maintaining its integrity and minimizing contamination from gDNA. ctDNA is the most studied, with a wide range of available stabilizing agents, some of which have also been evaluated outside the plasma compartment.[19] Time-to-processing and extraction impacts reagent choice. Samples collected in EDTA require processing within 6 hours, before leukocyte lysis, while collection using other preservatives can stabilize cfDNA and prevent cell lysis for ~7 days.[6,11,13,19] Notably, gDNA contamination via cell lysis may be of less importance in compartments with fewer contaminating cells.[8]

cfDNA quality may also be temperature dependent, with several studies suggesting that samples might benefit from storage at 4°C before extraction; this, however, is controversial, as other studies report storage of blood at this temperature does not prevent leukocyte lysis.[11] Regardless, collection tubes should be kept within their manufacturer-recommended temperature ranges and processing times. Both processed samples and extracted cfDNA can subsequently be stored frozen for 1 year at −80°C and −20°C, respectively, at the expense of ~30% degradation.[6] Multiple freeze–thaw cycles should be avoided to prevent further cfDNA degradation.[10,11]

BioFluid and Supernatant Processing and Cell-Free DNA Extraction

In the absence of cfDNA isolation standards, numerous lab-specific protocols using multiple commercially available extraction kits have been published.[19] Few methods have been systematically studied outside of peripheral blood, which hinders reproducibility and direct comparison of their yield, cfDNA fragment-size selection bias, and purity. However, while the optimal method of choice is unclear, the chosen method should be optimized for cfDNA to prevent further fragmentation and/or loss of smaller fragments.

As noted previously, biofluids contain cells and cellular debris that must be removed before cfDNA extraction, most commonly via a series of centrifugation and/or filtration steps (see **Fig. 1**). The reported number of centrifugations (1–3) and centrifugation conditions vary, but most studies use initial centrifugation between 800 and 2,000g followed by second centrifugation between 2000 and 16,000g.[6] Compartments with fewer contaminating cells, such as CSF, might dispense with a second centrifugation step.[6] Centrifugation temperature does not seem to influence cfDNA quality or quantity.[6]

cfDNA extraction methods range from conventional ethanol precipitation, phenol–chloroform, or triton-heat-phenol-based methods to commercial kits using silica-based technologies to promote binding and detachment of cfDNA under different chaotropic salt conditions, magnetic beads, or polymer mediated enrichment (PME) technology.[19] Approaches designed to extract total DNA (both cfDNA and gDNA) followed by size-selective enrichment of smaller cfDNA fragments have also been described; however, such enrichment strategies would reduce/remove gDNA not only from nonneoplastic cells, but from any tumor cells present within the sample extracted.[19] Of note, some manufactures provide different protocols for EDTA and cell-preserving tubes due to possible interactions between these commercial kits and the preservative conditions.[19]

Quantification and Characterization of Cell-Free DNA

Technologies for quantifying cfDNA include quantitative PCR (qPCR)-based methods, spectrophotometry, and fluorometry. qPCR, including real-time PCR (RT-PCR) and digital PCR (dPCR), uses intercalating dyes or hydrolysis probes to estimate cfDNA concentration. qPCR is accurate and capable of revealing PCR inhibitors, but may be expensive.[19] Spectrophotometry and fluorometry are inexpensive, reliable, effective, and fast, although residual organic solvents, salts, detergents, and/or other nucleic acids/free nucleotides may impact their accuracy.[6] For a more comprehensive evaluation, automated electrophoresis instruments offer the characterization of cfDNA size distribution in addition to quantitation.

cfDNA reference materials should mimic extracted cfDNA, especially fragment size.[21] Well-characterized patient samples are one potential standard, though limited volume and long-term storage are problematic.[21] Artificial standards generated from spike-in of synthetic or exogenous cfDNA fragments of different lengths are another option.[21] By comparing the quantitative signals of the extracted reference and clinical samples, extraction efficiency, and size-fragmentation bias can be assessed.

ANALYTICAL STRATEGIES FOR CELL-FREE DNA EVALUATION IN ONCOLOGY

The method chosen for cfDNA evaluation depends on several factors, including quantity and fragment-size distribution, the variants assessed, and the assay limit of detection (LOD), which is dependent on the depth of coverage and variant allele fraction (VAF). Assays may be allele-specific (targeted single or multi-locus) or broad (whole exome or genome). Allele-specific PCR, such as RT-PCR or dPCR, detects only targeted mutations, typically at lower VAFs than broader panels using standard next-generation sequencing (NGS) technologies, which do not require a priori variant knowledge.[6,11]

Cell-Free DNA Evaluation by Reverse Transcription-Polymerase Chain Reaction

RT-PCR monitors the amplification progression of specific variants and reference gene(s), allowing absolute or relative quantification, with multiple reference genes resulting in more reliable estimates of mutation concentration.[19] LODs of ~0.5% VAF are common, with a quick turnaround time (TAT) and reasonable cost at the expense of limited multiplexing capabilities.[6,11]

Cell-Free DNA Evaluation by Digital Polymerase Chain Reaction

dPCR transforms the exponential analog nature of PCR into a binary signal via physical separation of template alleles according to Poisson's distribution.[6,11,19] This allows for parallel but isolated amplification of single molecules of mutant or reference targets using end-point fluorescence detection.[6,11,19] Like qPCR, dPCR is only capable of assessing variants known *a priori* with limited ability to multiplex.[6,11,19] Advantages include reduced template input, relative cost-effectiveness, quick TAT, and reduced susceptibility to inhibitors. While dPCR LODs of <1%-0.001% VAF have been reported, this method is susceptible to cross-contamination, necessitating impeccable sample handling and consideration of replicate reactions to confirm the presence of low VAFs.[6,11]

Multiple methods of partitioning target templates have been developed, including solid dPCR (sdPCR), droplet dPCR (ddPCR), and BEAMing (beads, emulsion, amplification, and magnetics) dPCR. sdPCR uses individual reaction chambers, such as microwell plates or microfluidic systems, to accomplish the physical separation of target molecules, while ddPCR uses oil–water emulsion to partition targets into ~12,000 to 20,000 reaction droplets.[11] BEAMing binds biotinylated-oligos to streptavidin-coated magnetic beads, which are subsequently compartmentalized into droplets via oil–water emulsion.[22] After amplification and droplet-disruption, released beads are purified and bound to base pair-specific fluorescent probes before flow cytometry.[22] Individual techniques have advantages and limitations; ddPCR is susceptible to droplet breakage, which can decrease performance, while BEAMing is sensitive and specific, but expensive with a complicated workflow.[6,11]

Cell-Free DNA Evaluation by Next-Generation Sequencing

NGS assays, unlike variant-specific methods, can evaluate a broader range of targets, from small gene panels to whole exomes or genomes. Although increasing the number of targets typically increases expense and TAT while decreasing analytical sensitivity, techniques such as molecular barcoding and/or digital error correction can compensate.[6,23–25]

Molecular barcodes (AKA unique molecular identifiers, UMIs), are random oligomers ligated to single- or double-strand DNA.[23] Single-strand systems uniquely label individual DNA fragments, resulting in independent tagging of the forward and reverse strands; this can result in false-positive "jackpot errors" in the first round of amplification. Double-stranded DNA tagging prevents this problem by using complementary oligomers for the forward and reverse strands.[23] After sequencing, specialized bioinformatics pipelines recognize and collapse NGS reads containing the same- or complementary-UMIs.[23] Mutation are considered "true" only if present in multiple collapsed read families, with an ~20-fold error reduction; LODs of ~0.01% VAF have been reported with double-stranded tagging.[23]

Bioinformatic digital error suppression, such as cancer personalized profiling by deep sequencing (CAPP-Seq) or targeted error-correction sequencing (TEC-Seq) are comparable, with LODs as low as 0.02% to 0.00025% VAFs.[23,25]

POSTANALYTICAL CELL-FREE DNA CONSIDERATIONS IN ONCOLOGY

While tumor tissue testing is the gold standard for cancer profiling, cfDNA represents a promising noninvasive tool for diagnosing cancer, determining prognosis, monitoring disease burden, identifying therapeutic targets, and detecting evolution/resistance mutations. Consideration of the intended use(s) of specific assays is critical to setting decision thresholds and determining the clinical validity of detected variants. Notably, higher thresholds may be advisable for *de novo* (vs known) mutation calling to increase specificity.

Clinical Validity of Cell-Free DNA Evaluation in Biofluids and Supernatants

The evaluation of CSF-derived cfDNA is particularly intriguing for CNS lesions, as tumor mutations are difficult to detect in ctDNA, presumably secondary to the blood–

brain barrier.[8] Studies of CSF-derived cfDNA in patients with primary brain tumors have demonstrated sensitivities of 38% to 92% in the detection of genetic alterations, including tumor-defining 1p/19q codeletions, and *BRAF, IDH1/2*, Histone 3, and *TERT* mutations.[8,26] One retrospective study correctly classified 85% (17/20) of tested gliomas using a combination of ddPCR and targeted sequencing of 7 brain-tumor associated genes, failing only in the setting of low-grade tumors or those not in direct contact with CSF.[27] Another study sequenced 68 brain tumor-associated genes, and identified tumor-specific alterations in ~82% (47/57) of CSF samples, including all somatic findings in ~84% of cases (31/37) and at least one mutation in greater than 97% of cases (36/37).[28] Additionally, CSF-derived cfDNA may be useful in monitoring therapeutic response and/or identifying recurrent/residual disease per several studies.[8,29] The evaluation of cfDNA for metastatic lesions has been similarly successful, with moderate-high sensitivity (63%–100%) and high specificity.[8,26] One study of patients with CNS-metastatic lung adenocarcinoma demonstrated 87.5% sensitivity and 100% specificity in *EGFR*-mutation detection in CSF-derived cfDNA, while another reported improved sensitivity compared with ctDNA (100% vs 86.4%).[30,31] Tumor-derived cfDNA has also been reported in the CSF of patients with a wide range of CNS metastases despite the absence of malignant cells on cytologic examination.[32,33]

Early studies assessing saliva-derived cfDNA in patients with tumors arising in the oral cavity, oropharynx, hypopharynx, or larynx also reported moderate-to-high sensitivity in the detection of neoplasia.[34,35] Furthermore, the presence of tumor cfDNA in postsurgical saliva specimens seemed to predict disease recurrence.[35] Tumor mutations have also been reported in sputum (13%–80%) and bronchoalveolar lavage (BAL) specimens of patients with lung cancer, with one limited study reporting greater than 90% sensitivity in the identification of *EGFR*-mutations in BALs (compared with ~42% in ctDNA).[36–40]

Occasional observations of endometrial and ovarian cancer cells in routine papsmears prompted the evaluation of recurrently mutated genes in paired patients with endometrial and ovarian cancer, identifying at least one concordant mutation in 100% and 41% of cases, respectively.[41] A follow-up study, combining an 18 genepanel with an aneuploidy assay, demonstrated 81% and 33% sensitivity in 382 endometrial and 245 ovarian cancers, respectively, with 98.6% specificity (714 cancer-free women).[42] These metrics were further improved for a subset of patients who underwent intrauterine sampling by Tao brush (93% and 45% sensitivity, 100% specificity).[42] While uterine lavage has also been reported to increase sensitivity, it seems to come at the cost of specificity.[26,43,44]

Analysis of cfDNA in gastrointestinal fluids and urine has likewise shown promise, with several studies suggesting increased sensitivity of stool-derived cfDNA in patients with colorectal cancer (CRC) and utDNA in patients with urothelial-cell cancer (UCC) compared with ctDNA.[45–47] For example, cfDNA testing of stool samples from patients with CRC identified tumor mutations in 92% versus 50% of ctDNA, while utDNA testing of patients with UCC identified tumor mutations in greater than 85% versus ~10% of ctDNA.[45,47] utDNA also demonstrated superior sensitivity to cytology alone per one study, which evaluated 67 healthy adults and 118 early stage, predominantly noninvasive patients with UCC and achieved a sensitivity of 100% for histologically detected cancers and 82% in false-negative cytology specimens.[48] However, utDNA is not limited to UCC, as assays using utDNA for the detection of mutations in nongenitourinary tumors including lung, breast, gastric, colorectal, and liver cancers have also reported sensitives comparable to ctDNA.[20,49] For example, one assay using utDNA demonstrated 88% concordance between *EGFR* mutations present in patients with nonsmall cell lung cancer (vs 98% in ctDNA). Studies also demonstrated 100% and 77% concordance of KRAS-mutation-status between utDNA and CRC and polyps, respectively.[49] The presence of utDNA may also be predictive; per another study, TP53 mutations were identified in 100% of recurrent hepatocellular carcinomas up to 9 months before radiologically confirmed recurrence.[49]

Evaluation of supernatants from organ-cyst fluids (including ovarian, pancreatic, and thyroid), ampullary brushings, and effusions have also shown diagnostic and prognostic potential.[7,9,26] Two recent studies are noteworthy for their direct comparison between tissue and supernatants. Perrone and colleagues compared the molecular findings of 30 paired tissue and cytology samples (including 29 neoplastic samples, predominantly lung) to FNAs and effusions.[7] Using tissue as the gold standard, 90% of mutations (44/49) and 74% of samples (20/27) were concordant.[7] Moreover, mutations predicting therapeutic response, including an ETV6::NTRK3 fusion, were concordant in greater than 75% (13/17) of cases, with an additional 2 cases positive by supernatant alone.[7] Roy-Chowdhuri and colleagues, who evaluated a wider range of malignancies (including 25 tumors of the lung, pancreas, colon, bladder, and breast) and 10 benign lymph nodes, reported 100% sensitivity and specificity for tumor mutations (for those that could be confirmed using an orthogonal method and/or paired tissue testing).[9]

Limitations of Cell-Free DNA Evaluation

Variables resulting in both false negatives and false positives are a potential limitation of cfDNA testing. The former is usually the result of undetectable tumor cfDNA and/or the dilutional effects of nonneoplastic cfDNA and gDNA, while the latter poses a significant problem, and may be the result of improper specimen handling, processing, or other clonal processes—benign or malignant.

Analytically real, but unrelated genomic mutations are observed in clonal hematopoiesis of indeterminate potential (CHIP). CHIP incidence increases with age, with detectable mutations in 3% to 5% of individuals 50 to 69 years old, and increasing to greater than 10% among those 70 to 79.[26] Mutations occur not only in genes commonly mutated in hematological disorders but in oncogenes frequently associated with (adeno)carcinomas (eg KRAS, NRAS, BRAF, and PIK3CA).[26] One sensitive UMI assay reported CHIP mutations in 95% of individuals 50 to 60 years old, which could result in the misattribution of CHIP mutations to a malignant process, potentially decreasing assay specificity and impacting therapy selection.[26] Sequencing of matched white blood cells (WBCs) may allow the identification of CHIP interference, which should be detectable in both samples.

Benign clonal expansions in other nonhematopoietic tissues have also been described.[26] Driver mutations in NOTCH1 and TP53 have been reported in "normal" bronchial and esophageal epithelium, with increased prevalence associated with smoking, alcohol consumption, and age.[26] KRAS, PIK3CA, and PTEN mutations have also been reported in uterine lavage fluids of greater than 50% of patients without cancer and have been associated with the epithelial component of deeply infiltrating endometriotic lesions, postmenopausal status, and patient age.[26]

Given the risk of false positives, somatic mutations in benign cytologic samples require confirmation through the review of the anatomic specimen to verify the absence of malignancy, reproducibility of the results, confirmation by an orthogonal platform, and/or testing of the concurrent cytologic cell block. The possibility of CHIP must always be considered.

Benefits of Cell-Free DNA Evaluation

The benefits of cfDNA testing are manifold. Acquisition of cfDNA results in fewer surgical complications compared with tissue biopsy, and assays using biofluid and supernatant-derived cfDNA frequently demonstrate improved quality metrics and reduced TAT and cost.[8,9] Moreover, cfDNA assays may overcome issues of intratumor heterogeneity, that is, subclonal or region-specific mutations that might be missed during the sequencing of a small tissue biopsy, which would result in a false negative and suboptimal therapeutic selection.[6,8,26] The close proximity of most nonplasma biofluids to a communicating tumor may also result in improved sensitivity.[50] These biofluids can include CSF in the context of primary and metastatic CNS tumors, saliva for head and neck cancers, sputum for lung cancer, gastrointestinal fluids for their associated malignancies, and urine for genitourinary and nongenitourinary cancers. Additionally, assessing supernatant-derived cfDNA in lieu of tissue allows for the conservation of limited samples for histopathologic diagnosis and other necessary ancillary studies.[7,9]

SUMMARY

Tumor-derived cfDNA is a valuable substrate for assessing genetic alterations for multiple clinical applications, including prognosis, therapy prediction, and monitoring tumor evolution. Although low yield and limited specificity may preclude mutation detection in cfDNA from being the sole means of classifying neoplasms, cfDNA analyses spare patients the discomfort and morbidity associated with more invasive procedures, which are not only resource-intensive but can produce a less comprehensive molecular profile. Additional studies using larger cohorts and standardization of preanalytical approaches may allow for the development of evidence-based guidelines to expand the use of liquid biopsies to supernatants and nonplasma biofluids for the benefit of oncology patients.

CLINICS CARE POINTS

- The identification of tumor-derived cfDNA in asymptomatic individuals before a cancer diagnosis suggests the possibility of cfDNA as an analyte for cancer screening; this potential must be balanced with the risk for false negatives (and positives) and the identification of nonspecific tumor mutations.

- The era of targeted therapy requires assays capable of efficiently using samples obtained through minimally invasive procedures to identify biomarkers of therapeutic response and resistance; cfDNA has the added benefit of overcoming potential issues of tumor heterogeneity.

- The assessment of tumor burden, residual disease, and disease recurrence through serial cfDNA evaluation can identify and stratify patients requiring additional adjuvant therapy and spare low-risk patients from over treatment.

DISCLOSURE

Spouse of C.H. Lockwood is used by Bayer Health. V. Paulson and E.Q. Konnick have nothing to disclose.

FUNDING

Funding Source: Brotman-Baty Institute for Precision Medicine.

REFERENCES

1. Mandel P, Metais P. Nuclear acids in human blood plasma. C R Seances Soc Biol Fil 1948;142(3–4):241–3. Les acides nucleiques du plasma sanguin chez l'homme.
2. Kustanovich A, Schwartz R, Peretz T, et al. Life and death of circulating cell-free DNA. Cancer Biol Ther 2019;20(8):1057–67.
3. Leon SA, Shapiro B, Sklaroff DM, et al. Free DNA in the serum of cancer patients and the effect of therapy. Cancer Res 1977;37(3):646–50.
4. Stroun M, Anker P, Lyautey J, et al. Isolation and characterization of DNA from the plasma of cancer patients. Eur J Cancer Clin Oncol 1987;23(6):707–12.
5. Sorenson GD, Pribish DM, Valone FH, et al. Soluble normal and mutated DNA sequences from single-copy genes in human blood. Cancer Epidemiol Biomarkers Prev 1994;3(1):67–71.
6. Volckmar AL, Sultmann H, Riediger A, et al. A field guide for cancer diagnostics using cell-free DNA: from principles to practice and clinical applications. Genes Chromosomes Cancer 2018;57(3):123–39.
7. Perrone ME, Alvarez R, Vo TT, et al. Validating cell-free DNA from supernatant for molecular diagnostics on cytology specimens. Cancer Cytopathol 2021;129(12):956–65.
8. McEwen AE, Leary SES, Lockwood CM. Beyond the blood: CSF-derived cfDNA for diagnosis and characterization of CNS tumors. Front Cell Dev Biol 2020;8:45.
9. Roy-Chowdhuri S, Mehrotra M, Bolivar AM, et al. Salvaging the supernatant: next generation cytopathology for solid tumor mutation profiling. Mod Pathol 2018;31(7):1036–45.
10. Merker JD, Oxnard GR, Compton C, et al. Circulating tumor DNA analysis in patients with cancer: american society of clinical oncology and college of american pathologists joint review. J Clin Oncol 2018;36(16):1631–41.
11. Russo A, Incorvaia L, Del Re M, et al. The molecular profiling of solid tumors by liquid biopsy: a position paper of the AIOM-SIAPEC-IAP-SIBioC-SIC-SIF Italian Scientific Societies. ESMO Open 2021;6(3):100164.
12. Giacona MB, Ruben GC, Iczkowski KA, et al. Cell-free DNA in human blood plasma: length measurements in patients with pancreatic cancer and healthy controls. Pancreas 1998;17(1):89–97.
13. Wan JCM, Massie C, Garcia-Corbacho J, et al. Liquid biopsies come of age: towards implementation of circulating tumour DNA. Nat Rev Cancer 2017;17(4):223–38.
14. Snyder MW, Kircher M, Hill AJ, et al. Cell-free DNA comprises an in vivo nucleosome footprint that informs its tissues-of-origin. Cell 2016;164(1–2):57–68.
15. Mouliere F, Chandrananda D, Piskorz AM, et al. Enhanced detection of circulating tumor DNA by fragment size analysis. Sci Transl Med 2018;10(466):eaat4921.
16. Zheng YW, Chan KC, Sun H, et al. Nonhematopoietically derived DNA is shorter than hematopoietically derived DNA in plasma: a transplantation model. Clin Chem 2012;58(3):549–58.
17. Patel A, Hissong E, Rosado L, et al. Next-generation sequencing of cell-free DNA extracted from pleural effusion supernatant: applications and challenges. Front Med (Lausanne) 2021;8:662312.
18. Yu Y, Qian J, Shen L, et al. Distinct profile of cell-free DNA in malignant pleural effusion of non-small cell lung cancer and its impact on clinical genetic testing. Int J Med Sci 2021;18(6):1510–8.
19. Pos Z, Pos O, Styk J, et al. Technical and methodological aspects of cell-free nucleic acids analyzes. Int J Mol Sci 2020;21(22):8634.

20. Oshi M, Murthy V, Takahashi H, et al. Urine as a source of liquid biopsy for cancer. Cancers (Basel) 2021;13(11):2652.
21. Geeurickx E, Hendrix A. Targets, pitfalls and reference materials for liquid biopsy tests in cancer diagnostics. Mol Aspects 2020;72:100828.
22. Dressman D, Yan H, Traverso G, et al. Transforming single DNA molecules into fluorescent magnetic particles for detection and enumeration of genetic variations. Proc Natl Acad Sci U S A 2003;100(15):8817–22.
23. De Luca G, Dono M. The opportunities and challenges of molecular tagging next-generation sequencing in liquid biopsy. Mol Diagn Ther 2021;25(5):537–47.
24. Narayan A, Carriero NJ, Gettinger SN, et al. Ultrasensitive measurement of hot-spot mutations in tumor DNA in blood using error-suppressed multiplexed deep sequencing. Cancer Res 2012;72(14):3492–8.
25. Newman AM, Lovejoy AF, Klass DM, et al. Integrated digital error suppression for improved detection of circulating tumor DNA. Nat Biotechnol 2016;34(5):547–55.
26. Dudley JC, Diehn M. Detection and diagnostic utilization of cellular and cell-free tumor DNA. Annu Rev Pathol 2021;16:199–222.
27. Martinez-Ricarte F, Mayor R, Martinez-Saez E, et al. Molecular diagnosis of diffuse gliomas through sequencing of cell-free circulating tumor DNA from cerebrospinal fluid. Clin Cancer Res 2018;24(12):2812–9.
28. Pan C, Diplas BH, Chen X, et al. Molecular profiling of tumors of the brainstem by sequencing of CSF-derived circulating tumor DNA. Acta Neuropathol 2019; 137(2):297–306.
29. Liu APY, Smith KS, Kumar R, et al. Serial assessment of measurable residual disease in medulloblastoma liquid biopsies. Cancer Cell 2021;39(11):1519–30.e4.
30. Kawahara A, Abe H, Murata K, et al. Screening system for epidermal growth factor receptor mutation detection in cytology cell-free DNA of cerebrospinal fluid based on assured sample quality. Cytopathology 2019;30(2):144–9.
31. Li YS, Jiang BY, Yang JJ, et al. Unique genetic profiles from cerebrospinal fluid cell-free DNA in leptomeningeal metastases of EGFR-mutant non-small-cell lung cancer: a new medium of liquid biopsy. Ann Oncol 2018;29(4):945–52.
32. Swinkels DW, de Kok JB, Hanselaar A, et al. Early detection of leptomeningeal metastasis by PCR examination of tumor-derived K-ras DNA in cerebrospinal fluid. Clin Chem 2000;46(1):132–3.
33. Zhao Y, He JY, Zou YL, et al. Evaluating the cerebrospinal fluid ctDNA detection by next-generation sequencing in the diagnosis of meningeal Carcinomatosis. BMC Neurol 2019;19(1):331.
34. Wang Y, Springer S, Mulvey CL, et al. Detection of somatic mutations and HPV in the saliva and plasma of patients with head and neck squamous cell carcinomas. Sci Transl Med 2015;7(293):293ra104.
35. Boyle JO, Mao L, Brennan JA, et al. Gene mutations in saliva as molecular markers for head and neck squamous cell carcinomas. Am J Surg 1994; 168(5):429–32.
36. Hubers AJ, Prinsen CF, Sozzi G, et al. Molecular sputum analysis for the diagnosis of lung cancer. Br J Cancer 2013;109(3):530–7.
37. Wang Z, Li X, Zhang L, et al. Sputum cell-free DNA: valued surrogate sample for the detection of EGFR exon 20 p.T790M mutation in patients with advanced lung adenocarcinoma and acquired resistance to EGFR-TKIs. Cancer Med 2021; 10(10):3323–31.
38. Yanev N, Mekov E, Valev D, et al. EGFR mutation status yield from bronchoalveolar lavage in patients with primary pulmonary adenocarcinoma compared to a venous blood sample and tissue biopsy. PeerJ 2021;9:e11448.

39. Park S, Hur JY, Lee KY, et al. Assessment of EGFR mutation status using cell-free DNA from bronchoalveolar lavage fluid. Clin Chem Lab Med 2017;55(10): 1489–95.

40. Ryu JS, Lim JH, Lee MK, et al. Feasibility of bronchial washing fluid-based approach to early-stage lung cancer diagnosis. Oncologist 2019;24(7):e603–6.

41. Kinde I, Bettegowda C, Wang Y, et al. Evaluation of DNA from the Papanicolaou test to detect ovarian and endometrial cancers. Sci Transl Med 2013;5(167): 167ra4.

42. Wang Y, Li L, Douville C, et al. Evaluation of liquid from the Papanicolaou test and other liquid biopsies for the detection of endometrial and ovarian cancers. Sci Transl Med 2018;10(433):eaap8793.

43. Nair N, Camacho-Vanegas O, Rykunov D, et al. Genomic analysis of uterine lavage fluid detects early endometrial cancers and reveals a prevalent landscape of driver mutations in women without histopathologic evidence of cancer: a prospective cross-sectional study. PLoS Med 2016;13(12):e1002206.

44. Maritschnegg E, Wang Y, Pecha N, et al. Lavage of the uterine cavity for molecular detection of mullerian duct carcinomas: a proof-of-concept study. J Clin Oncol 2015;33(36):4293–300.

45. Diehl F, Schmidt K, Durkee KH, et al. Analysis of mutations in DNA isolated from plasma and stool of colorectal cancer patients. Gastroenterology 2008;135(2): 489–98.

46. Ou Z, Li K, Yang T, et al. Detection of bladder cancer using urinary cell-free DNA and cellular DNA. Clin Transl Med 2020;9(1):4.

47. Zhang R, Zang J, Xie F, et al. Urinary molecular pathology for patients with newly diagnosed urothelial bladder cancer. J Urol 2021;206(4):873–84.

48. Dudley JC, Schroers-Martin J, Lazzareschi DV, et al. Detection and surveillance of bladder cancer using urine tumor DNA. Cancer Discov 2019;9(4):500–9.

49. Jain S, Lin SY, Song W, et al. Urine-based liquid biopsy for nonurological cancers. Genet Test Mol Biomarkers 2019;23(4):277–83.

50. Durin L, Pradines A, Basset C, et al. Liquid biopsy of non-plasma body fluids in non-small cell lung cancer: look closer to the tumor! Cells 2020;9(11):2486.

Germline Testing for the Evaluation of Hereditary Cancer Predisposition

Ozge Ceyhan-Birsoy, PhD

KEYWORDS

- Genetic testing • Cancer • Hereditary cancer predisposition • Germline testing

KEY POINTS

- Expanded germline testing revealed that hereditary cancer predisposition is more common than previously anticipated.
- Germline testing can inform clinical management of patients with cancer and allow timely surveillance and interventions to reduce future disease risk for both patients and family members.
- Various testing strategies, specimen types, and analysis methods are available, but optimal approach may differ based on patient phenotype.
- Recent developments in resources for variant interpretation, data sharing, and paired tumor-normal sequencing strategies lead to improved germline genetic testing for patients with cancer.

INTRODUCTION

Germline testing for hereditary cancer predisposition has become increasingly important in the management of patients with cancer. Recent studies have demonstrated that hereditary cancer predisposition is more common than previously recognized and germline pathogenic variants may be actionable for patient treatment strategies.[1–12] This article reviews the significance of hereditary cancer predisposition assessment and highlights the current practices in germline genetic testing approaches.

DISCUSSION
Significance of Hereditary Cancer Predisposition Testing

Hereditary predisposition to develop solid tumors or hematologic malignancies has been considered to have a modest contribution to cancer incidence overall.[13–16]

Department of Pathology and Laboratory Medicine, Memorial Sloan Kettering Cancer Center, 1275 York Avenue, New York, NY 10065, USA
E-mail address: birsoyo@mskcc.org

Clin Lab Med 42 (2022) 497–506
https://doi.org/10.1016/j.cll.2022.04.007
0272-2712/22/© 2022 Elsevier Inc. All rights reserved.

labmed.theclinics.com

These estimates have long been biased because of the selection of individuals at high risk of having a hereditary cancer predisposition syndrome based on their clinical and family histories. In recent years, widening the pretest selection criteria led to the identification of cancer predisposition in individuals who do not meet current testing criteria, revealing that hereditary cancer predisposition is more prevalent than previously anticipated.[1–3,5–9,11,12] Germline pathogenic variants that confer high to moderate cancer risk have been identified in 3% to 12% of adult and 8.5% to 10% of pediatric patients with a range of tumor types.[3–5,8,12]

Determining whether an individual has a germline defect that increases their cancer risk and identifying the causative pathogenic variants have important implications for both patients and their family members.[17,18] First, discovering at-risk individuals can allow timely screening and interventions to reduce future cancer risk. Second, certain gene defects are associated with treatment implications, such as increased toxicity to radiation therapy in *TP53* carriers,[19,20] or predicting response to targeted therapies, such as PARP inhibitors in *BRCA1/BRCA2* carriers[21] or immune-checkpoint inhibitor therapies in carriers of mismatch repair pathway gene defects.[22,23] In a recent cohort of patients who have cancer with high-penetrance pathogenic germline variants, 28.2% had clinically actionable management changes indicated by their germline variant.[9] Another recent universal genetic testing approach uncovered a germline variant with therapeutic actionability in 8% of patients with advanced cancer,[10] suggesting that germline testing may be highly informative to guide treatment strategies for patients with cancer. Third, identification of germline variants that predispose to cancer necessitates testing of potential donors for patients with hematologic malignancies to avoid inadvertently selecting an affected family member.[18] Finally, patients and family members can receive appropriate genetic counseling for reproductive planning.

Genetic Testing Criteria

In current practice, patients are selected for hereditary cancer predisposition testing in a guideline-based manner. Only individuals who meet established criteria from national medical organizations are offered genetic testing based on their cancer type, age of onset, and other clinical and/or family histories.[17,18,24–26] These guidelines are not static and are updated periodically as new data becomes available regarding the utility and expected yield of genetic testing for different patient groups. Of note, many cancer predisposition genes have incomplete penetrance and variable expressivity with a wide age of onset range, which poses challenges in identifying at risk individuals before testing, as their personal or family histories may not be significant. Most genes are associated with risk for cancer only. Although certain genes such as *TSC2* and *FANCA* underlie syndromic presentations that may include developmental anomalies in addition to predisposition to cancer, carriers of such genes may have mild presentations that may be missed clinically. Therefore, universal testing strategies without pretest selection of patients have the potential to uncover hereditary cancer predisposition in individuals who do not meet current testing criteria.

Specimen Types

The choice of specimen type for germline testing may vary depending on the patient's current disease status. For individuals without a history of hematologic malignancy, testing is typically performed using peripheral blood or saliva as the "normal" tissue source to look for pathogenic variants that cause a known cancer predisposition syndrome. Although blood has traditionally been the gold standard specimen type for many genetic tests and is the most commonly used specimen type used for hereditary cancer predisposition testing currently, saliva is another specimen that is increasingly used by clinical laboratories. The fact that saliva can be collected in a noninvasive manner by the patients themselves and can be mailed to the laboratory without an in-person clinic visit makes it a convenient alternative specimen type for many molecular assays.

In individuals with active circulating hematologic malignancies, deoxyribonucleic acid (DNA) isolated from peripheral blood samples may include somatic mutations that are not representative of the patient's constitutional genetic composition and may interfere with the germline analyses.[27] In addition, somatic reversion, when a pathogenic variant undergoes reversion to a functional allele, may occur in lymphocytes and confound germline testing in certain disorders such as Fanconi anemia.[28] Saliva and buccal swab are also often contaminated with lymphocytes and therefore may not be suitable for germline testing in individuals with hematologic malignancies. Therefore, the preferred specimen type for these patients is skin fibroblasts, which can yield high quality and quantity of DNA expected to represent their constitutional genome. Fibroblast testing has the disadvantage that it requires an invasive skin punch biopsy and culturing of fibroblast cells for several weeks to obtain a pure culture, delaying the time to diagnosis.[27] The invasive nature of obtaining this specimen type and the long turn-around time led laboratories to search for other samples that may be suitable for germline testing in patients with hematologic malignancies, such as nails or hair bulbs, although none of these specimen types are widely used for clinical genetic testing at the moment.

Testing Options

When hereditary predisposition to cancer is suspected, the choice of testing strategy may vary based on the individual's pretest likelihood of carrying a variant, specificity of clinical history for a particular diagnosis, genetic heterogeneity of disease, and cost or turn-around time considerations.

Targeted variant testing: Targeted variant testing is performed for a specific variant or variants if the patient has a relatively high prior probability of being a carrier. For instance, a known pathogenic variant in the family often justifies testing for the familial variant in an individual regardless of their clinical history and disease status. In addition, founder mutations that have high prevalence in certain populations may suggest targeted testing for these variants, such as *BRCA1* and *BRCA2* founder mutations in the Ashkenazi Jewish population.[29–31] Targeted testing is typically performed with a rapid turn-around time (often 1–2 weeks) and using inexpensive methods, such as Sanger sequencing for single nucleotide variants (SNVs) and small indels or multiplex ligation-dependent probe amplification for gene- or exon-level deletion/duplications.

Single gene analysis: Testing a single gene may be reasonable when there is high clinical suspicion for a specific gene defect based on the patient's personal or family history. This strategy is most helpful for diseases without genetic heterogeneity, such as retinoblastoma. However, testing may be complicated for diseases with wide phenotypic spectrum or when features overlap between multiple different disorders. In such instances, a negative single gene analysis may lead to sequential testing, which may delay diagnosis and may not be cost-effective.

Multigene panels allow simultaneous testing of multiple genes that may be associated with a patient's phenotype and is highly effective for diseases with genetic heterogeneity or phenotypic overlap. For a comprehensive evaluation of SNVs and large deletion/duplications, multigene panel analyses often include both next-generation sequencing (NGS) and a copy number detection method, which may be based on NGS data or using a targeted oligonucleotide array.[32] Currently, a wide range of diagnostic multigene panels is offered by clinical laboratories for various categories of hereditary cancer predisposition syndromes. It is important to note that the gene content of any particular disease test may vary widely across different laboratories.[33] Differences may also exist in the targeted regions of each gene, such that specific exons or noncoding regions that may harbor pathogenic variants may be variably included by different laboratories (**Fig. 1**). Although multigene panels provide a highly comprehensive analysis for many syndromes, their limitations to detect certain types of variants, such as large transposable element insertions, inversions, or mosaicism should be kept in mind.[33] Testing for genes that have regions with high homology to pseudogenes (ie, *PMS2* and *CHEK2*) is typically supported with additional assays such as long-range polymerase chain reaction to detect and distinguish variants that occur on the authentic gene.

Whole-exome sequencing (WES) may be considered when targeted testing options have been exhausted and there is high suspicion for hereditary basis of disease. Although WES allows analyzing most medically relevant disease genes with a single test, coverage may vary across different genomic regions. In addition, analysis methods, including gene or variant filtration and prioritization of reported variants, may also differ between laboratories. WES is particularly useful in discovery of new disease genes or previously unknown gene-disease associations, although variants of uncertain significance may pose challenges in results interpretation.

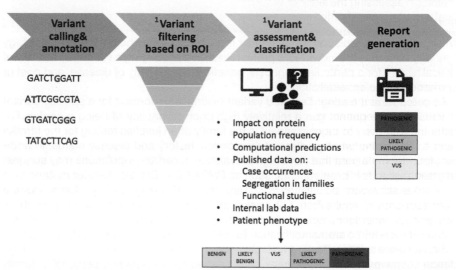

Fig. 1. Laboratory processes in multigene panel testing from variant annotation to reporting. Annotated variant calls are filtered based on the target region of interest that may be restricted to coding exons and splice regions only or may include noncoding regions that may harbor known pathogenic variants. Variants are assessed based on data such as their impact on protein function, frequency in population databases, computational predictions to affect the protein or splicing, published data on occurrence in cases versus controls, segregation in families, functional studies, internal laboratory data on occurrence in affected individuals, and patient phenotypes. Using this information, variants are classified in a 5-tier system according to their likelihood to cause disease from benign to pathogenic. In diagnostic testing, variants classified as pathogenic, likely pathogenic and uncertain significance are returned in the report. [1]Indicates processes that may have notable differences between different laboratories. ROI, region of interest; VUS, variant of uncertain significance.

Germline Variant Classification and Results Interpretation

Clinical laboratories performing germline genetic testing typically use the criteria developed by the American College of Medical Genetics and Genomics and the Association for Molecular Pathology[34] for assessment and classification of a variant's clinical significance (see **Fig. 1**). Although these guidelines provide a standardized framework for germline variant classification, interpretation of variants may require disease- or gene-specific adjustments. For this purpose, the Clinical Genome Resource (https://clinicalgenome.org) has established working groups and expert panels that provide guidance and specifications to variant classifications for various genes and disease categories. For hereditary cancer predisposition, multiple expert panels have been formed and published variant interpretation recommendations for different genes.[35–39] Laboratories also take advantage of their expertise and internal data while assessing variants. Many clinical laboratories share their variant classifications and supporting evidence in the ClinVar database (https://www.ncbi.nlm.nih.gov/clinvar/), which is a useful resource that facilitates access to information about variants evaluated by different laboratories. Phenotypic data from the patient being tested are an important piece of information in understanding the clinical significance of identified variants. For instance, when reviewing an *MSH2* variant detected in a patient with colorectal cancer, knowledge about their tumor profile including immunohistochemistry for mismatch repair pathway proteins, microsatellite instability, second-hit mutations in the gene or loss of heterozygosity (LOH) for the variant would be very helpful in assessing the likelihood of pathogenicity. Therefore, providing available clinical and tumor profile information from the patient to laboratories performing the germline genetic test is important for accurate results interpretation.

Germline Analysis Based on Tumor Sequencing Data

Tumor sequencing results include a mixture of germline and somatic variants. In current practice, in the absence of direct germline testing using a nonmalignant "normal" tissue, tumor sequencing results are occasionally used by clinicians to identify variants that are likely to be of germline origin based on their allele fractions.[7] It is important to determine whether a pathogenic variant identified in tumor sequencing is a somatic versus a germline variant. However, using tumor sequencing data to identify germline variants is problematic for both germline and somatic assessment purposes.

Various strategies are used to predict variants that are likely to be germline from tumor sequencing results.[40–43] The most frequently used approach relies on the allele fraction of variants in tumor sequencing data, such that allele fractions close to ∼50% (∼35–65%) are assumed to likely represent heterozygous germline variants, whereas allele fractions lower than ∼35% are predicted more likely to be somatic mutations.[4] However, tumor purity and changes in variant allele fractions in the tumors due to deletions or amplifications may affect the fraction of a germline variant in the tumor. In addition, the fraction of a variant in NGS mapped reads may not be representative of its true allele fraction depending on its genomic location or its size (if it is a deletion/insertion variant). Therefore, many germline variants may be misinterpreted as somatic mutations and those that confer hereditary cancer risk may be missed using this approach.

Patients need to receive appropriate genetic counseling before having germline testing, which is not standard before tumor sequencing. When a variant identified in tumor sequencing is suspected to be germline and may be pathogenic for hereditary cancer predisposition, genetic consultation and follow-up testing of a "normal" tissue are needed to confirm whether the variant is germline. Distinguishing somatic mutations from germline variants is important to avoid unnecessary genetic testing in the patient and extended family members, as somatic mutations are not inherited. For these reasons, laboratories performing tumor sequencing often attempt to filter out variants that have a high likelihood of being germline from the results, so that only mutations that are likely to be somatic are returned. One such filtering method is to exclude variants that are present in large population databases such as 1000 Genomes[44] and the Genome Aggregation Database,[45] assuming that they are more likely to be of germline origin.[4,40,41,46] However, rare variants often cannot be filtered out using this method. Owing to these limitations, predicting germline variants from tumor sequencing remains challenging and may lead to false positive and false negative variant calls.[4,46,47]

Paired Tumor-Normal Sequencing

Paired tumor-normal sequencing is a comprehensive strategy for precise interpretation of both germline and somatic results.[43] Although blood is the standard source of constitutional DNA for germline analyses, DNA isolated from blood may include mutations that the individual is mosaic for or somatic mutations in the hematopoietic lineage [referred to as clonal hematopoiesis (CH)] in addition to germline variants.[48–53] CH is common in patients with cancer and may be detected in the absence of any evidence for a hematologic malignancy.[54,55] Incorrect designation of a CH variant as germline may have implications for the patient's clinical care,[56] as the incorrect designation of a CH-related mutation as a germline variant may lead to a false diagnosis of a hereditary cancer syndrome, leading to long series of screening tests for a range of cancers for the patient and cascade testing for family members.[20] On the other hand, mosaicism is the presence of a variant in some but not all cells of an individual.[52] Depending on the timing of occurrence and tissue of origin, a mosaic variant may be present at varying levels in different tissues, and predicting its clinical consequences may be challenging.[53] Determining whether a variant occurs as mosaic or a heterozygous germline variant is important for appropriate clinical management. Sequencing DNA isolated from the blood alone may be unable to distinguish true germline variants from mosaic and CH-related variants.[48,50,57] In a test that involves sequencing DNA isolated from the blood only, allele fractions lower than expected for true germline variants may suggest mosaicism or CH.[50,51] However, true germline variants, particularly large deletions/insertions or those occurring near homopolymers or regions with high homology, may also be detected at lower allele fractions. In addition, high-level mosaic variants or CH-related mutations that arose early or were amplified in clonal expansion may occur at higher allele fractions and may be misinterpreted as germline variants.[49] To understand whether a variant detected in blood-only sequencing is germline, mosaic, or CH-related, a different tissue specimen, such as skin fibroblasts, may be tested. A paired tumor analysis often helps in predicting potential mosaic or CH-related variants, as the tumor represents another tissue specimen from the tested individual.[43] Variants that are present in the blood but not in the tumor in the absence of deletion/amplification or LOH in the region are highly suggestive of CH-related mutations in the blood,[49] whereas those detected at a low allele fraction both in the blood and the tumor may be suspected of being mosaic.

Paired tumor-normal sequencing also has advantages over tumor-only sequencing for somatic analyses. Pairing tumor sequencing analysis with data from a "normal" tissue DNA allows to correctly subtract germline variants from tumor sequencing variant calls, resulting in improved accuracy in returning somatic mutations only.[58] Filtering out the germline variants from somatic mutations also allows more reliable estimations of tumor attributes such as mutation burden, microsatellite instability, or mutation signatures[59–61] and gives the opportunity to assess somatic biallelic inactivation through LOH or a second mutation ("second hit").[62–64]

SUMMARY AND FUTURE DIRECTIONS

Germline genetic testing can guide the treatment of patients with cancer and allow surveillance and/or prophylactic interventions to reduce future disease risk in patients and their family members. Offering universal genetic testing to wider groups of patients with cancer may allow more larger groups of patients to take advantage of these benefits. However, questions and challenges remain regarding the cost-effectiveness of comprehensive testing in individuals with different types of cancers and the impact of inconclusive test results due to variants of uncertain significance. Further studies on broader cohorts will elucidate the optimal testing strategies for diverse patient populations.

CLINICS CARE POINTS

- Germline testing for cancer predisposition is currently offered to patients selected based on established guidelines.

- Expanded testing approaches uncovered hereditary cancer predisposition in patients who do not meet established testing criteria.

- Germline testing can impact treatment of patients with cancer and allow surveillance and prophylactic interventions to reduce future disease risk in patient and family members.

- Germline testing may be performed using different "normal" DNA sources depending on patient's disease status and feasibility of sample collection.

- Using tumor sequencing data to predict germline variants may result in inaccurate interpretations and additional confirmatory testing.

- Paired tumor-normal sequencing has many advantages for both germline and somatic interpretation purposes.

DISCLOSURE

The author has nothing to disclose.

REFERENCES

1. AlDubayan SH, et al. Inherited DNA-repair defects in colorectal cancer. Am J Hum Genet 2018;102(3):401–14.
2. Carlo MI, et al. Prevalence of germline mutations in cancer susceptibility genes in patients with advanced renal cell carcinoma. JAMA Oncol 2018;4(9):1228–35.
3. Huang KL, et al. Pathogenic germline variants in 10,389 adult cancers. Cell 2018; 173(2):355–70.e14.
4. Jones S, et al. Personalized genomic analyses for cancer mutation discovery and interpretation. Sci Transl Med 2015;7(283):283ra53.
5. Lu C, et al. Patterns and functional implications of rare germline variants across 12 cancer types. Nat Commun 2015;6:10086.
6. Mandelker D, et al. Mutation detection in patients with advanced cancer by universal sequencing of cancer-related genes in tumor and normal DNA vs guideline-based germline testing. JAMA 2017;318(9):825–35.

7. Meric-Bernstam F, et al. Incidental germline variants in 1000 advanced cancers on a prospective somatic genomic profiling protocol. Ann Oncol 2016;27(5): 795–800.

8. Parsons DW, et al. Diagnostic yield of clinical tumor and germline whole-exome sequencing for children with solid tumors. JAMA Oncol 2016;2(5):616–24.

9. Samadder NJ, et al. Comparison of universal genetic testing vs guideline-directed targeted testing for patients with hereditary cancer syndrome. JAMA Oncol 2021;7(2):230–7.

10. Stadler ZK, et al. Therapeutic implications of germline testing in patients with advanced cancers. J Clin Oncol 2021;39(24):2698–709.

11. Whitworth J, et al. Comprehensive cancer-predisposition gene testing in an adult multiple primary tumor series shows a broad range of deleterious variants and atypical tumor phenotypes. Am J Hum Genet 2018;103(1):3–18.

12. Zhang J, et al. Germline mutations in predisposition genes in pediatric cancer. N Engl J Med 2015;373(24):2336–46.

13. Garber JE, Offit K. Hereditary cancer predisposition syndromes. J Clin Oncol 2005;23(2):276–92.

14. Lichtenstein P, et al. Environmental and heritable factors in the causation of cancer–analyses of cohorts of twins from Sweden, Denmark, and Finland. N Engl J Med 2000;343(2):78–85.

15. Rahman N. Realizing the promise of cancer predisposition genes. Nature 2014; 505(7483):302–8.

16. Stadler ZK, et al. Cancer genomics and inherited risk. J Clin Oncol 2014;32(7): 687–98.

17. Robson ME, et al. American society of clinical oncology policy statement update: genetic and genomic testing for cancer susceptibility. J Clin Oncol 2015;33(31): 3660–7.

18. Godley LA, Shimamura A. Genetic predisposition to hematologic malignancies: management and surveillance. Blood 2017;130(4):424–32.

19. Kasper E, et al. Contribution of genotoxic anticancer treatments to the development of multiple primary tumours in the context of germline TP53 mutations. Eur J Cancer 2018;101:254–62.

20. Kratz CP, et al. Cancer screening recommendations for individuals with Li-Fraumeni syndrome. Clin Cancer Res 2017;23(11):e38–45.

21. Mateo J, et al. A decade of clinical development of PARP inhibitors in perspective. Ann Oncol 2019;30(9):1437–47.

22. Le DT, et al. Mismatch repair deficiency predicts response of solid tumors to PD-1 blockade. Science 2017;357(6349):409–13.

23. Sun BL. Current microsatellite instability testing in management of colorectal cancer. Clin Colorectal Cancer 2021;20(1):e12–20.

24. Hampel H, et al. A practice guideline from the American College of medical genetics and genomics and the national society of genetic counselors: referral indications for cancer predisposition assessment. Genet Med 2015;17(1):70–87.

25. Daly MB, et al. NCCN guidelines insights: genetic/familial high-risk assessment: breast and ovarian, version 2.2017. J Natl Compr Canc Netw 2017;15(1):9–20.

26. Gupta S, et al. NCCN guidelines insights: genetic/familial high-risk assessment: colorectal, version 3.2017. J Natl Compr Canc Netw 2017;15(12):1465–75.

27. Furutani E, Shimamura A. Germline genetic predisposition to hematologic malignancy. J Clin Oncol 2017;35(9):1018–28.

28. Gross M, et al. Reverse mosaicism in Fanconi anemia: natural gene therapy via molecular self-correction. Cytogenet Genome Res 2002;98(2–3):126–35.

29. Hartge P, et al. The prevalence of common BRCA1 and BRCA2 mutations among Ashkenazi Jews. Am J Hum Genet 1999;64(4):963–70.
30. Oddoux C, et al. The carrier frequency of the BRCA2 6174delT mutation among Ashkenazi Jewish individuals is approximately 1%. Nat Genet 1996;14(2): 188–90.
31. Struewing JP, et al. The carrier frequency of the BRCA1 185delAG mutation is approximately 1 percent in Ashkenazi Jewish individuals. Nat Genet 1995; 11(2):198–200.
32. Rehder C, et al. Next-generation sequencing for constitutional variants in the clinical laboratory, 2021 revision: a technical standard of the American College of Medical Genetics and Genomics (ACMG). Genet Med 2021;23(8):1399–415.
33. Bean LJH, et al. Diagnostic gene sequencing panels: from design to report-a technical standard of the American College of Medical Genetics and Genomics (ACMG). Genet Med 2020;22(3):453–61.
34. Richards S, et al. Standards and guidelines for the interpretation of sequence variants: a joint consensus recommendation of the American College of medical genetics and genomics and the association for molecular Pathology. Genet Med 2015;17(5):405–24.
35. Fortuno C, et al. Specifications of the ACMG/AMP variant interpretation guidelines for germline TP53 variants. Hum Mutat 2021;42(3):223–36.
36. Lee K, et al. Specifications of the ACMG/AMP variant curation guidelines for the analysis of germline CDH1 sequence variants. Hum Mutat 2018;39(11):1553–68.
37. Mester JL, et al. Gene-specific criteria for PTEN variant curation: recommendations from the ClinGen PTEN expert panel. Hum Mutat 2018;39(11):1581–92.
38. Wu D, et al. How I curate: applying American society of Hematology-clinical Genome resource Myeloid malignancy variant curation expert panel rules for RUNX1 variant curation for germline predisposition to myeloid malignancies. Haematologica 2020;105(4):870–87.
39. Luo X, et al. ClinGen myeloid malignancy variant curation expert panel recommendations for germline RUNX1 variants. Blood Adv 2019;3(20):2962–79.
40. Hiltemann S, et al. Discriminating somatic and germline mutations in tumor DNA samples without matching normals. Genome Res 2015;25(9):1382–90.
41. Sukhai MA, et al. Somatic tumor variant filtration strategies to optimize tumor-only molecular profiling using targeted next-generation sequencing panels. J Mol Diagn 2019;21(2):261–73.
42. Teer JK, et al. Evaluating somatic tumor mutation detection without matched normal samples. Hum Genomics 2017;11(1):22.
43. Mandelker D, Ceyhan-Birsoy O. Evolving significance of tumor-normal sequencing in cancer care. Trends Cancer 2020;6(1):31–9.
44. Genomes Project C, et al. A global reference for human genetic variation. Nature 2015;526(7571):68–74.
45. Karczewski KJ, et al. The mutational constraint spectrum quantified from variation in 141,456 humans. Nature 2020;581(7809):434–43.
46. Garofalo A, et al. The impact of tumor profiling approaches and genomic data strategies for cancer precision medicine. Genome Med 2016;8(1):79.
47. Mandelker D, et al. Germline-focussed analysis of tumour-only sequencing: recommendations from the ESMO precision medicine working group. Ann Oncol 2019;30(8):1221–31.
48. Coombs CC, et al. Identification of clonal hematopoiesis mutations in solid tumor patients undergoing Unpaired next-generation sequencing assays. Clin Cancer Res 2018;24(23):5918–24.

49. Ptashkin RN, et al. Prevalence of clonal hematopoiesis mutations in tumor-only clinical genomic profiling of solid tumors. JAMA Oncol 2018;4(11):1589–93.
50. Slavin TP, et al. Prevalence and characteristics of likely-somatic variants in cancer susceptibility genes among individuals who had hereditary pan-cancer panel testing. Cancer Genet 2019;235-236:31–8.
51. Weitzel JN, et al. Somatic TP53 variants frequently confound germ-line testing results. Genet Med 2018;20(8):809–16.
52. Biesecker LG, Spinner NB. A genomic view of mosaicism and human disease. Nat Rev Genet 2013;14(5):307–20.
53. Forsberg LA, Gisselsson D, Dumanski JP. Mosaicism in health and disease - clones picking up speed. Nat Rev Genet 2017;18(2):128–42.
54. Coombs CC, et al. Therapy-related clonal hematopoiesis in patients with non-hematologic cancers is common and associated with adverse clinical outcomes. Cell Stem Cell 2017;21(3):374–82.e4.
55. Jaiswal S, et al. Age-related clonal hematopoiesis associated with adverse outcomes. N Engl J Med 2014;371(26):2488–98.
56. Mitchell RL, et al. Misdiagnosis of Li-Fraumeni syndrome in a patient with clonal hematopoiesis and a somatic TP53 mutation. J Natl Compr Canc Netw 2018; 16(5):461–6.
57. Ceyhan-Birsoy O, et al. Paired tumor-normal sequencing provides insights into TP53-related cancer spectrum in Li-Fraumeni patients. J Natl Cancer Inst 2021. https://doi.org/10.1093/jnci/djab117.
58. Zehir A, et al. Mutational landscape of metastatic cancer revealed from prospective clinical sequencing of 10,000 patients. Nat Med 2017;23(6):703–13.
59. Mandal R, et al. Genetic diversity of tumors with mismatch repair deficiency influences anti-PD-1 immunotherapy response. Science 2019;364(6439):485–91.
60. Van Hoeck A, et al. Portrait of a cancer: mutational signature analyses for cancer diagnostics. BMC Cancer 2019;19(1):457.
61. Samstein RM, et al. Tumor mutational load predicts survival after immunotherapy across multiple cancer types. Nat Genet 2019;51(2):202–6.
62. Diaz-Gay M, et al. Integrated analysis of germline and tumor DNA identifies new candidate genes involved in familial colorectal cancer. Cancers (Basel) 2019; 11(3):362.
63. Kanchi KL, et al. Integrated analysis of germline and somatic variants in ovarian cancer. Nat Commun 2014;5:3156.
64. Knudson AG. Two genetic hits (more or less) to cancer. Nat Rev Cancer 2001; 1(2):157–62.

Moving?

Make sure your subscription moves with you!

To notify us of your new address, find your **Clinics Account Number** (located on your mailing label above your name), and contact customer service at:

Email: **journalscustomerservice-usa@elsevier.com**

800-654-2452 (subscribers in the U.S. & Canada)
314-447-8871 (subscribers outside of the U.S. & Canada)

Fax number: **314-447-8029**

Elsevier Health Sciences Division
Subscription Customer Service
3251 Riverport Lane
Maryland Heights, MO 63043

*To ensure uninterrupted delivery of your subscription, please notify us at least 4 weeks in advance of move.

Printed and bound by CPI Group (UK) Ltd, Croydon, CR0 4YY

03/10/2024

01040484-0001